SPEECH AND COMMUNICATION PROBLEMS IN PSYCHIATRY

D0140917

FORTHCOMING TITLES

Occupational Therapy for the Brain-Injured Adult
Jo Clark-Wilson and Gordon Muir Giles

Physiotherapy in Respiratory Care
Alexandra Hough

Management in Occupational Therapy
Zielfa B. Maslin

Speech and Language Problems in Children
Dilys A. Treharne

THERAPY IN PRACTICE SERIES
Edited by Jo Campling

This series of books is aimed at 'therapists' concerned with rehabilitation in a very broad sense. The intended audience particularly includes occupational therapists, physiotherapists and speech therapists, but many titles will also be of interest to nurses, psychologists, medical staff, social workers, teachers or volunteer workers. Some volumes are interdisciplinary, others are aimed at one particular profession. All titles will be comprehensive but concise, and practical but with due reference to relevant theory and evidence. They are not research monographs but focus on professional practice, and will be of value to both students and qualified personnel.

Speech and Communication Problems in Psychiatry

ROSEMARY GRAVELL
Chief Speech Therapist, Riverside Health Authority, London

and JENNY FRANCE
Chief Speech Therapist, Broadmoor Hospital, Crowthorne, Berks.

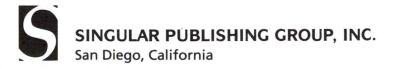

SINGULAR PUBLISHING GROUP, INC.
San Diego, California

Singular Publishing Group, Inc.
4284 41st Street
San Diego, California 92105

First edition 1992

© 1992 Rosemary Gravell and Jenny France

This edition is only available for sale in the United States of America
and Canada.

Typeset in Great Britain by Intype, London
Printed in Great Britain by Page Bros, Norwich

ISBN: 1–879105–58–6

A catalogue record for this book is available from the British Library

Library of Congress Catologing-in-Publication data available.

Contents

Contributors

Judith Chaloner, MCST
Speech Therapist,
West Middlesex Hospital and Gender Clinic, Charing Cross Hospital,
London

Jenny France, MCST
Chief Speech Therapist,
Broadmoor Hospital, Crowthorne, Berks.

Rosemary Gravell, B.Med.Sci. MCST
Chief Speech Therapist,
Riverside Health Authority, London

Helen Griffiths, B.Sc. MCST
Speech Therapist,
Central Manchester Health Authority

Niki Muir, MCST
Speech Therapist,
Long Grove Hospital, Epsom

Pauline Tanner, M.Sc. MCST
Chief Speech Therapist, Horton Hospital, Epsom

Acknowledgements

The authors would like to thank the following for their assistance and support in the preparation of this volume: The Committee of the Special Interest Group in Psychiatry; Alice Thacker; Jo Parton; Lyn Gregory; Phil Dylak and Lisa Ibbetson.

Foreword

This volume represents a painstaking and scholarly introduction to the management of children and adults who have problems of communication related to, or in addition to, mental disorder.

It is a relatively unexplored field having received scant attention until recent years, but the quality of the work included here gives a clear indication that the area should move from the periphery into a mainstream position in the education and practice of speech therapists. Although all students in training receive some teaching in the area of psychiatry it tends to be limited to a brief consideration of the role of the psychiatrist, and clinical psychologist – very rarely the speech therapist.

It has been proposed that the education of the speech therapist who intends to enter this difficult but rewarding field should be developed at post graduate level and there are strong arguments given in this volume to support the idea. Claims that the field is neglected during initial training are, however, well founded and this volume should alert those responsible for the education of speech therapists to this deficiency.

The current volume includes a number of important areas which receive only superficial treatment in most other textbooks dealing with disorders of speech and language. Difficulties encountered in management of the deaf child or adult who also has a psychiatric condition deserve to be considered in a single text as do such major areas as acquired language disorder and cognitive disability. The book should act as a watershed in the academic development of the subject and we must look forward with interest to major developments in the future.

Professor Robert Fawcus

1

Mental disorders and speech therapy: an introduction

Rosemary Gravell and Jenny France

Psychiatry is the branch of medical science that is concerned with mental health in the widest sense, although mental illness is often seen as synonymous. In practice this means that the field of psychiatry will encompass mental illness, personality disorders and areas of mental handicap. This book will consider these various aspects, and it is therefore most appropriate to begin by defining what may be described as mental disorder, before dealing more specifically with mental illness.

MENTAL DISORDER

Mental disorder is defined by statute in England and Wales (Mental Health Act 1983) as 'mental illness, arrested or incomplete development of the mind, psychopathic disorder and any other disorder or disability of the mind'. In the Act from which this definition is taken there are four categories, of which the largest is mental illness. This is not defined by the Act but will be the focus for subsequent discussion within this chapter, and in later chapters particular conditions will be considered. The second group is psychopathic disorder, which is defined as a persistent disorder or disability of the mind which results in abnormally aggressive or seriously irresponsible misconduct and is therefore viewed solely in terms of its being antisocial behaviour. The inclusion of this in mental health legislation has raised much controversy. This will be considered later in this volume. The third and fourth categories are mental impairment and severe mental impairment, terms created for the Act and not clinical syndromes – thus 'mental handicap' does not appear in this definition of mental disorder. These terms are used for forms of mental handicap in which there is significant impairment of social functioning associated with abnormally aggressive or seriously irresponsible conduct.

Consideration will be given in more detail to mental handicap and psychopathy later in this volume, but the topic of mental illness warrants some introductory comments as it is mentally ill people with which this book will be most concerned.

MENTAL ILLNESS

To understand the causes and even to define mental illness satisfactorily is far from easy, and within medicine it is considered an elusive concept. Definition, diagnosis and measurement lack the precision of somatic illnesses, yet it is recognized that mental illness is prevalent. Estimates suggest that one in eight women and one in twelve men in Great Britain will enter hospital for treatment for mental illness at some point in their lifetime (Ineichen 1979); these figures represent only a small proportion – perhaps 5–10% – of the total psychiatric morbidity in a community. The larger proportion are treated by general practitioners, and the prevalence at this point has been quoted by Dean (1989) as between 9% and 15% in different centres, with women outnumbering men in much the same ratio as is seen for hospital admissions.

The fact that women do appear to be more likely to suffer from psychiatric illness than men, in all levels of society, suggests that social factors play an important part in the aetiology of mental illness. This is supported further by evidence that people lower on the social scale are also more vulnerable to mental illness, and the search for the causes of mental illness has thus led into examination of relationships within families, local communities and places of work.

What is mental illness?

There has been debate as to whether there is such an entity as mental illness. Szasz (1960) states that, in his opinion, the concept of mental illness does not exist as illness can only be defined in terms of physical pathology and most mental disorders have no such demonstrable pathology. Szasz goes on to say that mental disorders are therefore not the province of doctors. Variously people have proposed that these 'patients' are not ill but showing the effects of the problems of living or that some people are responsible and others not. Trower, Bryant and Argyle (1978) suggest that some forms of mental disorders are caused or exacerbated by lack of social competence and that this can be cured or alleviated therefore by means of social skills training.

Historically the understanding and treatment of mental illness has evolved slowly over the centuries and has been the focus of much controversy. In the Middle Ages it was commonly thought that if anything went wrong in the mind the devil was in some way responsible, in some cases because of the influence of witches who were agents of the devil. Sufferers were often referred to as lunatics, changes in the illness being associated with changes in the phases of the moon. Writers of the Renaissance period regarded all mental abnormality as a 'species of melancholy'. By the nineteenth century it was thought that insanity could be overcome, if not prevented, by the exercise of will-power and the cultivation of character.

The present-day concept of mental illness is still complex, but modern theories – some of which will be discussed in subsequent chapters – demonstrate that the definition and treatment of mental disorders have undergone radical change, due in part to the discoveries and new approaches in and to both medical and social sciences.

Diagnosis

Diagnosis of mental illness is difficult for a variety of reasons, and some argue for the abolition of the use of diagnostic categories in this field. The language of psychiatry contains as much jargon as any specialized subject, but psychiatric terms have frequently become part of everyday speech – for example, terms like neurotic, psychotic, paranoid and deluded are used quite freely by lay people, and have thus assumed in the public mind sometimes quite different and misleading meanings from those intended when used in psychiatric circles. However, in psychiatry the meaning of the word is most important since the psychiatrist relies predominantly on language to arrive at a diagnosis. The centrality of language and communication to diagnosis will be addressed later in this chapter. Most psychiatrists do make use of diagnostic categories, despite the controversy referred to earlier and the belief held by some that psychiatric diagnoses are not vital for successful intervention and may indeed be harmful.

One reason why psychiatric diagnoses are held in low esteem is that they cannot be confirmed by laboratory tests or on autopsy, and patients may be given different diagnoses by different psychiatrists. Kendell (1988) identifies the shortcomings of diagnosis as fourfold. Firstly they convey relatively little information about aetiology, symptomatology, treatment and prognosis. Secondly that few patients fit neatly into textbook categories and as a result reliability of diagnosis is low. Thirdly the diagnosis often influences other people's behaviour towards the patient and his own attitude towards himself in unhelpful ways, and finally that labelling creates a spurious impression of understanding and encourages naive assumptions about disease entities. Those who would abolish diagnoses argue that each person is unique and their individual problems should be formulated in detail and treated on their own merits.

Kendell (1988) discusses in detail the question of diagnosis and classification, speaking of features each patient shares with all other patients, those he shares with some but not all and those which are unique to himself. In the first case classification is unnecessary as apart from superficial differences all patients will require the same treatment. In the case of unique features being dominant, classification is impossible and nothing useful can be learnt from textbooks, colleagues or the accumulated wisdom of previous workers in the field. Indeed even personal experience would have no value if there were no significant similarities between patients. Attention must therefore focus on the features shared by some, in order to recognize, identify and distinguish the important aspects – which is the process of diagnosis. If more than one type of treatment is available and to be desired it is essential to distinguish between types of patients. Thus Kendell argues that some classification is inevitable, but stresses that it is impossible not to lose sight of the fact that all diseases and diagnostic categories are simple concepts. Certainly it is true that while diagnoses may exclude issues that might otherwise have arisen, they do allow better communication between and within disciplines. It is widely agreed that classifications of disorders should, whenever possible, be based on aetiology.

Classification of mental illness

Mental illnesses are usually divided into two major groups – the psychoses and the neuroses. At times it is difficult to distinguish between the two, but it has been suggested that 'neurotics live in our world partly or wholly but the psychotic is not only out of his mind, but also out of our world' (Roth and Kroll, 1986). Psychoses are the major mental illnesses and involve distorted perception of reality whereas the neurotic conditions do not. Psychotic conditions are fewer and are considered more serious, the most severe of them being schizophrenia.

Neurotic conditions are often milder and more common, including such feelings as tension and anxiety, unreasonable fears and phobias, hysteria and obsessional behaviour. Unless severe these are less likely to be treated by a psychiatrist and patients are rarely admitted to hospital. The psychotic conditions are more likely to be referred to formal psychiatric services and patients admitted to hospital. These groups will be discussed more fully in subsequent chapters but classification of mental illness is more complex than mere mention of the major categories suggests. Mental disorders have been classified in various ways but the most commonly accepted protocols are considered below.

CLASSIFICATION OF MENTAL DISORDERS

So far no practical alternative to a classification system based on symptoms has been found, but there are obvious disadvantages which influence the reliability of such systems, and classification is very complex. The two alternative systems which are thought to learn from each other and grow closer with subsequent revisions are the *International Classification of Diseases*: ninth revision (ICD–9, 1977), which is widely used in the UK, and the *Diagnostic and Statistical Manual*: third edition (DSM-III-R, 1987), which is used in the USA. Both systems are multiaxial, familiar to those in the field, and easy to understand, remember and use.

DSM-III

It has been said that the DSM-III system conveys more information, is more flexible and does not impose boundaries where none exist. When published in 1980 it was stated 'DSM-III is only one still frame in the ongoing process of attempting to better understand mental disorders'; however, the impact of this system was remarkable. Soon after publication it was accepted widely in the USA as the common language of mental health clinicians and researchers for communicating about disorders for which they have professional responsibility. DSM-III was intended primarily for use in the USA but it has had considerable international influence.

In 1987 a revised version was drawn up (DSM-III-R), brought about by the need to keep abreast of the increasing volume of literature in the field and the recognition that revisions would be needed long before the anticipated publication of DSM-IV in the 1990s. The basic feature of DSM-III-R is that it provides classification of mental disorders, each disorder being conceptualized as a clinically significant behaviour or psychological syndrome or pattern that occurs in a person and that is associated with present distress or disability or with significantly increased risk of suffering, death, pain, disability or an important loss of freedom. Whatever its original cause it must currently be considered a manifestation of a behavioural, psychological, or biological dysfunction in a person. DSM-III-R can be said to be descriptive in that the definitions of the disorders are generally limited to descriptions of their clinical features. It has a multi-axial system for evaluation to ensure that information that may be of value in planning treatment and predicting

5

outcome for each person is recorded on each of the five axes, which are mental disorder (axes I and II), physical disorders and conditions (axis III), and severity of psychosocial stresses and global assessment of functioning (axes IV and V). Thus the multi-axial system approach provides a biopsychosocial approach to assessment.

ICD–9

The publication of DSM-III coincided with that of the ICD–9 system, and DSM-IV is planned to coincide with ICD–10. The International Classification of Diseases was developed by the World Health Organization and is revised every ten years. It is a classification and not a nomenclature of diseases, and is organized into 17 major sections, each of which is in turn subdivided into a defined set of categories, although the structure is such that the axes are not consistent within each of the 17 sections. The fifth major section is concerned with mental disorders.

The international community of psychiatrists was dissatisfied with the classification of mental disorder in previous versions of the ICD and it was therefore not widely used. However, the recognition of the importance of the study of mental disorders led to an acceptance of the need for an internationally agreed classification and this became a priority in order to minimize the discrepancies among diagnostic concepts by establishing a uniformly understood terminology.

Other classifications are used, particularly in research, but the ICD–9 and DSM-III-R are the most used classifications among psychiatrists. It needs to be emphasized that classification is used to complement other clinical skills and that care should be taken in the way descriptions are used, whether talking or writing about a patient. The way labels are used is not only the responsibility of psychiatrists, but of all those working in mental health, thus all must recognize the potential stigma attached and the risk of stereotyping based on a label. Those suffering from mental disorders are people no less than others.

A HISTORICAL PERSPECTIVE TO CARE

In the UK before the eighteenth century, mentally ill people were left in the community with no organized care, reflecting the views of contemporary society about 'madness'. The famous Bethlehem Hospital was a noted exception, but it was only after an Act of Parliament distinguished between lunatics and paupers that other institutions sprang up to cope with the former by means, largely, of constraint. The 1890 Lunacy Act regulated the use of mechanical restraint, but it was not until the 1920s that a hospital solely for voluntary patients was founded. The 1930 Mental Treatment Act developed the trend towards a more liberal approach by emphasizing the view that such people were *ill* rather than evil and encouraging more out-patient care.

After the Second World War, with the creation of the National Health Service and more accepting social attitudes, there were great changes culminating in the 1959 Mental Health Act. This assumed there was an illness and that people would, if able, cooperate in treatment – most of which by then was hospital based. It was the development of psychotropic drugs in the 1950s that most radically influenced care of the mentally ill population. This opened the possibility of community care on a much wider scale, and as a result split provision of services between the health and social services. A transfer of resources began from the large Victorian institutions to units within general hospitals, although not all districts followed this trend and there was great variability in the speed with which change was brought about. Psychiatry remained a relatively neglected field in terms of finance and development, and especially services for chronic long-stay patients assumed a 'second-class' air. Even in 1976 Downham and Walker pointed out the enormous difference in funding for staff and hotel/support services between psychiatric and acute hospitals.

The trend to community care has continued apace over recent years, although not without problems. The difficulties that have been experienced in resettling people from hospital to community accommodation suggest that early planning failed to consider the ramifications for mentally ill people of moving out of a known environment.

PRACTICE AND PRINCIPLES OF CARE

Psychiatric services must be organized through the spectrum of dependency, covering the primary care team (which often acts as the 'gate-keeper' to specialist services), acute, residential and long-stay facilities. They must consider all the patient's needs, from medical to sociocultural, and also the need to provide a support service to the families of these people. This can only happen given the full support of administrators and planners, and there are perhaps even more difficulties due to limited budgets than in other medical services.

'The ultimate aim of treatment is to reestablish patients as well integrated members of society able to meet the demands of normal family life, and to pursue their work and leisure interests fully' (Davies and Grove, 1976). Obviously there are those for whom this aim will be unrealistic as their abilities are too severely impaired and some – particularly older patients with organic syndromes – face only deterioration. The aim must be to achieve the individual's potential for social and daily functioning, by rehabilitative or maintenance activities. Lewis (1981) indicates the need to pull back from too enveloping care: 'the elimination of all risk is the negation of the patient's responsibility and leads to the chronic living death of some of our long stay patients'.

The service must be able to respond to impaired function due to the psychiatric illness itself, to secondary social disadvantages (such as poverty and homelessness) and to adverse personal reactions to their situation. Treatment may involve the use of medication (and people should receive counselling in relation to this as there are problems of compliance), physical treatments such as electroconvulsive therapy (ECT), psychotherapy, behaviour modification, social therapy and other rehabilitative intervention.

The Royal College of Psychiatry (1980) stressed the need to plan, provide and coordinate services locally to meet the specific needs of that locality. This is important as there are undoubtedly national and regional differences in service needs – for example, some areas have a high proportion of elderly residents, other areas show rapid demographic changes due to mobile younger populations, some rural areas face problems in providing accessible services, and so on. Furthermore as Scott *et al.* (1976) point out, demand is not simply equatable with prevalence but is affected by attitudes, cultures, expectations and numerous other factors.

Good practice must not neglect the need to evaluate services, both as they exist and in terms of the unmet needs within a locality. This will involve evaluation of the services offered in different care settings. Before considering these settings in more detail attention will be given to some of the legal aspects of providing comprehensive psychiatric services, particularly when the need arises to order compulsory treatment – which is not at odds with the concept of good practice *if* the guidelines are adhered to conscienciously.

LEGAL ASPECTS OF CARE

While different countries will have their own specific legislation relevant to the care of mentally ill people, there will be many shared principles – among which is provision for compulsory treatment. In the United Kingdom the Mental Health Act (1983) regulates the care of mentally abnormal persons, providing three main groups of compulsory order for assessment and intervention, for instance if a person's illness puts themself or others at risk. These groups are for admission for assessment (sections 2, 4, 5, 135, 136), for treatment (section 3) and for admission and transfer of patients concerned with clinical proceedings (sections 37, 41, 47, 49). Each relevant section of the Act specifies strict procedural restrictions and allows certain time-spans over which they are valid. In addition very occasionally the Public Health Act (1968) may be used if there is a state of serious 'squalor or self-neglect'.

The Mental Health Act also introduced increased safeguards for detained patients, more opportunity to appeal against detention, new laws relating to consent to treatment for detained patients, more stringent conditions for compulsory admission and detention, and new measures for admitting offender patients to hospital. It also established a Mental Health Commission. There is also a responsibility upon the health authority to seek out those in need of treatment, a requirement that links in with the stated concern of good practices with assessing unmet need.

SETTINGS OF PSYCHIATRIC CARE

Comprehensive psychiatric services will provide care in closed institutions and hospitals, residential facilities, day/out-patient clinics or centres and in community settings including the patient's own home when this is appropriate. Attention needs to be given to when each care facility is most appropriate to the individual's needs – and this may of course vary with time.

Community: primary care

As has already been indicated, most people with mental disturbances do not reach beyond the primary health care team, which is usually headed by the general practitioner/family doctor. Some will present at that point with specific psychiatric needs, while others will be socially in need (for example, unemployed or isolated). Resources to allow effective primary care in the community are very limited and often liaison between the community and hospital services is difficult – both when care is state provided or privately funded. There may be some bias in the ages and conditions referred on for formal psychiatric help – for instance, fewer elderly patients are referred despite high incidences of both functional and organic disorder in older age groups (Karmer, Taube and Redick 1973). Shepherd *et al.* (1966) state that only 5% of all who present to the primary care team are referred on.

Community: social service provision

Local authorities have been involved in various community schemes for psychiatric patients either who do not need hospitalization or who have been discharged from hospital. This includes day centres, which aim to provide social care (and relief for families); sheltered residential accommodation in hostels providing varying intensity of supervision and short- or long-term support; group homes for more independent people and, rarely seen in the United Kingdom but common in other parts of Europe, boarding out with families.

Short- and long-term residential accommodation is needed for patients who are well enough not to need hospital care but not well enough to live with their families or alone. It is thought that there are many mentally disordered people living destitute in the community, in prison or causing problems to their families who would be better accommodated in hostels (Gelder *et al.*, 1986). Supervision varies and may be provided by a resident warden or, particularly in the case of hostels situated in or near hospitals in order to act as stepping stones to less closely supervised accommodation, by medical or nursing staff. Group homes provide the opportunity for small groups of patients to be more independent and to take responsibility for their daily lives, usually with a community nurse visiting regularly to ensure all is well.

Educational establishments are also an important provision both for children and for adults with special needs, and may be on a day or residential basis.

Hospital services: out-patient and day care

Out-patient clinics serve a similar purpose in psychiatry as they do in other fields of medicine, seeing patients after referral by the family doctor, to follow up after discharge from hospital care or to monitor progress. These clinics are in most cases the first link with formal psychiatric services and may be based in hospitals or – occasionally – in community clinics.

Day hospital facilities aim to provide medical as well as social care, unlike the local authority day centres. However, in practice clients and staff often see their purposes as the same and in both instances a sizeable proportion of users become long stay – Edwards and Carter (1979) found over 50% of centre and 33% of hospital users had been attending for over one year. In the UK day places are provided separately by the health service, social services and some voluntary or private bodies. This is the case also in other countries.

The advantages of day care are in increasing contact with the community, decreasing risks of institutionalization (not removing this risk, however, as day units and families can foster such behaviours), and reducing the stigma for the patient and their family which sadly so often accompanies psychiatric illness. It allows a more normal family life in many cases, although the stresses on the family should not be under-estimated. If day care can provide employment training it is very valu-able as a major problem for this population is in being under-occupied after discharge from hospital. Sometimes past hospital experience was actually more stimulating for them and – particularly for younger patients – Wansborough's comment (1981) that work is the 'corner stone of rehabilitation' is no exaggeration.

Hospital services: in-patient care

In-patient facilities are necessary for short-term admissions and for long-term care. There must also be provision for those whose criminal actions are associated with mental illness or whose behaviour may put themselves or others at risk. Care may be within psychiatric hospitals or units within general hospitals. The former are often, in the UK, remote Victorian buildings and this limits or frustrates opportunities to mix more with other medical disciplines. However, in the units, while liaison is easier, it can be more difficult to create informal environments and to provide for occupational and leisure activities.

There has been a decrease in long-stay hospital provision since the 1950s as a result of the belief that whenever possible people should be maintained in the community rather than in an institutional setting. This has resulted in a higher proportion of elderly, frail patients – either with dementia or hospitalized for schizophrenia many years ago – in the hospitals as their conditions did not allow them to be relocated to their former communities. There have been resultant problems in motivating staff as active rehabilitation is seen as limited. About 50% of women and 30% of men in psychiatric hospitals are over 65 years old (Pitt, 1982) and the chance of admission increases sharply in later life.

Wards must have clear policies and keep good records to enable good communication between staff. The setting must provide an accept-able social environment and good practice demands intensive day-long programmes (formal or informal) involving all those in contact with the patient, and an awareness of the risks of institutionalization in order to adapt accordingly. The physical setting, equipment and staffing must allow full support for the most dependent while not limiting the more independent.

11

In addition to local services there may also be regional units which are able to provide specialized in- and out-patient services for specific groups of patients, such as adolescents, drug-dependent people or potentially violent individuals.

Community: resettlement

Over-optimistic assumptions may have been made originally when the benefits of resettlement in the community were discussed and undoubtedly some patients have suffered adversely as a result of being discharged from hospital. There will be a proportion of chronically handicapped mentally ill people who will need some form of long-term institutional care and support. At the same time there were and are those who were inappropriately placed in long-term hospital care. A great deal of consideration must be given to the individual's need for time to adjust to their new status and develop appropriate skills, especially if resettlement follows a long period in hospital. Morris (1981) suggests that 'the first six months may be a time of "unsettlement" ', and much support is needed in this adjustment time. Different people will have different needs in terms of the type and amount of support necessary – hostel, group home, lodgings, day care and so on, and there must also be attention to the problem of finding employment for this population. Other difficulties may revolve around a person's inability to organize a daily routine, to the effects of stigma and segregation and to financial problems.

COMMUNICATION

Having 'set the scene' by introducing the topic of mental disorder and discussing briefly the ways in which mentally ill people are managed in general terms, it seems appropriate to introduce at this point the subject of communication, which will of course be the focus of many of the following pages of this volume.

Successful communication is to do with the ability to set up and maintain the full interaction of utterance and response which achieves a mutually acceptable outcome. It is a social process, used for the flow of information, the circulation of knowledge and ideas and to achieve shared meanings. Language is the most important tool of communication as it permits people to exchange tremendous ranges of attitudes and information, biases and truths. It allows people to communicate via a mutually accepted pattern of rules and conventions, be they verbal or non-verbal, and is a continuing process, a constantly changing dynamic function. Speaking well (that is, the use of verbal language) is usually associated with effective living, allowing people to make links with others and to effect mutual change, by solving problems and influencing each other.

Burgoon and Ruffner (1978) state that when a person is isolated they may become prey to delusions and fantasies about themselves in relation to the rest of the world, but that through interaction with others they can be made aware of reality.

Human communication is a complex phenomenon and one that most people take for granted, but satisfactory social relationships go hand in hand with effective communication.

Psychiatry and communication

Diamond (1981) states that psychiatrists are interested in the speech content and the linguistic aspects of the patient's communication, which are most important in establishing the psychiatric diagnosis. They rely on what their patients tell them of their history, feelings, complaints, present thoughts, hopes and fears. These are the verbal communications that predominate among the diagnostic criteria, but non-verbal communications are also of importance. Body language, gestures, mannerisms, unusual or odd behaviour and activities, facial expression and signs of emotion in expression or tone of voice all communicate to experienced diagnosticians information about the patient's psyche, whether used intentionally as communicative devices or not. Similarly appearance and such behaviours as how close a person stands to the person with whom they are communicating are relevant. Psychiatrists are trained to recognize such signs and to interpret their significance as evidence of psychopathology or of normal mental processes.

People generally are becoming more aware of and interested in communication, which has become a major topic of conversation and is thought to be at the root of many problems. However, there is still a lack of consensus regarding the nature of competence in communicating or the best way to identify the ability to communicate well. Communicative competence is the yardstick for measuring the quality of interpersonal relationships and is necessary to fulfil the general need of all people to exert control over their environment. Effective environmental control requires successful interface with other people who are an integral part of that environment. Today's communicative environment presents many challenges that make this competence an important and highly relevant concern and, although many seem to believe that they need no training or education in an activity they are performing adequately every day, a variety of indicators suggest that some people's communicative needs are not always necessarily being met. It has been suggested that 7% of the 'normal' adult population have fairly serious difficulties with social behaviour and therefore skill in communicating is not something that should be taken for granted (Argyle, 1981).

Sullivan (1950) was among the first to elaborate an entire psychiatric theory of human development in which the interpersonal system was the primary unit of analysis and in which competence was a central notion. He identified stages of psychosocial development (infancy, childhood, juvenile, pre-adolescence, late adolescence and maturity) in which relations with others provided the basis for developing 'mature competence for life in a fully human world'. If an individual is prevented from fully developing in any stage, later stages will be impaired, resulting in mental disturbances (such as anxiety) and incompetence. He presented evidence that competent people were less likely to manifest certain psychopathological symptoms, were less likely to be institutionalized and for shorter periods of time, and were less likely to be reinstitutionalized than socially incompetent people. He therefore felt that the concept of mental health is strongly grounded in the way people interact in social contexts. Obviously this is one theory and others have taken other approaches, ranging from the purely biological to the psychoanalytical; however, social behaviour – and this necessarily implicates communicative ability – does seem to be crucial at some level of involvement with the mentally ill, whether or not it is seen as a causative factor – for example, in diagnosis, intervention and so on.

There are a great number of human activities that cannot usually be avoided, one of which is interaction with others. It is by talking to others that personality is conveyed and there is no way a person can avoid being evaluated on the way he or she speaks. Sullivan (1950) suggests that personality is nothing more than the regular interpersonal contacts that a person carries on by talking. With all the communicative devices available, it is almost impossible not to communicate; even trying not to communicate itself communicates something!

Psychiatrists are interested not only in interpersonal communication but equally importantly in intrapersonal communication, otherwise referred to as the 'inner voice'. Ultimately all communicative responses take place within a person as he reacts to various communicative cues. Intrapersonal communication can take place without communication in other areas, but communication in those other areas cannot take place without intrapersonal communication.

Ruesch (1987) states that 'almost all phenomena included under the traditional heading of psychopathology are disturbances of communication and that such disturbances are in part defined by the culture in which they occur'. He goes on to say that 'Psychiatric theories are implicitly theories of communication', thus psychiatric therapy aims at improving the communicative system of the patient. Restoration of a broken-down system of interpersonal communication on a semantic or interactional level is achieved either by reducing the number of incoming messages and preventing 'jamming', or by increasing the numbers of messages in transition and preventing isolation and starvation. It is thought that once the communication of the patient with himself and with others is improved correction and self-correction of information will provide the foundations for a change in the conduct of the patient. Therapies all take place in a social context and all use communication as a method of influencing the patient. Reusch goes on to state that the psychiatrist's work is aimed at helping the patient to acquire a communication system which is similar to that of the core group and to prevent disturbances of communication which in turn are responsible for disturbed behaviour.

SPEECH THERAPY AND PSYCHIATRY

Speech therapists who work with the mentally ill are aware of subtle changes in communication and these changes may be among the first signs of the onset of mental illness, thus it is through the way in which people begin to communicate differently that it becomes apparent that all is not well (France 1985). Speech therapists are interested in the quality, quantity, content and use of language and the identification, diagnosis, observation and treatment of all speech and language pathology. Towards this latter aim they have highly trained listening skills. Over recent years they have moved away from the earlier limited view of speech/language to consider 'communication' – that is, the overall skills, disorders, dysfunctions and inadequacies of communication, recognizing that non-verbal skills are as much part of human communication as verbal.

The rest of this chapter will briefly outline the current status of speech therapy in psychiatry.

The international picture

In general there is a dearth of information regarding current provision of speech and language rehabilitation services, although there are signs that national associations are beginning to establish task forces and working parties to consider the service as it stands and necessary developments.

In the UK there has been a recent survey of speech therapy in psychiatry (France, 1987) conducted by postal questionnaire. Although only small numbers were involved some interesting facts were made apparent. Of those who worked in formal psychiatric settings (psychiatric hospitals or units) most were only involved part time and the client group with which most were involved was elderly people. Other groups covered were adult general psychiatry, child psychiatry, mental handicap, forensic units, adolescent units and dependency units. Often one therapist was involved with a variety of these groups. However, it must be stressed that the numbers of speech therapists in formal psychiatry are small – in 1972 the College of Speech Therapists provided figures of 5.10 therapists working with the mentally ill, out of a register of one thousand. This number has risen dramatically since but remains small within the profession as a whole.

More therapists are involved outside a formal setting, but with regular input to psychiatric services, most being based in clinics or general hospitals, or in a purely advisory/occasional way, responding to referrals when necessary.

Most services had been established by district speech therapy managers, although some had stemmed from district planning initiatives and other disciplines, and aimed at general psychiatry or the elderly mentally ill population. There are some specialist services to the mentally handicapped and hearing impaired. It is evident that there are difficulties in retaining the funding for some posts once they become vacant, and France attempted to look at why speech therapists left posts in psychiatry. She highlighted two main reasons – one to gain more general experience and the other due to dissatisfaction relating mostly to lack of time and poor working conditions. Other reasons for dissatisfaction included the lack of valid assessment and therapy equipment for use with this population, difficulty organizing treatment around other staff (due to shift work, for example) and a lack of support from other professions. The lack of relevant training was apparent and will be discussed later in this volume.

In the USA the American Speech–Language–Hearing Association has recently established a task force on psychiatric and correctional institutions to develop a prevalence report of communication disorders in this population. At present however there is no detailed information on the state of speech therapy services to psychiatric patients and it is therefore not possible to attempt to compare the problems that exist in socialized health care systems, such as in the UK, and a predominantly private system.

Similarly there has as yet been no formal compilation of data related to this question in Canada. Some provinces admit to having no specialized service for psychiatric patients while others have minimal cover. For example, in New Brunswick (Ough, 1989) there is a single therapist working in a formal psychiatric setting as a member of the multidisciplinary team and providing both in- and out-patient services for adults, including elderly people. No service exists for adolescents or children with mental illnesses. Problems identified in the UK are also seen here as in other countries, particularly in relation to recruitment difficulties.

Heine (1989) conducted an informal survey of speech therapy in psychiatry in New Zealand and found few therapists working specifically in the field, although there were posts with psychogeriatric services, attached to child assessment units and working with mentally handicapped people. In general referrals were accepted by speech therapy departments and input varied depending upon staffing levels, with most work on an out-patient basis. It was generally agreed that a more comprehensive service should be available, if staffing could allow such development to take place. The situation appears similar in Australia, although again there are no formal data available.

Establishing a speech therapy service

Speech therapists are comparative newcomers to the field of psychiatry and face the difficulties in establishing themselves that are inherent in that statement. It is true in general of the remedial professions that limited staffing levels and a lack of awareness of their role on the part of more established professions in the field have contributed to an underestimation of their potential contributions. This is very much the case in speech therapy and those attempting to establish services face numerous difficulties *en route*.

The greatest stumbling block is finding funding sources, be it within a stretched public health service or a private system. Contributing to this problem is the lack of a voice at appropriate levels of management to allow remedial professions to be wholly involved in planning and developing services. General management aims will influence which posts are approved – for example, services for elderly people have been set as priorities in many areas, resulting in an imbalance of provision. In some instances funding may be more difficult to locate within private health care systems, as the role of speech therapists is very much in the development stage and awaits further empirical evaluation of its worth, making justification in monetary terms difficult at the present time.

Posts must be planned to fit in with the multidisciplinary team and allow full participation. Skill mix has been a topic for discussion over recent years and particularly in psychiatry there is often considerable overlap of skills. Whether this becomes a barrier to effective work seems largely to rest on the personalities involved, but this question will be addressed more fully in Chapter 11. The team must appreciate the role and the value of speech therapy if the service is to be used effectively, and this necessitates – at the planning stage – considerable energies being put into a public relations role. Often, as Parton (1989) has pointed out, there are preconceptions as to the speech therapist's role based on 'the received notions of what she ought to be doing in a general hospital', and it is important therefore to represent the special skills of the speech therapist with the mentally ill. Such a role also allows the therapist to gain information about the structure of the unit and the roles of other professionals.

Recruitment in this field is not easy, partly due to the lack of training received at undergraduate level which makes people wary of entering an unknown area and necessitates a high training input initially. Posts should include clinical involvement (including appropriate family work), teaching and research elements in order to provide opportunities to develop and extend the role. Accountability must also be clearly established prior to appointment, and in the UK will usually be to the district speech therapy manager.

Legal issues cannot be overlooked in establishing a service to mentally ill patients and all involved need to be aware of the rights of patients and their own professional and safety needs. This can be a high-risk area in which to work and insurances and local policies need to be carefully investigated.

These issues will arise whether the post is intended to cover health or social service settings, although there may be differences in account-ability, for example, if working outside the health service. Prisons and voluntary institutions may differ similarly. There is a risk that in these settings posts may become isolated from colleagues in the same pro-fession, and care should be taken to provide or encourage such links to be established.

Once a therapist is in post they will face the problem of how to generate a manageable case-load (Parton, 1989) and this must be done by prioritizing not just in terms of the greatest client need but also in relation to other factors that may 'operate to reduce the speech thera-pist's effectiveness' – such as staffing levels, attitudes of other members of the team, other activity plans for the clients, personal preferences of the therapist and likely levels of cooperation and feedback. This field can generate a great deal of stress and support is crucial, but at the same time rewards can be high. As Parton says: 'breaking new ground depends on a re-alignment of old skills and the emergence of new skills which can be filtered back into the profession at all levels'.

THE AIMS OF THIS VOLUME

This introductory chapter has sought to provide an overview of what is meant by mental disorder and mental illness and of the approaches taken in providing services for this population. It has linked this to the importance of communication and given a brief outline of current speech therapy involvement.

The aim of this volume is to provide descriptions of the main categories of disorder and how communication is affected; to discuss the role of the speech therapist with reference to the different skills, approaches and knowledge needed in working with particular client/patient groups (for example, hearing impaired, mentally handicapped or adolescents) with mental disorder; to provide practical management suggestions and information; and to consider two areas of particular interest in terms of the speech therapist's role in more detail – that is, work with elderly mentally ill people and with those who have gender identity problems. The latter is included because it is a population that usually comes to the speech therapist via psychiatric services, although it is not of course an *illness*.

It is hoped this volume will introduce the reader to the speech, language and communication problems faced by mentally disordered people and their carers and to the range of approaches and techniques of intervention that a speech therapist (or other professional) might employ in relation to these disorders or inadequacies. Such involvement has been a late addition to psychiatric services, but this should not detract from its value. It would be impossible to offer a comprehensive discussion of all aspects of this topic and whenever possible suggestions for further information sources will be made. However, it is true to say that very little has been written specifically on this subject and all too often clinicians have been left to fall back on experience and clinical anecdotes. It is hoped this volume will go a small way towards filling that gap, but it will be stressed throughout that intervention must be constantly evaluated. The lack of research in the field means that there will be suggestions, particularly related to management issues, which are not yet backed by available references – the reader is advised to be aware of this and to evaluate carefully the worth of particular techniques they might attempt with individual patients. It is only by doing this and sharing the information that the role of speech therapists in psychiatry will be properly defined.

REFERENCES

Argyle, M. (1981) The contribution of social interaction research to social skills training, in *Social Competence* (eds J. Wine and M. Smye), Guildford Press, New York, p. 264.
Burgoon, M. and Ruffner M. (1978) *Human Communication*, Holt, Rinehart and Winston, New York.
College of Speech Therapists (1972) Unpublished figures.
Davies, M. and Grove, E. (1976) Contributions of the remedial professions, in *Comprehensive Psychiatric Care* (ed. A. A. Baker), Blackwell Scientific Publications, London, pp. 92–116.
Dean, C. (1989) Psychiatry in general practice, in *Companion Guide to Psychiatric Studies* (eds R. E. Kendell and A. K. Zealley), Churchill Livingstone, Edinburgh, pp. 634–59.
Diagnostic and Statistical Manual of Mental Disorders (1980) DSM-III, American Psychiatric Association, Washington, DC.
Diagnostic and Statistical Manual of Mental Disorders (1987) DSM-III-R, American Psychiatric Association, Washington, DC.
Diamond, B. (1981) The relevance of voice in forensic psychiatric evaluations, in *Speech Evaluation in Psychiatry* (ed. J. K. Darby), Grune and Stratton, New York.
Downham, D. J. and Walker, P. R. (1976) The role of the administrator, in *Comprehensive Psychiatric Care* (ed. A. A. Baker), Blackwell Scientific Publications, London, pp. 141–64.
Edwards, C. and Carter, J. (1979) Day services and the mentally ill, in *Community Care for the Mentally Disabled* (eds J. Wing and R. Olsen), Oxford University Press, Oxford.
France, J. (1985) 'Broadmoor: venture into the unknown' in *Speech Therapy in Practice 1* (2), 4–5
France, J. (1987) *A National Survey of Speech Therapy in Psychiatry*, unpublished.
Gelder, M., Gath, D. and Mayou, R. (1986) *Oxford Textbook of Psychiatry*, Oxford University Press, Oxford.
Heine, M. (1989) *Speech Therapy and Psychiatry in New Zealand*, personal communication.
Ineichen, B. (1979) *Mental Illness*, Longman Press, London.
International Classification of Diseases (1977) *Manual of the International Statistical Classification of Diseases, Injuries and Causes of Death*, Vol. 1, WHO, Geneva.
Karmer, M., Taube, C. A. and Redick, R. W. (1973) Patterns of use of psychiatric facilities by the aged, in *The Psychology of Adult Development and Aging* (eds C. Eisdorfer and M. P. Lawton), APA, Washington, DC.
Kendell, R. E. (1988) Diagnosis and classification, in *Companion Guide to Psychiatric Studies* (eds R. E. Kendell and A. K. Zealley), Churchill Livingstone, Edinburgh, pp. 207–23.
Lewis, S. (1981) The role of the nurse, in *Handbook of Psychiatric Rehabili-*

tation Practice (eds J. K. Wing and B. Morris), Oxford University Press, Oxford, pp. 33–7.

Lunacy Act (1890) HMSO, London.

Mental Health Act (1959) HMSO, London.

Mental Health Act (1983) HMSO, London.

Mental Treatment Act (1930) HMSO, London.

Morris, B. (1981) Residential units, in *Handbook of Psychiatric Rehabilitation Practice* (eds J. Wing and B. Morris), Oxford University Press, Oxford, pp. 99–121.

Ough, D. (1989) *Speech Therapy and Psychiatry in Canada*, personal communication.

Parton, J. (1989) *Setting Up a Service*, personal communication.

Pitt, B. (1982) *Psychogeriatrics: An Introduction*, Churchill Livingstone, Edinburgh.

Public Health Act (1968) HMSO, London.

Roth, M. and Kroll, J. (1986) *The Reality of Mental Illness*, Cambridge University Press, Cambridge.

Royal College of Psychiatry (1980) *Psychiatric Rehabilitation in the 1980s*, RCP Publication.

Reusch, J. (1987) Values, communication and culture, in *Communication in the Social Matrix of Psychiatry* 3rd edn (eds J. Reusch and G. Bateson), Norton, London, pp. 3–20.

Scott, P. McI., Kolvin, I., Tweddle, E. G. and McLaren, M. (1976) Psychiatric care of children and adolescents, in *Comprehensive Psychiatric Care* (ed. A. A. Baker), Blackwell Scientific Publications, London, pp. 214–38.

Shepherd, M., Cooper, B., Brown, A. C. and Kalton, G. (1966) *Psychiatric Illness in General Practice*, Oxford University Press, Oxford.

Sullivan, H. S. (1950) Tensions interpersonal and international: a psychiatrist's view, in *Tensions That Cause Wars* (ed. H. Cantrill), University of Illinios Press, Champaign.

Szasz, T. (1960) The myth of mental illness. *American Psychologist*, **15**, 113–18.

Trower, P., Bryant, B. and Argyle, M. (1978) *Social Skills and Mental Health*, Methuen, London.

Wansborough, S. N. (1981) The place of work in rehabilitation, in *Handbook of Psychiatric Rehabilitation Practice* (eds J. Wing and B. Morris), Oxford University Press, Oxford, pp. 79–94.

21

2

From childhood to old age

Jenny France and Rosemary Gravell

As has already been made apparent this is a relatively new field for speech therapists and as such there have been difficulties in defining and establishing a role. These difficulties begin at the level of undergraduate training with little recognition of the importance of this area on the part of course administrators and planners, although there has been recent evidence of an increased awareness of the need to include the broad field of psychiatry and mental health in the training of speech therapy students. However, it is not uncommon for courses on abnormal psychology/psychiatric disorders to fail to discuss communication in any depth and not even to attempt to outline the specialist role of the speech therapist. There is a body of opinion that suggests such an approach should take place at a postgraduate level.

At present this means speech therapists are entering the field and learning from their own and others' experiences and the sparse literature that directly discusses the communicative needs of mentally ill patients. Undoubtedly this is reflected in the difficulties speech therapists have experienced in defining their role in relation to other professionals. This is a problem not confined to psychiatry, as therapists in many fields face often confusing overlaps of expertise with psychologists, counsellors, occupational therapists and others. This question will be addressed in greater detail in Chapter 11.

A major factor in establishing speech therapy, not surprisingly, is that other disciplines fail to recognize the need for specialist advice or input regarding individuals' communicative abilities. Perhaps the best example of this is seen in the cases of pre-school children whose language disorders are not diagnosed when they present as referrals to psychiatric clinics and who are then improperly placed in units/schools for general learning difficulties (e.g. Love and Thompson, 1988). Other examples are seen in the approach adopted towards the management of mentally handicapped children and adults, where there is a high proportion of both language and psychiatric/behavioural problems, and in working with brain-damaged individuals with communication and other psychological difficulties. In all these cases it is sadly not unusual for treatment to be instigated without considering the possible links between communicative impairment and psychological well-being. When speech therapists *are* involved with these populations they often feel as if they are breaking new ground, without sufficient background training/education on the psychiatric/psychological needs of their patients, that may directly or indirectly relate to communication difficulties. In France's survey (1987) approximately a third of those working in formal psychiatric settings summarized their main problem as uncertainty about their own role.

However, there does seem to have been an increase in interest shown by the profession as a whole and as more clinicians move into the field it is important that these needs are more carefully considered and addressed. It is important that specific attention is paid to the need to research and evaluate the role and skills of speech therapists working in psychiatry.

SPEECH THERAPY SPECIALISMS

Although most speech therapists working in psychiatry tend to cross the boundaries between psychiatric specialisms, there does appear to have been some degree of specialization – often as a result of nebulous or accidental factors (such as the interest shown by other members of particular teams) rather than because of deliberate planning. There are certain areas in which specialism is written into a post when established – such as working solely in units for elderly mentally ill (EMI) patients, child or adolescent psychiatry units and in forensic establishments.

This chapter and the following one focus on the main areas in which speech therapists have developed or perceive the need to develop further a special role. The need for specialist knowledge, as will become apparent, is not limited to those within formal psychiatric settings or teams. Often a general clinician or a clinician specializing in other fields (such as mental handicap, hearing impairment or neurology) which have a marked overlap with psychiatry will be faced with clients or situations when such background information would be invaluable. Indeed it is quite likely that the lack of this knowledge has led and will continue to lead therapists into courses of management that are less than optimally effective for individual patients.

The areas that will be addressed are those of child, adolescent, adult and old-age psychiatry; and in Chapter 3 hearing loss; mental handicap; acquired brain damage and forensic psychiatry. As space prohibits an attempt to cover these areas comprehensively it is hoped the following discussion will highlight needs and direct readers to further study. Detailed descriptions of communication allied to particular mental disorders and of specific management techniques may be found elsewhere in this volume.

CHILD PSYCHIATRY

Purser (1982) pinpoints the beginnings of specific psychiatric services for children as being in 1909 in Chicago, a movement which grew into the now well-established child guidance clinics. Psychological and psychiatric services for children are now part of mainstream medical provision in both socialized and private health care systems. As in other areas of psychiatry movements and models have progressed and changed, thereby affecting treatment and management approaches adopted by all disciplines, including speech therapy.

Classification and diagnostic categories

In Chapter 1 there was a brief description of some of the difficulties and advantages of psychiatric diagnostic classifications. The main codes used are the DSM-III-R and the ICD–9, to the latter of which Rutter, Schaffer and Sturge (1975) proposed the addition of a fifth axis – abnormal psychosocial situations – specific to child psychiatry, which has proved invaluable. The other axes are clinical psychiatric syndromes, specific delays in development, intellectual level, and medical conditions. The DSM-III classification uses five axes – clinical syndromes, developmental and personality disorders, physical disorders, severity of psychosocial stressors, and global assessment of functioning (GAF). Assessment should consider each of these areas/axes to allow a complete evaluation of the child's condition. The main classes of clinical psychiatric syndromes seen in children are mentioned below, but are discussed more fully in the relevant chapters on specific disorders.

Psychoses of childhood

This category includes schizophrenia, disintegrative psychoses and early infantile autism, all of which are characterized by 'severe and extensive disturbance in intellectual, social and emotional functioning in children between birth and puberty' (Purser, 1982). Recently some prefer to describe autism as a 'pervasive developmental disorder' rather than a psychosis (e.g. Rutter and Garmezy, 1983). Disintegrative psychoses may, when established, present like autism; onset is a sudden profound deterioration in abilities and behaviour between the ages of 3 and 6 years. Some stabilize, while others continue to deteriorate and occasionally it may be that an atypical presentation of a specific disease process is underlying this decline – Wilson's disease, for example, has been implicated.

Disruptive behaviour/conduct disorders

Conduct disorders are characterized by persisting antisocial behaviour, which is not part of another psychiatric disorder and in which 'age appropriate societal norms or rules are violated' (Barker, 1988). Conduct disorders are more common in older children and often occur with attention deficit, hyperkinetic disorder, reading disability, depression and dysthymic disorder. (The first two of these co-occurring conditions are usually seen with other diagnoses, such as autism or developmental delay). A mild form of conduct disorder is sometimes described as oppositional deficit disorder. In the past minimal brain dysfunction was linked to these disorders, but it is hard to define and is rather a controversial concept – indeed some have discarded it, such as Barker (1988), although others continue to make use of it.

Neurotic, anxiety and emotional disorders

The primary feature of all these disorders is an abnormally high anxiety level. There is evidence that some may be context dependent (Rutter *et al.*, 1970; Offord *et al.*, 1987) and that there may be cultural differences (Barker, 1988). In children phobic states are often related to school (that is, school phobia or school refusal).

Major affective disorders

This category includes depression, bipolar mood disorders and adjustment reactions. Suicidal thoughts often occur, but completed suicide is rare before 10 years of age – in the USA Shaffer (1985) found a prevalence of less than 1 in 100 000 and this figure is lower in Britain.

Other axes on which each child is assessed include specific delays in development and intellectual level. The former are distinguished from cases of general retardation or below-average ability and may occur, for example, specifically in reading, arithmetic, speech/language or motor abilities. Specific speech and language difficulties are the most likely to come to the child psychiatrist (Wolff, 1988). Intellectual level is linked with psychiatric disorder, to the extent that Rutter *et al.* (1970) found the latter three to four times more common in children with IQs two or more standard deviations below the norm; with a particularly high incidence of hyperkinetic syndrome and psychosis (Corbett, 1979). The question of mental handicap and psychiatry will be addressed later in this volume.

Incidence of mental illness in childhood

There have been several studies of the incidence of mental illness in childhood, of which the best known are those based on populations in the Isle of Wight (Rutter et al., 1970), London (Rutter et al., 1975) and Ontario, Canada (Offord et al., 1987).

The first of these found 6.8% of 10- and 11-year-olds in a rural population had some psychiatric disturbance, with twice as many boys as girls affected – a trend which is reversed in adulthood. The London-based study, of an inner city urban area, found double this prevalence rate. Even higher figures were given in the Ontario study of 4–11-year-olds – 19.5% in boys and 13.5% in girls. The most common diagnoses in children were conduct and behaviour disorders and specific developmental delay, but the proportions of diagnoses alter as puberty is passed, at which point more girls than boys are diagnosed with psychiatric disorder, particularly of the neurotic, anxiety or emotional type (Offord et al., 1987).

These studies have looked at general populations within certain age bands and therefore would not necessarily reflect either the numbers receiving formal psychiatric help or indeed those needing such intervention. Various explanations have been offered for the higher incidence of problems in boys, with sociocultural factors thought to play a part, via parental and teacher role models and expectations of behaviour/achievement. The different prevalence between rural and urban populations is also of interest.

There is considerable evidence for a high incidence of psychiatric disorder in speech/language-impaired children and vice versa (e.g. Cantwell et al., 1979), a situation to which this discussion will return.

Causes of mental illness in childhood

It is now generally accepted that a detailed knowledge of normal development and of family/social development is necessary to any professional working in this field. Few childhood disorders have single clear-cut causes, but reflect complex reactions to a variety of factors – constitutional (genetic/chromosomal, pre- or peri-natal damage); physical (Rutter et al., 1970, found psychiatric disorder was five times more likely in brain-damaged children and three times as common in physically handicapped children as in a normal population); temperamental; and environmental (including family, social and physical environmental factors).

The recognition of multifactorial causes has affected theoretical approaches to therapy and intervention, by increasing the range of explanations. As Purser (1982) summarizes, the three major models to have provided the basis of therapy have been psychoanalytical, behaviourist and cognitive. Many psychiatrists now adopt a case-centred eclectic approach formulating management plans on the basis of as full an assessment as is possible and seen to be valuable.

General management

Obviously a full description of the management of mental illness in childhood is outside the scope of this book, but as the theories and principles are of direct relevance to those working with the communicatively impaired it seems useful to offer a brief outline of approaches to and types of intervention.

Assessment

Assessment of children encompasses interviews with and testing of the child and of the family and environment. Psychiatric interviews depend on gaining rapport with the whole family. Knowledge of the child's presenting complaint and current functioning is needed and a full history will also need to consider the family's development, structure and current functioning. There would normally be a physical examination (including motor behaviour, activity and skills) and a psychological evaluation (e.g. of play, mood, attention skills, modes of thinking and perception). Form and level of speech and language, intellectual level, personality and social adjustment assessments should also be included. This will involve information about any events of importance in the child's life such as illness, separation, bereavements, moving house or school and so on. Occasionally special investigations may be ordered, for instance EEGs or brain scans. The diagnostic process must operate flexibly, adjusting to the child's developmental levels, as the significance of certain behaviour patterns alters with the age of the child.

It will be useful to determine the parent's expectations of treatment, as these may be of interest both for assessment and management planning. Once the necessary information has been gathered, this leads to a formulation of all the relevant factors and to specific treatment plans.

Infants and young children are harder to diagnose and classification systems are often inappropriate. One reason for the diagnostic difficulties that arise is that these very young children are pre-verbal. It is also not properly known yet what factors link to early resolution or presage later psychiatric problems – although there does seem to be evidence that early speech or language disorder results in greater risk of later problems (e.g. Lerner *et al.*, 1985).

Treatment and intervention techniques

Numerous techniques have been tried with children diagnosed as having a psychiatric disorder. Some are based on the child at home, within the family or as an individual, and others upon removal from the home environment. The latter course may be necessary because of the complexity of their symptoms, the belief that home life is maintaining or causing their symptoms, severe behavioural disturbance or risk of injurious behaviour either to self or others. There may furthermore be cases where children are removed legally from parental care which is deemed harmful to their psychological or physical development.

Individual therapy may be psychotherapy, behaviour therapy/modification, hypnosis or pharmacotherapy – the latter is used especially cautiously with children as there may be risks in suppressing symptoms, thus masking underlying problems, apart from the recognized difficulties of side effects. Play therapy (Klein, 1963) enables therapists to overcome the constraints on verbal communication imposed by the immaturity of younger children. Group therapy may be appropriate for the child and/or parents. These therapies may be offered on an outpatient basis, within day care settings or as in-patient treatment. Educational measures may be utilized, such as remedial teaching, transfer between classes or schools, or placement in a special unit or centre.

Parental therapy and counselling may be used to help the parents understand their child's condition, appreciate their own role (be it in cause or management) and cope with the current situation. There may be value in undertaking formal family therapy (see Chapter 10) which involves the therapist as an active participant in the family system. Wolff (1988) states that treatment of the majority of children with behaviour disorders should also involve treatment of the parents and it is probably safe to say that all disciplines accept that work with the parents of these children is crucial, even when limited to offering explanations, advice and support, rather than expecting their active participation in programmes.

The role of the speech therapist

It must be stressed that the speech therapist's role should be defined within the multidisciplinary team and the value of the team approach should be accepted as underlying this discussion. The multidisciplinary team will be considered more fully in Chapter 11.

The speech therapist's role may be within formal psychiatric services, thus working with children who already have psychiatric diagnoses, or that of a generalist working with a case-load of pre-school or school-aged children who are initially referred for specific speech/language assessment. The relevance and importance of a knowledge of the psychological needs of this latter group of children will first be addressed.

General speech/language therapy

Gordon (1987) states that 'among all the disabilities that can affect children, difficulties with communication are among the most severe and distressing'. Language delay can have consequences for numerous other aspects of development – including cognition, educational attainment, social, emotional and behavioural development (Howlin and Rutter, 1987; Paul, Cohen and Caparino, 1983) and may sometimes be linked to later psychosis. This last statement is subject to contradictory claims in the literature, partly due to difficulties in diagnosis, as Howlin and Rutter point out, and it may be that there is a subgroup which has related antecedent causes (Lewis and Mezey, 1985).

There is a growing body of literature outlining research and providing evidence for a link between psychiatric disorder and speech/language impairment. Several of these studies have looked at the prevalence of psychiatric illness in pre-school-aged children or in children referred to speech/language clinics. Using the definition of psychiatric disorder adopted by Rutter *et al.* (1970) as a 'disorder of behaviour, emotions or relationships sufficiently prolonged and/or severe to cause distress to the child and/or a disturbance in his environment', Cantwell, Baker and Mattison (1979) looked at 100 consecutive speech/language clinic referrals of children (ranging in age from 2 to 13) and found over half to have at least one psychiatric diagnosis. The most common were attentional deficit disorder (with or without hyperactivity), oppositional disorder and anxiety, but no specific psychiatric diagnosis was uniquely associated with speech/language impairment.

Beitchman *et al.* (1986) felt that selective attendance, for example in terms of social class or ethnicity, at clinics was a possible cause of bias. However, when they studied 5-year-olds at English language schools in a Canadian municipal region via screening and when appropriate more intensive speech/language and psychiatric assessments, they found 49% of the speech/language impaired to have some psychiatric disorder (most often attention deficit or emotional disorder) as opposed to 12% of a control group. It is interesting that parent/teacher ratings of psychiatric disorder indicated double the prevalence found by the use of formal psychiatric assessment.

It is not too difficult to see that these results have direct implications for speech therapy services. Firstly there is the need to recognize that a significant number of children referred will have psychiatric disturbances that may need referral to and possible intervention by a specialist. Specific types of language disability may be implicated – for example Rutter and Lord (1987) suggest that poor comprehension increases the risk. Future research will, it is hoped, reveal more about the characteristics of particular children that put them at risk of psychiatric illness.

Secondly speech therapists must address the need to consider such aspects in their use of assessment materials and interpretation of results. Coombes (1987) cautions care with current test batteries, many of which are not psychometrically sound. The need to involve the parents and teachers in systematic enquiry in order to arrive at a reliable diagnosis should be stressed.

Implications for management go beyond taking the decision to refer to other disciplines, although this may be appropriate. Management programmes must include consideration of the family's needs, the stage of development at which the child is in all aspects (for instance, the timing of introducing group work will depend on appropriate social adjustment and skills as well as upon linguistic development) and when possible educational services should be involved. There is a pressing need to identify these children and offer them support, as Beitchman et al. (1986) indicate.

Finally there are implications for the speech therapist in terms of preventative intervention. This will be influenced by the evidence regarding causal links in the relationship between speech/language and psychiatric disorder. There are three possibilities according to Baker and Cantwell (1987) – the psychiatric disorder may cause the communication loss, the latter may directly or indirectly lead to psychiatric sequelae or the two may share antecedent factors. To these it must be added that it is likely that over time the relationship will become less clear cut and the two disorders may well interreact. It seems well borne out that shared causative factors are implicated in many instances of brain damage, hearing impairment and mental handicap. However, the high incidence of psychiatric disorder in a general communicatively impaired child population suggests there may well be a role for the therapist to help prevent later psychiatric distress in cases where the communication difficulty is primary. Early diagnosis and intervention would then be crucial, and the approach may well be to work through families, helping them to understand their child's speech-language level and needs, particularly when there are more subtle problems, for instance in receptive language skills, and teaching them appropriate strategies to adopt in communicating with their child. Parents need time to accept any handicap in a child and thus to adapt their expectations and hopes accordingly.

Child abuse

A subject which has led to much public and professional discussion over recent years is child abuse. Many speech therapists working with children will have in their case-loads some at risk of abuse, which is defined as deliberate action on the part of an adult which injures the child, or of neglect, which is deliberate omission of care. It is mentioned here as some evidence suggests a link between abuse and/or severe neglect and language disability. Normal language acquisition theory emphasizes the importance of parent-child interaction (e.g. Weiss and Lillywhite, 1981) and studies of abuse in families suggest the involvement of factors in the parent's personality and in the child (for example, minimal dysfunction, poor health, developmental disorder) and in the interaction of these. There is some evidence of poor language ability in abused (Blager, 1979) and neglected (Allen and Oliver, 1982) children, particularly of poor language comprehension (Fox et al., 1988). Again, although this is patently not the whole story, there are implications for speech therapy interventions.

Speech therapy within formal psychiatric services

Unlike the therapist working in a general clinic, within a psychiatric service most children will already have been seen by the psychiatrist and other members of the team. This will lead to a greater number of certain diagnostic groups being referred – notably autism, psychosis and elective mutism. However, before the role with these conditions is considered in more detail, there is evidence for a high incidence of speech/language disordered in a general child psychiatric population that warrants the speech therapist's attention.

Gualtieri et al. (1983) looked at children referred for psychiatric services and found a strong association with developmental language disorders. Of their admittedly small sample of 40 referrals over half had speech/language problems. Of 26 who were given full language evaluations 20 had moderate or severe impairments, 4 mild and only 2 were found to have no language problems. Love and Thompson (1988) felt that previous studies had methodological errors and attempted to rectify these in their study of 200 children referred to psychiatry, excluding those with mental retardation or pervasive developmental disorder; 48% had both speech/language and attention deficit disorders, but only 16% had solely the former and 25% the latter, suggesting a strong relationship with the possibility of shared antecedents, perhaps for subgroups of both broad categories. They concluded, in agreement with other papers, that pre-schoolers referred to psychiatric services 'are at high risk for language disorders'. They further state that there is 'convincing evidence that problems associated with language disorders in young children often persist into adolescence and even adulthood, and have a negative impact on personal relationships, academic success, vocational and professional achievement and learning power'.

Gualtieri *et al.* (1983) state that 'speech and language therapists seem to be much more aware of psychiatric problems in their clients than psychiatrists and psychologists are of language disorders in theirs' – despite the fact that so many psychiatric techniques are strongly language based. They speak of implications for psychiatric management in terms of the need to consider language level in assessment and choice of therapy techniques. This leads to a role for speech therapists in informing other team members of the importance of language evaluation and subsequently advising others involved in the care of an individual child of the appropriate level and style of language or non-verbal communication to use.

Love and Thompson (1988) suggest that all children referred to psychiatric services, or if this is unrealistic all those with attention deficit disorder, should be screened by the speech therapist, who would then direct appropriate intervention levels – a suggestion also made by Cantwell *et al.* (1979), who stress the need for early intervention as a preventative measure, decreasing the risk of later or persisting psychiatric disorders.

It seems important for an assessment to be made of these children's language environments and consideration of adaptations to these if there are barriers to communication or unmet needs. Strategies need to be developed for training parents and professional carers in more effective interactions with children who are language impaired. There is a crucial role for speech therapists in working with the relevant education services. Lambert *et al.* (1978) point out how often pre-school language disorder was 'likely to be redefined as a learning disability once the child entered the school system'. This may result in children receiving inappropriate education rather than the specialist help they require.

It is worth mentioning that hearing loss, which will be discussed in Chapter 3, has also been found to have a strong association with psychiatric disorder, as well as with speech/language difficulties (e.g. Funk and Ruppert, 1984; Gualtieri *et al.*, 1983).

Various texts have looked at therapeutic considerations in working with speech- and language-impaired children and this is obviously outside the scope of this volume. However, it is worth stressing certain points in relation to the speech therapist's role with children who also have some psychiatric disturbance. Firstly the parents must be involved and the therapist endeavour to gain an understanding of how they perceive the problem. A consultative role may be most appropriate (Coombes, 1987). Both language and psychiatric disorders to an extent are 'hidden handicaps' and the latter in particular carry a stigma even today.

Specific structured language programmes may have a value but there is a risk that they may not use language for 'social, control, information, affective or expressive functions' as happens in natural language acquisition. This social view of language is crucial in working with psychiatrically disturbed children and therapists need to build this into structured programmes or behaviour modification methods (e.g. by using 'natural' rewards which have functional significance in everyday life). As Wells and Gutfreund (1987) suggest, parents may be led by abnormal cues from the child to modify their language in inhibitive rather than facilitatory ways. The speech therapist can act as a model, demonstrating effective interaction techniques and can also explain and offer support when parents feel rejected and guilty over their child's disabilities. As Gath (1987) stresses, 'time spent understanding the family and respecting their individuality is time well spent'.

As has already been suggested, assessment results may be difficult to interpret with children who have psychiatric disorders – for example, is a child failing because of a specific language disorder, as a result of attention deficits or because of psychotic distancing? This is an area for future study, aiming to develop appropriate procedures. Consideration must also be given to psychosocial stressors in the child's environment, abuse and neglect have been mentioned but numerous other factors may be relevant and although they are looked at with all children who present for therapy, they are particularly important if there is psychiatric disturbance of some description. Goals in therapy must be clear and functional, especially in conditions where progress is limited by the disorder/disease process, and set for short- and long-term guidance.

Specific conditions relevant to speech therapy

This discussion of the role of the speech therapist in psychiatry with children has stressed the high prevalence of speech and language disorders in this population and therefore the need for speech therapy services to be used particularly in assessing and advising. Of course the specialist therapy role will not always be appropriate and input may well best be judged 'in terms of the extent to which it facilitates the work of parents and teachers in fostering children's normal development' (Rutter and Lord, 1987). There will, however, be certain conditions with which the speech therapist will have a particular role to play – with the hearing impaired or mentally handicapped child who is disturbed, for example. Of particular relevance is the condition of infantile autism, which is touched on in this chapter but more fully described and discussed in Chapter 5. Childhood psychosis is also addressed in more detail in Chapter 5, but it is worth at this point mentioning that such children may be referred to the speech therapist. Speech and communication symptoms vary, but there are marked deviations from normal, probably without a specific clustering of defects (Ostwald, 1981).

Elective mutism

This condition will be referred to again in the section of adult psychiatry, but onset is usually between 3 and 5 years of age although referral is often after school age is reached (Rutter and Lord, 1987) and symptoms rarely persist for more than one year. There are some cases of adolescent onset which differ somewhat in pattern. Although elective mutism was thought to be situation specific, most of these children are very shy and have poor peer relationships across a variety of situations. They may also show mild cognitive delays and behavioural immaturities and often come from disturbed families (Kolvin and Fundudis, 1981). Diagnosis depends on the ability to understand and to speak in *some* situations. The prognosis is worse if symptoms continue after 10 years of age. Elective mutism may be a fairly common reaction to starting school (Brown and Lloyd, 1975).

There has been some attempt to identify subgroups in terms of onset or personality type, but treatment is usually based on behavioural intervention with occasional use of psychodynamic therapy and family work. The value of frequent, brief therapy sessions is remarked upon by Rutter and Lord (1987). Speech therapists have a role to play which should extend beyond merely obtaining speech and thus decreasing maladaptive behaviour in specific situations, to a more systematic consideration of treatment goals.

Other conditions

The speech therapist may well be called upon in a variety of other conditions and situations. For example, some attempt has been made to correlate articulation errors with psychosexual immaturity (Rousey and Moriarty, 1965) which may be an area warranting further study. Gender identity problems are considered in Chapter 9. There may also be a role in working with children of psychiatrically disturbed parents, when their disorder affects interaction and thus the child's normal development is put at risk – preventative work could prove very valuable in such cases. Finally stuttering is included in some texts as a psychiatric disorder of childhood – a debatable placement, but one that must be acknowledged. Numerous texts exist which discuss the possible causes of stuttering and other dysfluent behaviours, including psychiatric theories, such as that by Dalton and Hardcastle (1977). The reader is referred to those texts for consideration of treatment approaches, which is outside the scope of this volume.

ADOLESCENT PSYCHIATRY

Adolescence is the period of life between childhood and adulthood. Puberty marks the onset of adolescence during which time there is rapid physiological and psychological development, but there is no clear ending – various ages from 16 into the twenties have been accepted by different authors, and in some cases well into adult life personal development is not yet complete. Adolescence is a time of increased awareness of personal identity and individual characteristics, which is accompanied by physical, psychosexual, emotional and social changes. Adjustment to the rapid physiological changes, especially in weight and height, may lead to social awkwardness, clumsiness and social discomfort; if there is difficulty coping with these bodily changes, over which there is no voluntary control, negative self concepts may be induced, particularly if there is thought to be a deviation from cultural stereotypes. Occasionally handicapping social anxiety results in selective or total withdrawal from the public eye (Hill, 1986).

Most adolescents begin to spend more time with their peer groups and so less with the family and a wider age range of social contacts is developed, offering a wider repertoire of social roles and experiences.

Dependency on the family reduces as independence develops. The adolescent develops adult forms of thought, including the ability to manipulate abstract concepts and set up hypothetical propositions. Language is mostly conscious, controlled and censored; style being influenced by intellectual, social, ethnic and sexual differences. The adolescent will develop his own individual style of communication and speech and be able to moderate these depending on the listener, if he or she has enough flexibility of grammar and vocabulary to be able to choose between speech codes and the social awareness to know that different listeners will have different needs in conversation. For example, certain modes of address are more polite than others and this must be recognized in particular settings or in interaction with particular people.

Adolescence is also a time of rapid changes of mood, varying from serious contemplation to being childish and impulsive. Behaviours may become unsociable, unpredictable, unpleasant and even destructive, but if transient and mild they may fall within the normal range of behaviour. When more marked they can underline conduct and emotional disorders in younger, or conduct and neurotic disorders in older, adolescents. Some develop such major problems in the way they feel, their attitudes and their capacity to form relationships that these problems pervade most or all aspects of their personality development (Steinberg, 1987).

Classification and diagnostic categories

Previous confusion in describing young people's problems was somewhat overcome when the multi-axial classification systems were introduced. Both ICD–9 and DSM-III contain schemes for classifying the psychiatric disorders of childhood, as has been stated, and those of adult life. Disorders of adolescence are classified in part as are those of childhood and in part as those seen in adults. However, there are difficulties in classifying adolescents' disorders – as has already been said everyone is unique and labelling the disorder can become confused with labelling the person, and not all problems, of course, fit neatly into the available categories. Making a diagnosis should be the start but not the conclusion when dealing with patients of any age.

It is especially crucial in both child and adolescent psychiatry that family and social circumstances are taken into account, particularly perhaps in relation to conduct disorders. Steinberg (1983) draws attention to the need to differentiate between true psychiatric disorders (such as a conduct disorder) and problems described for other purposes (for example, delinquency is a legal term, not a psychiatric condition).

ICD–9 makes use of five axes, as outlined in the preceding section on child psychiatry, and Steinberg stresses that this was designed to be a reliable descriptive system, without aetiological implications. The DSM-III identifies disorders first evident in infancy, childhood or adolescence as being developmental (e.g. mental retardation, autism, specific disorders); disruptive behaviour disorders; anxiety disorders (e.g. separation anxiety); eating disorders; gender identity disorders; tic disorders; elimination disorders; speech disorders not classified elsewhere (e.g. cluttering, stuttering); and others, such as elective mutism and identity disorders.

It is obviously important that healthy reactions are not confused with symptoms, thus grief, depression and euphoria, for example, should be evaluated within day-to-day functioning. The diagnostic categories of particular relevance to disciplines working with an adolescent case-load include the following.

Delayed development

Problems caused by delayed development, when the individual displays precocity, delay or fixation at an earlier stage or in a specific area (e.g. motor, speech/language, cognitive, social, sexual, affective or integrative) may persist into adolescence from childhood.

Neurotic disorders

A similar pattern occurs in adolescence as is seen in adult life and this is discussed more fully in Chapter 4.

Psychotic disorders

Many adult psychoses begin during adolescence but the reported incidence is much greater in adult life, which is partly a result of reluctance to diagnose psychosis in the young. All types of psychosis produce impairment of reality testing; that is, inability to test the reality of the external world. Contact with others is influenced to an excessive degree by the individual's internal world and by the extent to which he or she is out of contact with reality (Evans 1982). Psychoses relevant to this age group include manic-depression, schizophrenia and drug-induced.

Manic-depressive psychosis is very rarely diagnosed in adolescence due to the pronounced mood swings at this time and the risk of confusion with some of the features of schizophrenia. The mood swings must be very intense to justify an 'illness' label. In other respects the presentation of this condition is similar to that seen in adults.

Schizophrenia may onset insidiously or in acute form. The age of onset of catatonic and hebephrenic forms, which are insidious in onset, tends to be during adolescence or early adulthood. Acute schizophrenia is dramatic, lasting any length of time from days to weeks, and may appear following a change in lifestyle or after anxiety or depression induced by stress, the person withdrawing to an inner world. However, it may just 'happen' with no evident precipitating influence. Acute forms respond to treatment better than insidious and the earlier antipsychotic drugs are prescribed when new symptoms appear, the less likelihood there is of another florid breakdown.

Drug psychoses are the most common psychoses in this age group, because of adolescent misuse of drugs. The resulting psychosis may last for hours but more often for days; and the majority recover within two weeks, although some continue for months and can then be difficult to distinguish from schizophrenia. There are reports in the literature of adolescents who have shown a psychotic reaction following ingestion of drugs which has progressed into a classical schizophrenic illness, but there is debate as to whether the drug caused the illness or precipitated symptoms during what was in fact an early phase of that illness (Evans, 1982).

Organic brain syndrome

This area includes minimal cerebral dysfunction, which was referred to in the preceding section, and all types of neurotic and disruptive behaviour resulting from a primary organic cause or due to the prolonged psychosocial effects of the disability. There may be restlessness, irritability, dizziness, poor concentration, epilepsy and specific learning difficulties such as dyslexia. The latter two symptoms particularly will necessitate special educational and vocational intervention and guidance.

Personality disorder

This is difficult to diagnose in adolescence, but the most common forms seen by psychiatrists seem to be the impulsive, disorganized, frustrated acting-out type and the antisocial or delinquent individual. In the latter case the behaviour may be in reaction to maturational or neurotic conflict with a life-long pattern of personality disorder (Peterson, 1988). In recent years there has been a considerable increase in alcoholism and drug addiction in this age group and many of these adolescents are thought to display personality disorders.

The incidence of mental illness in adolescence

Only a minority of adolescents suffer from handicapping psychiatric disorder and prognostic features seem to be comparable with those for other age groups. Before puberty emotional problems occur equally between the sexes, while depression is more common in boys. Rutter *et al.* (1970) quote 20% of 14-year-olds in the Isle of Wight study as having some degree of psychiatric disturbance. After puberty girls are more likely to have depression or anxiety than boys. Adult-type symptoms are seen in adolescence with classic signs of depressive illness, anxiety, phobic and obsessional states, as well as the less well-differentiated mood disorders of childhood. There appears to be an increase in the prevalence of psychiatric disorder from around 10% in childhood to 10–15% in mid-adolescence, rising with age, but which reduces to 10% again in adult life. The incidence is higher in urban areas.

In adolescence a distinction must be made between a true disorder and maturational problems. It has been stated that there are no conditions that are only found in adolescence although anorexia nervosa seems to be specially related to the maturational tasks of this time of life and antisocial behaviour peaks during adolescence – a fact reflected in the phenomenon of juvenile delinquency (Hill, 1986).

Causes of mental illness in adolescence

Individual predisposition is partly shaped by genetically based vulnerability factors and as these apply to personality, intelligence and mental illness they should be taken into account when considering disorders.

Neurological causes might include brain damage of varying degrees, including the possibility of minimal cerebral dysfunction, which is difficult to diagnose as there are no neurological signs as may be seen, for example, in cases of head injury and encephalitis. A history of problems in the pre- and post-natal period lends some support to studies which suggest that minimal cerebral dysfunction contribute to adolescent difficulties more frequently than has been generally acknowledged, although as has been stated the concept is not accepted at all by some researchers and psychiatrists.

Mental handicap, epilepsy (which may or may not be associated with brain damage), chronic illness, physical disability or abnormality are all factors that may render an adolescent at risk of psychiatric complications – perhaps as a result of perceiving themselves to be different.

Chronic illness in other members of the family also produces problems for the adolescent, and other family and social influences may be important. The adolescent who has been separated from his or her family in early life is often more vulnerable, tending to be over-dependent, compliant, depressed, antisocial or aggressive – reactions which demonstrate the importance of early attachment to a constant person to provide a secure base for later development (Bowlby, 1969).

Parental factors may be important, for example – the older parent may have more difficulty adapting to the adolescent (Peterson, 1988); unwanted children show higher incidences of delinquency, school failure and psychological ill health in adolescence; parental mental illness reduces their effectiveness as parents; and parental criminal behaviour and delinquency may produce poor parenting skills and family discord (Steinberg, 1987). Family disharmony or deviance of any kind makes the adolescent more vulnerable, be it due to death, separation, divorce or illegitimacy (Peterson, 1988). Children from stable homes withstand loss better than those from disturbed homes. Extremes of parental behaviour – permissiveness, negligence, over-protectiveness or over-strict discipline – may produce problems.

As well as these, such factors as family size, structure and patterns of behaviour, adoption, being fostered and institutional care all add to the risk of psychiatric disorder. Unresolved conflicts from childhood, perhaps arising from child guidance intervention, may re-emerge later in life. Finally there needs to be recognition of the possible effects of communication defects and difficulties upon mental health.

Management

The proportion of adolescents in the population who are seen in specialist psychiatric clinics is less than for other age groups, partly because some of the less mature are seen in child psychiatry clinics and older, more mature are seen by adult services. However, care for the majority should ideally be provided by a specialist service and as yet there is no generally agreed model for this. Most units accept out-patient referrals and in-patient facilities are limited.

Assessment

The need for assessment is to discover whether the person is disturbed or simply maturing in a way that is different and so difficult for others to tolerate. It is often reported that examination of adolescents is 'fraught with hazards' (Peterson, 1988), as few see the psychiatrist willingly and many have difficulty expressing themselves verbally and they may be frightened by the idea that they must be insane to see a psychiatrist and try hard to prove their sanity.

Special skills are needed for interviewing adolescents and it is thought that ideally the patient should be seen before the parents and other members of the family so that he or she realizes they are being treated as an independent person. The usual psychiatric history is taken, including information about home life, school, work and relationships with peers.

The measurement of family communication presents great problems, Rutter (1979) points out that discussions in a family with a disturbed child or adolescent tend to give rise to more tension and disagreement than they do in normal families. There are apparently more negative feelings when the families are talking together and there are more conflicting messages. They may feel that communication with this disturbed adolescent is likely to be inefficient and to give rise to fruitless disputes and few agreed solutions. Thus communication problems at this level are not just experienced by the patient but are shared with the family and those at work or school.

There are three possible outcomes to assessment – no diagnosis may be reached but reassurance offered; no diagnosis but formal help is given to the disturbed family; or finally a psychiatric disorder may be diagnosed and the appropriate intervention agreed.

Treatment and intervention techniques

Following assessment the first question after deciding whether to treat is who to treat – the adolescent, the parents or the whole family. It is accepted that it is important to work with relatives and teachers, and to offer a tripartite approach involving the psychiatrist, social worker and clinical/educational psychologist. Generally it is felt that the team approach has a great deal to offer and one or more members of the team may be involved in a particular case.

Various treatments may be offered, depending on the facilities available in a particular setting, including out-patient family therapy, individual psychotherapy or psychoanalysis, group psychotherapy, multifamily group therapy, supportive therapy, behaviour therapy, marital therapy for parents, drug or physical therapies, remedial education, counselling, residential care/schooling, hospital admission, or local authority placement for care and protection. Rehabilitation therapies may be offered, among them – of course – speech therapy.

Psychotherapy with children and adolescents grew out of psychoanalytic theory and practice (Garfield, 1980) which approach has been modified to meet varying demands. Psychotherapy is determined by a number of factors but the emphasis is placed on the quality of the interaction between therapist and patient. The theoretical standpoint of the therapist has least to do with the effectiveness of therapy; it is the level of experience, style and other personal qualities that have an important bearing on the outcome. An eclectic approach is increasingly adopted integrating affective, cognitive and behavioural means of promoting change.

The role of the speech therapist

Some forms of language deficiency are camouflaged until the child has shown many instances of failure and frustration. As the child reaches the end of school life these problems are interfering with achievement. Language production in both oral and written forms may be noticeably inadequate, affecting reading, comprehension and arithmetical skills. These inadequate language skills may begin to take their toll on social interactions, affecting the ability to interpret subtle aspects of conversation – such as hints or unstated intentions. As the child progresses demands increase in terms of the need to be able to interpret abstract material, understand linguistic ambiguities and relate previously learned information to new materials. Failure in these aspects can be described as failure to develop communicative competence. If there is the additional complication of mental illness communication is likely to be even more impaired.

A number of adolescents who are seen by psychiatrists in the community might also have been referred for speech therapy and thus links are formed with the team in order to liaise on decisions about the advisability of pursuing treatment and to share information. In residential units the speech therapist is likely to work with the rest of the clinical team, either providing an individual programme or organizing and planning group treatments with other professionals. These groups may include one or more of the treatment techniques outlined earlier.

While the majority of traditional therapy is likely to be with stutterers (which does not necessarily mean the dysfluency is a primary psychiatric disorder), by far the most common problem is that of dysfunctional communication. Patients themselves often refer to long-term communicative difficulties, particularly with their families and those in authority at school. Parents will also often agree that their child has been 'difficult' or 'impossible' to communicate with. Each side will see the situation as the other's problem. School teachers also report that many of these young people are quiet or withdrawn at school, do not take part willingly in verbal activities in class and possibly have further difficulties with written comprehension and reading. Occasionally poor motor skills add to the picture.

Within this age group there will be some who have received formal speech therapy in the past, possibly before starting or during their early years at school. These early language learning problems may have continued or re-emerged, resulting in their arrival at specialist psychiatric units – patients often report increasing difficulty throughout secondary education. Some – not wishing to appear different – may suffer in silence whilst others present with more conspicuous behavioural problems.

A useful foundation for treatment in these cases is to encourage the keeping of a daily diary, stressing that grammar and spelling are unimportant to this exercise and accepting entries at the person's own level – which may be single words – and using a simple layout. The diary can be expanded – which often happens spontaneously – and will include feelings, reactions and attitudes as well as daily events. As vocabulary increases and language develops an individual creative style will emerge and there will be indications of areas for improvement and for further support and intervention. This technique might be viewed as introspective and solitary in a therapy designed to expand and develop communication, but during therapy sessions the diary will be shared and a communicative link is formed through which a therapeutic relationship can develop.

ADULT PSYCHIATRY

Adult psychiatry covers all aspects of adult psychiatric care with some overlap with late adolescent services and those for elderly mentally ill people. It is the major psychiatric service and extends to community care, out-patient clinics and hospitals, wards and units for day or in-patient care. As was seen in Chapter 1, the largest proportion of patients treated are seen in the community by their general practitioner. About 5–10% are referred to specialist services and seen in psychiatric clinics or hospitals. There are variations in the rates of psychiatric morbidity found in different surveys, but approximately 15% women and 10% men appear to suffer psychiatric illness (Dean, 1988), figures which reveal the size of the problem. Most people in health or social services are likely to encounter patients suffering from mental illness during the course of their work and are likely also to know colleagues, relatives, friends and neighbours who suffer from psychiatric conditions of some description.

Classification and diagnostic categories

The main DSM-III headings for adult disorders relevant to this volume are organic (e.g. dementia, psychoactive substance induced and those associated with physical disorders); psychoactive substance use disorder; schizophrenia; delusional (paranoid) disorder; other psychotic disorders; mood disorders (bipolar and depressive); anxiety and phobic disorders; somatoform disorders; and personality disorders.

ICD–9 categories to which attention should be drawn are labelled slightly differently as psychoses (including senile and pre-senile organic, alcoholic, drug induced, transient organic, schizophrenic, affective, paranoid and other chronic organic psychoses) and neurotic disorders, personality disorders and other non-psychotic mental disorders (including as well as the obvious categories, alcohol and drug dependency, organic conditions and depressive and conduct disorders not classified elsewhere). Chapters 4–7 will elaborate these categories further.

Incidence of adult mental disorder

People with psychiatric and emotional problems are increasingly being treated out of hospital and admission, when it does become necessary, is likely to be short rather than long term and in a district general hospital rather than a psychiatric institution (Williams and Clare, 1986). The general practitioner is well placed to monitor psychiatric disorder in the community as it is known that in the National Health Service in Great Britain 60–70% of registered patients will consult the GP at least once in a year and 90% in any two years (Williams and Clare, 1986). The GP has access to the medical history and often knows the social background of his patients, giving an advantage in gaining cooperation and eliciting personal information that may be essential to a complete appraisal of the patient's complaints (Shepherd et al., 1966).

Estimates of the extent of psychiatric disorder in the community vary widely and there is evidence that psychiatric morbidity seen in general practice often occurs in association with physical morbidity and is associated with a wide variety of social disabilities and dysfunctions. In a general practice serving a population of about 2500 the major acute disorders seen in any year are listed in Table 2.1, and total about 380 cases. Of those diagnosed as psychiatrically ill 87% are assigned to categories of neurosis, insomnia, tension headache and physical disease presumed to be psychogenic in origin, while only 5.5% are diagnosed as psychotic (Dean, 1988). Dean goes on to state that GPs refer 5.5% of those they feel are psychiatrically ill to psychiatric services and a further 4.4% to other medical services for investigation. Patients with

Table 2.1 Psychiatric disorders in an average general practice population of 2500

Acute major disorders	Cases per annum
Severe depression	13
Suicidal attempts	3
Completed suicide	1 in 3 years
Chronic mental illness	55
Severe mental handicap	10
Neurotic disorders	300

Based on Royal College of General Practitioners (1986)

severe symptoms are more likely to be referred but there is also a tendency for better-educated patients to be referred to the psychiatric services as they request it more often.

The numbers of those patients admitted to mental health hospitals or units in Great Britain, either for the first time or as a readmission, during 1986 are given in Table 2.2. These figures demonstrate that psychotic patients are more likely than neurotic to receive hospital care, although many psychotics are successfully treated in the community. There are more patients readmitted than admitted for the first time,

Table 2.2 Patients admitted to mental health hospitals/units in the UK, 1986

Diagnostic group	Male	Female	Both sexes
Schizophrenia/paranoia	15 271	14 148	29 419
Affective psychoses	8 107	16 526	24 633
Senile/pre-senile dementia	7 624	13 234	20 858
Alcoholic psychoses	509	266	775
Other psychoses and drugs	7 455	10 537	17 992
Neurotic disorders	4 978	10 291	15 269
Personality and behaviour disorders	6 531	7 667	14 198
Depressive disorders not elsewhere classified	11 740	23 469	35 209
Mental retardation	305	284	589
Other psychiatric conditions	287	346	633
Mental illness – diagnosis not stated	65	48	113

Based on *Mental Health Statistics for England*, DHSS (1986)

and other trends include an increase in the number of elderly mentally ill people requiring the services of mental illness hospitals and an increase in the numbers of new patients attending out-patient clinics.

Causes of adult mental illness

Reference to the possible causes of mental disorders and in particular mental illness has been made in the sections on child and adolescent psychiatry. Much of this information is also relevant to adults. Further discussion will be found in the chapters on specific disorders – depression, psychoses, neuroses and personality disorder.

Management

Services are divided between those for acute and for chronic patients, and include those facilities described in Chapter 1.

Table 2.3 gives the figures for the duration of in-patient care in England up to 1986 and Table 2.4 for deaths and discharges from mental illness hospitals or units.

Table 2.3 Duration of in-patient care until December 1986

Durations	Numbers
Under 1 year	25 790
1 year	6 560
2 years	3 640
3 years	4 580
5 years +	19 710
Total	60 280

Based on *Mental Health Statistics for England*, DHSS (1986)

Table 2.4 Discharges and deaths from mental illness hospitals and units 1986

Durations	Numbers
Under 1 month	118 258
1 month	52 110
3 months	19 100
1 year	3 659
3 years	1 650
5 years	1 590
10 years	548
15 years +	1 915

Based on *Mental Health Statistics for England*, DHSS (1986)

Assessment

During the course of taking a history, observations will be made by the psychiatrist or by other professionals in a formal interview or informal setting. A mental state examination will take into account observations in both settings of the patient's appearance, behaviour, what is said and the way in which the person communicates. The psychiatrist is particularly interested in the patient's mood, concentration, insight and whether there are obsessional phenomena, delusions, depersonalization/derealization, illusions, hallucinations, disorientation, memory problems and attentional deficits.

A physical examination will be given and possibly a full neurological assessment, if an organic syndrome is suspected, which would include evaluation of language, constructional abilities and agnosias, for example. Psychological tests, usually administered by clinical psychologists, may be standardized or take the form of quantified observations of behaviour (for example, rating scales). Intelligence testing might be necessary and tests of reading ability, personality and thought disorder may also be used.

Treatment

Treatment will vary according to the type and severity of illness and the location of the patient. The main areas to consider are drug treatments, electroconvulsive therapy, psychosurgery and psychotherapy, the latter of which will be discussed in Chapter 10. Due to the fast increasing numbers of drugs prescribed in psychiatry a committee of the World Health Organization, in 1967, suggested a classification of psychotropic drugs into six groups. Antipsychotics are drugs with therapeutic effects on psychoses and other types of psychiatric disorder, but extrapyramidal side-effects such as tremor and rigidity frequently result. Antidepressants are used to treat pathological depressive states. Antianxiety drugs reduce pathological anxiety, agitation and tension without therapeutic effect on disturbed cognitive or perceptual processes and, while they do not lead to extrapyramidal effects, they can produce drug dependency. Psychostimulants increase the level of alertness and/or motivation. Psychodysleptics produce abnormal mental phenomena, particularly in the cognitive or perceptual spheres. Finally neoceptive drugs improve cognitive functioning and memory (Silverstone and Turner, 1988).

It has been observed that there is considerable variation from patient to patient in the response to a fixed dose of almost any drug and therefore in some cases a drug may produce a satisfactory response, in others there may be no response and in others there may be intoxication.

Electroconvulsive therapy (ECT) is known to be an effective treatment for severe depressive disorders and is used to bring about rapid improvement, but because of the effectiveness of modern psychotropic medication fewer courses of ECT are now given. The strongest indications are if there is risk of suicide, depressive stupor or danger to physical health, for example if the patient is not drinking (Gelder *et al.*, 1986). ECT is usually given as a course of about six treatments, administered twice weekly. One of the immediate side-effects of ECT is the loss of memory for events before the treatment and some impaired retention of information acquired soon afterwards. Normally there is no permanent memory disorder, except in a small minority and even in those cases it is difficult to know whether this effect was due to the ECT or to continuation of the depressive illness. ECT is discussed in detail by Taylor (1986).

Psychosurgery is the use of neurosurgical procedures to modify symptoms of psychiatric illness and involves operating on the nuclei of the brain or on the white matter. Surgery should only be used after failure of all other methods of treatment and even then rarely. Some clinicians state that it should never be used and others support its use for a very few intractable disorders, such as obsessional and severe chronic depressive disorders. Other forms of psychiatric intervention are referred to throughout this volume and will be given more specific attention in Chapter 10.

The role of the speech therapist

Communication problems abound in mental illness, varying in severity according to the illness or condition they accompany. Many of the problems are of long standing and often motivation to improve is limited. All aspects of speech (e.g. voice, articulation, prosody) and language can be affected, therefore pathology is diverse and this may be as a result of mental illness/disorder or as an accompanying factor. The quality and quantity of change in a person's communicative abilities may only really be evaluated by others who have known the patient prior to the onset of the illness – family, friends, colleagues, teachers, or perhaps the general practitioner – but the most important person of all, the patient, might be able to describe any changes and all professions must learn to listen to them. The speech therapist will be employed to assess, diagnose and treat all forms of speech pathology encountered in an adult population, but naturally in this context the most important area is that of diagnosis of such pathology in relation to mental illness. In particular the area of differential diagnosis is crucial and is discussed in Chapter 10. Emphasis needs to be placed on the importance of audiometric assessment because of the high incidence of hearing impairment in the mentally ill, as well as the normal deterioration in hearing ability as part of the ageing process. Such information will assist future management and treatment.

There are certain aspects of behaviour associated with mental disorder that have particular relevance to the speech therapist's role, as they are significantly linked to speech and communication. These include the phenomenon of self-mutilation, which is in fact quite common, especially in mentally handicapped and general psychiatric populations, and occurs as a result of emotional disturbance. People suffering from personality disorders, schizophrenia, borderline personality disorder, depression and hysteria might have a history of self-mutilation.

Self-mutilation

These patients are usually women who are young, attractive, have low self-esteem, express a dislike of their own body and often use drugs and alcohol in excess. Often linked are problems of confused sexual identity; a background of broken homes and parental deprivation through distancing and inconsistent maternal warmth; and there is a possibility that they have been involved in incestuous relationships. It has been emphasized that the difficulties these patients seem to have is in expressing needs – they show significant difficulties in verbalization and an improvement in verbal expressive ability is often associated with clinical improvement and cessation of the self-mutilating behaviour. It has been found that among schizophrenic children, for example, the more verbally fluent are significantly less likely to mutilate themselves (Simpson, 1976).

Elective mutism

This is a rare occurrence in adulthood but is nevertheless apparent. In this condition, discussed more fully in the section on child psychiatry, the mechanisms for the production of speech and language are usually intact but the patient chooses not to communicate and in so doing is communicating this negative decision. It is a very powerful way to involve and attempt to control or manipulate the people responsible for and caring for the individual, although most communicate effectively with their families. Problems often start during the early days at school.

Occasionally there may be conflict in differentiating elective mutism from true mutism.

Voice disorders

Traumatic voice disorders may result from suicide attempts by strangulation, swallowing corrosive substances or severe burning. Functional voice disorders due to vocal abuse are surprisingly rare, despite prolonged shouting and screaming during disturbed behaviour – sometimes for years, not just weeks or months and more often seen in women than men. Observers in such cases will often expect irreparable vocal damage to result, but the voice is a most resilient 'weapon' and usually no vocal harm is in fact found to occur.

THE PSYCHIATRY OF OLD AGE

It is probably true to say that more attention has been paid to the speech therapist's role with elderly mentally ill people than with any other age group in relation to mental health. It is included at this point only for the sake of completeness, following as it does sections on childhood, adolescence and general adult psychiatry, and is dealt with in detail in Chapter 8 of this volume, by Griffiths.

Classification and diagnostic categories

The psychiatric illnesses found in old age are the same as the disorders seen in a general adult population, and similarly are usually classified by use of either the DSM-III or ICD–9 systems. Certain disorders are more likely in old age (such as dementia of the Alzheimer's type) and others may have different characteristics/presentation when compared with a younger group.

The incidence of mental illness in old age

The emphasis that has been placed on old-age psychiatry has focused on the dementias and in many disciplines has been in reaction to the demographic changes that are resulting in increased numbers and higher proportions of older people in society – particularly of the very old who need more resources both socially and medically. In terms of psychiatric need there have been few epidemiological studies going beyond the prevalence of dementia, but Gianturco and Busse (1978) did look at a sample of elderly volunteers, apparently well functioning, and found 20–25% were depressed at any time (only 30% had no depressive episode over the twenty-year course of the study), over 50% had hypochondriacal ratings at some point, and at the last testing there were 38% with mild and 12% with moderate/severe organic brain syndrome. Arie and Isaacs (1978) quote incidences, also for a community-based sample, of 12% neuroses/character disorders, 2% major functional psychoses and 10% dementia (in residential care this last figure went up to 40%). Overall 25% of elderly people in the community and 40% of all over–65-year-olds (Pitt, 1982) are thought to have significant psychiatric disorder, but little attention has been paid to the needs of this population in terms of research or clinical management.

Causes of mental illness in old age

The causes of mental illness and disorder in old age are multifactorial, as indeed at any age, although there is more risk of organic brain syndrome. Some conditions onset in old age and the stresses and losses experienced by people as they age may well be implicated, while other conditions are long standing and individuals have grown old while suffering from them – for example, there are many elderly schizophrenics in psychiatric hospitals who were originally admitted as younger adults and often mentally handicapped people who have psychiatric or behavioural problems have been in care for many years. The underlying causes are probably the same as in younger life.

Management and the role of the speech therapist

Services for elderly people developed first as a medical speciality and subsequently as a specialism within psychiatry. Responsibility is taken by the psychiatry service for elderly people who have functional mental illness or dementia – although in the latter event in the UK mild cases are dealt with largely by the primary care team or local authority. In addition there is the group of patients who have grown old in long-stay psychiatric hospitals, a group decreasing in number with the trend to the community and early discharge.

Elderly mentally ill (EMI) people face, in Western society, a dual stigma of being 'old' and 'mad' and services need to be offered sensitively and to cover also issues of public education. Adverse attitudes towards these people are common even among those who work with them and can result in a nihilistic approach to rehabilitation.

Pitt (1982) suggests treatment principles of preventative work, attitudinal change, early identification of illness and early intervention, maintenance in the community and not to over-treat organic or under-treat functional illness. Baker and Clark (1976) ask for 'the provision of services which will give the elderly person just the amount of support needed without removing his independence'.

Speech therapists, as well as other professionals, can seek to follow these principles as members of the multidisciplinary team. General management suggestions for work with older people are offered by Gravell (1988) and specific involvement with EMI patients is covered later in this book.

REFERENCES

Allen, R. E. and Oliver, J. M. (1982) The effects of child maltreatment on language development. *Child Abuse and Neglect*, **6**, 299–305.

Arie, T. and Isaacs, A. D. (1978) The development of psychiatric services for the elderly in Britain, in *Studies in Geriatric Psychiatry* (eds. A. D. Isaacs and F. Post), Wiley, Chichester, pp. 241–61.

Baker, L. and Cantwell, D. P. (1987) Comparison of well, emotionally disordered and behaviourally disordered children with linguistic problems. *Journal of the American Academy of Child and Adolescent Psychiatry*, **26**, (2), 193–6.

Baker, A. A. and Clark, M. L. (1976) Mental illness in the elderly, in *Comprehensive Psychiatric Care*, (ed. A. A. Baker), Blackwell Scientific Publications, London, pp. 270–87.

Barker, P. (1988) *Basic Child Psychiatry*, 5th edn, Blackwell Scientific Publications, London.

Beitchman, J. H. Nair, R., Clegg, M. *et al.* (1986) Prevalence of Psychiatric disorders in children with speech and language disorders. *Journal of the American Academy of Child Psychiatry*, **25** (4), 528–35.

Blager, F. B. (1979) The effect of intervention on the speech and language of abused children. *Child Abuse and Neglect*, **5**, 991–6.

Bowlby, J. (1969) *Attachment and Loss*, Vol. 1, Hogarth Press, London.

Brown, B. and Lloyd, H. (1975) A controlled study of children not speaking at school. *Journal of the Association of Workers for Maladjusted Children*, **3**, 49–63.

Cantwell, D. P., Baker, L. and Mattison, R. E. (1979) The prevalence of psychiatric disorder in children with speech and language disorder: an epidemiological survey. *Journal of the American Academy of Child Psychiatry*, **18**, 450–61.

Coombes, K. (1987) Speech therapy, in *Language Development and Disorders*, (eds. W. Yule and M. Rutter) MacKeith Press, London, pp. 350–66.

Corbett, J. A. (1979) Psychiatric morbidity and mental retardation, in *Psychiatric Illness and Mental Handicap* (eds. F. E. James and R. P. Snaith), Gaskell Press, London.

Dalton, P. and Hardcastle, W. J. (1977) *Disorders of Fluency and their Effects on Communication*. Edward Arnold, London.

Dean, C. (1988) Psychiatry in general practice, in *Companion Guide to Psychiatric Studies*, 4th edn. (eds. R. E. Kendell and A. K. Zealley), Churchill Livingstone, Edinburgh, pp. 634–47.

DSM-III-R (1987) *Diagnostic and Statistical Manual of Mental Disorders* 3rd edn – revised, American Psychiatric Association, Washington, DC.

Evans, J. (1982) *Adolescents and Pre-adolescent Psychiatry*, Academic Press, London.

Fox, L, Long, S. H. and Langlois, A. (1988) Patterns of language comprehension deficit in abused and neglected children. *Journal of Speech and Hearing Disorders*, **53**, 239–44.

France, J. (1987) *A National Survey of Speech Therapy in Psychiatry*, unpublished paper.

Funk, J. B. and Ruppert, E. S. (1984) Language disorders and behavioural problems in pre-school children. *Developmental and Behavioural Paediatrics*, **5** (6), 357–60.

Garfield, S. (1980) *Psychotherapy: An Eclectic Approach*, Wiley, New York.

Gath, A. (1987) The social context: communication in families with a handicapped child, in *Language Development and Disorders* (eds W. Yule and M. Rutter). MacKeith Press, London, pp. 262–70.

Gelder, M., Gath, D. and Mayou, R. (1986) *Oxford Textbook of Psychiatry*, Oxford University Press, Oxford.

Gianturco, D. T. and Busse, E. W. (1978) Psychological problems encountered during a long term study of normal ageing volunteers, in *Studies in Geriatric Psychiatry* (eds A. D. Isaacs and F. Post), Wiley, Chichester, pp. 1–17.

Gordon, N. (1987) Developmental disorders of speech and language, in *Language Development and Disorders* (eds W. Yule and M. Rutter), MacKeith Press, London, pp. 189–205.

Gravell, R. (1988) *Communication Problems in Elderly People: Practical Aproaches to Management*, Croom Helm, London.

Gualtieri, C. T., Koriath, J., Van Bourgoridien, M. and Saleeby, N. (1983) Language disorders in children referred for psychiatric services. *Journal American Academy of Child Psychiatry*, **22** (2), 165–71.

Hill, P. (1986) The psychiatry of adolescence, in *The Essentials of Postgraduate Psychiatry*, 2nd edn (eds P. Hill, R. Murray and A. Thorley), Grune and Stratton, London, pp. 139–40.

Howlin, P. and Rutter, M. (1987) The consequences of language delay for other aspects of development, in *Language Development and Disorders* (eds W. Yule and M. Rutter), MacKeith Press, London, pp. 271–94.

International Classification of Diseases, 9th edn (1977) WHO, Geneva.

Klein, M. (1963) *The Psychoanalysis of Children*, Hogarth Press, London.

Kolvin, I. and Fundudis, T. (1981) Elective mute children: psychological development and background factors. *Journal Child Psychology and Psychiatry*, **22**, 219–32.

Lambert, N. M., Sandoval, J. and Sassone, D. (1978) Prevalence of hyperactivity in elementary school children as a function of social system definers. *American Journal of Orthopsychiatry*, **48**, 446–63.

Lerner, J. A., Inui, I., Trupin, E. W. and Douglas, E. (1985) Preschool behaviour can predict future psychiatric disorders. *Journal American Academy of Child Psychiatry*, **24** (1), 42–8.

Lewis, M. and Mezey, G. (1985) Clinical correlates of septum pellucidum cavities: an unusual association with psychosis. *Psychological Medicine*, **15**, 43–54.

Love, A. J. and Thompson, M. G. G. (1988) Language disorders and attention deficit disorders in young children referred for psychiatric services. *American Journal of Orthopsychiatry*, **58** (1), 52–64.

Offord, D. R., Boyle, M. H., Szatman, P. *et al.* (1987) Ontario child health study: prevalence of disorder and rates of service utilisation. *Archives of General Psychiatry*, **44**, 832–6.

Ostwald, P. F. (1981) Speech and schizophrenia, in *Speech Evaluation in Psychiatry* (ed. J. K. Darby), Grune and Stratton, New York, pp. 329–48.

Paul, R., Cohen, D. and Caparino, B. (1983) A longitudinal study of patients with severe developmental disorders of language learning. *Journal of the American Academy of Child Psychiatry*, **22**, 525–34.

Peterson, E. B. (1988) Psychiatric disorders of adolescence, in *Companion Guide to Psychiatric Studies*, 4th edn (eds R. E. Kendell and A. K. Zealley), Churchill Livingston, Edinburgh, pp. 535–54.

Pitt, B. (1982) *Psychogeriatrics: An Introduction to the Psychiatry of Old Age*, Churchill Livingstone, Edinburgh.

Purser, H. (1982) Clinical child psychology, in *Psychology for Speech Therapists* (ed. H. Purser), British Psychological Society/Macmillan Press, London, pp. 101–40.

Rousey, C. L. and Moriarty, A. E. (1965) *Diagnostic Implications of Speech Sounds*, Charles C. Thomas, Springfield, Illinois.

Rutter, M. (1979) *Changing Youth in a Changing Society*, Nuffield Provincial Hospitals Trust.

Rutter, M., Cox. A., Tupling, G. *et al.* (1975) Attainment and adjustment in two geographical areas – the prevalence of psychiatric disorder. *British Journal of Psychiatry*, **126**, 493–501.

Rutter, M. and Garmezy, N. (1983) Developmental psychopathology, in *Socialisation, Personality and Social Development Handbook of Child Psychiatry*, 4th edn, Vol. 4 (ed. E. M. Hetherington), Wiley, New York.

Rutter, M. and Lord, C. (1987) Language disorders associated with psychiatric disturbance, in *Language Development and Disorders*, (eds W. Yule and M. Rutter), MacKeith Press, London, p. 206–33.

Rutter, M., Schaffer, D. and Sturge, C. (1975) *A Guide to a Multiaxial Classification Scheme for Psychiatric Disorders in Childhood and Adolescence*, Institute of Psychiatry, London.

Rutter, M., Tizard, J. and Whitmore, K. (1970) *Education, Health and Behaviour*, Longman, London.

Shaffer, D. (1985) Depression, mania and suicidal acts, in *Child and Adolescent Psychiatry: Modern Approaches*, 2nd edn (eds M. Rutter and L. Hersov), Blackwell Scientific Publications, Oxford.

Shepherd, M., Cooper, B., Brown, A. C. and Kalton, G. (1966) *Psychiatric Illness in General Practice*, Oxford University Press, Oxford.

Silverstone, T. and Turner, P. (1988) *Drug Treatment in Psychiatry*, 4th edn Routledge Press, London.

Simpson, M. A. (1976) Self-mutilation. *British Journal of Hospital Medicine*, October, 430–8.

Steinberg, D. (1983) *The Clinical Psychiatry of Adolescence*, Wiley, Chichester.

Steinberg, D. (1987) *Basic Adolescent Psychiatry*, Blackwell Scientific Publications, London.

Taylor, P. J. (1986) Electroconvulsive therapy, in *Essentials of Postgraduate Psychiatry*, 2nd edn (eds P. Hill, R. Murray and A. Thorley), Grune and Stratton, London.

Weiss, C. and Lillywhite, H. S. (1981) *Communication Disorders: Prevention and Early Intervention*, 2nd edn, Mosby, St Louis.

Wells, G. and Gutfreund, M. (1987) The conversational requirements for language learning, in *Language Development and Disorders* (eds W. Yule and M. Rutter), MacKeith Press, London, pp. 90–102.

Williams, P. and Clare, A. (1986) Psychiatry in general practice, in *Essentials of Postgraduate Psychiatry*, 2nd edn (eds P. Hill, R. Murray and A. Thorley), Grune and Stratton, London, pp. 597–622.

Wing, L. and Gould, J. (1979) Severe impairments of social interaction and associated abnormalities in children: epidemiology and classification. *Journal of Autism and Developmental Disorders*, **9**, 11–29.

Wolff, S. (1988) Disorders of childhood, in *Companion Guide to Psychiatric Studies*, 4th edn (eds R. E. Kendell and A. K. Zealley), Churchill Livingstone, Edinburgh, pp. 505–34.

World Health Organization (1967) Research in psychopharmacology. *WHO Technical Report Series 371*.

3

Hearing loss, mental handicap, acquired brain damage and forensic psychiatry

Rosemary Gravell and Jenny France

HEARING LOSS AND PSYCHIATRY

While the effect of hearing loss on communication has been well documented and much discussed it is considered here from the often neglected angle of mental health. This is an area that should be recognized as of crucial significance in assessment and treatment by all team members. General reviews of the role of the speech therapist with hard of hearing and deaf people can be found, for example, in Parker (1983) and Gravell (1988).

Many comments have been made in the literature about the stigma associated with being deaf and it is worth briefly stressing this before discussing the relationship with mental health in a more systematic way. Ashley (1973) in his account of his own experiences discusses the lack of recognition and sympathy offered and his isolation from past pleasures and present social opportunity. Beethoven, in 1802, wrote of being 'obliged to seclude myself and live in solitude' and stated 'there can be no relaxation in human society'. The effect of social stigma is probably more apparent in individuals with acquired deafness and may lead to long delays in coming forward for help (Vernon, Griffin and Yoken, 1981) thus compounding later problems. In the public mind there seems to be a link between deafness and old age and/or lack of intelligence and major public education is needed to have any effect on this potentially harmful stereotype.

Social sequelae are common, indeed inevitable, for deaf or hard of hearing individuals – deafness alters experience and may force detachment or social isolation. However, there are studies that suggest social interaction may not necessarily decrease (e.g. Norris and Cunningham, 1981) and it may be that isolation and withdrawal mark out those who come forward to clinics, rather than a random sample. Within the family there are important issues to consider, both when a deaf child

56

is born into a hearing family and – more neglected in the literature – when deaf parents have a hearing child (Frankenburg *et al.*, 1985).

It is important to be aware of the difference between those who are congenitally or pre-lingually deaf and those who have later acquired deafness, as will be made apparent later in this discussion.

Classification and diagnostic categories

The classification of mental disorder in the case of hearing-impaired people follows the same systems as for others in any age group suffering from mental disorder and has therefore been discussed earlier in this chapter. However, two major diagnostic categories have been the focus of attention of researchers looking at the mental health of deaf people and it is therefore worth outlining the conclusions of these studies.

Psychoses

Various papers over recent years have considered the relationship between deafness and psychosis, a link often referred to perhaps with more anecdotal than empirical basis. Thomas (1981) felt there was little support for paranoia in deaf people but that there does appear to be a high incidence of hearing loss in paranoid psychotics – a phenomenon also alluded to by Post (1966) for instance – and stressed the need for more systematic study. Cooper (1976) discussed ways in which paranoia and long-standing hearing loss may be linked, by presenting several theories: firstly there may be personality characteristics which predispose to psychiatric illness – but studies are inconclusive. Psychosocial consequences of deafness may lead to withdrawal and isolation – but this may be due to pre-morbid personality. Sensory deprivation may be relevant from study of its effects in experiments on hearing people, but this is not established as a cause of mental disorder in the deaf population. Communication disorder may be the mediating factor and there does seem to be some evidence of 'an impairment in the perception of speech sounds' in schizophrenia, not revealed on pure-tone testing and of lateral asymmetries in sensitivity (e.g. Kugler *et al.*, 1982). Misunderstandings and misperceptions often occur and may lead to psychiatric sequelae. Finally Cooper suggests deafness may enhance in schizophrenics the screening out of environmental stimuli already due to attentional/perceptual deficits.

Roth and McClelland (1971) suggest that in predisposed individuals deafness may aggravate the tendency to withdrawal and disrupt reality testing, leading to misinterpretation of the outside world. Early onset, long duration and severity of hearing loss are probably implicated, but the links with psychosis remain controversial.

There has been some debate as to whether paranoid illness associated with sensory deficits is more common in elderly people – Cooper (1976) suggests it is, for example, while Moore (1981) found no link and felt that the hearing impairment needs to be of longer duration to cause psychosis. The variable of age obscures issues in relating sensory defects to psychiatric diagnoses, particularly when study is made of elderly in nursing homes where nihilistic attitudes in both staff and residents towards the rehabilitation of hearing disorders exist (Alpiner, 1978).

Depression

Harry (1986) suggests psychiatric depression and bipolar disorders are rare in deaf people; however, he does add that symptomatic expression rather than prevalence may be what is reflected. In the *British Medical Journal* (1977) meanwhile it states that depression, neuroses and psychosomatic sequelae are common, while Eastwood *et al.* (1986) found a link between severity of hearing loss and functional psychiatric disorder in their elderly subjects.

It is not difficult to postulate as to how pre- or post-lingual deafness could cause depressive symptoms, via social isolation, disorientation (partly due to the loss of background sounds), difficulty forming relationships and so on. Beethoven (1802) stated that he was 'on the point of putting an end to my life' and other personal reports have drawn attention to the depressed mood of some who become deaf. However, there appears to be little evidence of how prevalent depression is in acquired or congenital deafness and again there is need for further study, particularly as depression is in many cases a treatable condition.

Other psychiatric disorders

Diagnoses of personality disorders may have been made inappropriately in the light of deaf people's communication difficulties. Harry (1986) summarizes descriptions given of the 'deaf personality' – impulsive, aggressive, egocentric, isolated, lacking confidence and suspicious are just some of the terms used – and the debate as to whether there is a specific 'deaf personality' continues.

Denmark (1985) comments on a high number of referrals to a specialist clinic for the deaf who had committed criminal offences, many of a sexual nature. He postulates that this stems from poorly developed knowledge and experience of relationships.

Psychogenic deafness may occur although it is 'quite rare' (Harry, 1986) and can be discovered by inconsistencies of behaviour and by special audiometric testing.

The incidence of mental illness in hearing-impaired people

There have been a variety of studies of the prevalence of psychiatric disorder in hearing impairment but most have suffered from methodological problems that affect their value. Many studies have failed to take account of differences between congenital and acquired deafness, as Thomas (1981) points out, and Denmark stresses that the two groups cannot be equated – acquired deafness leads to sensory deprivation and congenital to sensory deficit. Other factors that need to be considered in attempting to study the relationship between deafness and mental health include the presence of associated disorders (e.g. tinnitus), shared causative factors (e.g. brain damage), severity of hearing loss, age and time since onset.

Past studies have tended to use biased questions in psychiatric assessment, for example relating to feelings of isolation which may be attributable either to the deafness or the psychiatric disorder. Samples have been unrepresentative, with high proportions of women and of single or widowed people or limited to clubs for hearing-impaired people rather than using random populations (Thomas, 1981). Hearing assessment has also not always been appropriate – for instance Mahapatra (1974) looked only at one frequency criterion, which was outside the speech range.

Bearing in mind these provisos in data interpretation it is accepted that there are higher prevalences of mental disorder in those with pre- and post-lingual deafness when compared to hearing populations. Eastwood *et al.* (1986) studied older nursing home residents and found 66% with clinically significant hearing loss and 52% with psychiatric disorder – results congruent with a community survey of elderly people conducted by Gilhome-Herbst and Humphrey (1980). Mahapatra (1974) looked at conductive deafness and in bilaterally affected people 41% and in unilaterally affected 18% were identified as psychiatrically ill. His use of only one frequency may have led to underestimation of disorder especially as it failed to cover speech frequencies, as has been stated. Another study of acquired deafness found 19% adults of working age to have mental disorder compared to 5% controls (Thomas and Gilhome-Herbst, 1980).

There is a need for properly planned epidemiological study of the prevalence of psychiatric disorder in acquired and in congenital/prelingual deafness, in order to plan effective management. As will become apparent this population has been sadly neglected clinically.

Causes of mental illness in hearing-impaired people

In the *British Medical Journal* (1977) it was stated that 'Deafness may contribute to the development of mental disorder through its association with sensory deprivation, communication disorder, perceptual distortion, and attention deficit or as a non-specific stress' and Denmark (1985) made the point that any degree of deafness at any age can lead to psychosocial sequelae. However, the mechanisms linking hearing loss and mental disorder are unclear and likely to be highly complex.

Some possible links have been discussed in relation to the specific conditions of psychosis and depressive illness but there have been attempts to simulate deafness (for example by using earplugs) to study the effect on people. These studies revealed emotional reactions, irritability, withdrawal, poor concentration and what Hebb *et al.* (1954) described as a 'slight personality disorder'. Clinical observations are rife, particularly since the Second World War (Thomas, 1981), noting tendencies to suspiciousness, anxiety, depression, hysteria and psychosomatic symptoms (e.g. Knapp, 1948; Ramsdell, 1962). Experimental studies in which, as has been mentioned, methodological problems abound have suggested decreased sociability and emotional stability, neuroses and paranoia. There has also been considerable attention paid to the question of whether there is a characteristic 'deaf personality'.

Harry and Farazza (1984) present a case study of a pre-lingually deaf adult presenting with a brief reactive psychosis and suggest as a possible aetiological factor the sociocultural conflict experienced by those who belong to the deaf culture and thus face problems relating to the hearing culture in which, to a certain extent, they must function. This perhaps parallels the difficulties faced by immigrants within a new society. People who become deaf later in life do not tend to be part of the often well-established deaf culture that exists, therefore this factor is less likely to be relevant in acquired deafness.

It has already been stated that there are possible links between mental illness and hearing impairment with family life, when deaf children are born to hearing parents or vice versa. Deaf children may have increased behavioural problems because of communicative deprivation rather than deafness *per se*. Family reactions range from denial to over-protectiveness and interaction is often decreased, causing the child to feel isolated. If a hearing child is born to deaf parents (deaf adults tend to intermarry) there may be problems due to the lack of 'distance contact' usually provided auditorially when out of sight, to lack of appropriate communication, to embarrassment or resentment in older children needed to interpret for their parents – and possible jealousy on the part of the parents, and to cultural differences as the child faces the conflict between the parents' deaf culture and the outside hearing society.

The effects of tinnitus

Tinnitus is a noise heard in the ear which does not have an external source; it is a symptom, not a disease (Davis, 1983). Severe tinnitus affects 2.5% of the population and of those in 20% it is disabling (MRC, 1985); however, usually help is only sought when the condition is a major aggravation (Harrop-Griffiths et al., 1987). Tinnitus may be experienced in one ear or both or as a head noise, there may be a single sound or several, and on testing Hawthorne et al. (1987) found only 12% did not have a significant hearing loss (although many of their subjects did not report this).

These last two studies both looked at psychiatric morbidity and found depression to be common in tinnitus sufferers – Hawthorne et al. quote 41% of their sample as having mental illness and Harrop-Griffiths et al. 80% as having major psychiatric illness at some time in their life, with depression the main differentiating factor. This depression may be a primary disorder with tinnitus as a secondary (psychosomatic) complaint or may be secondary due to the aversive affects of tinnitus. Referrals do tend to suggest certain patient characteristics (e.g. age and sex) are implicated, but it may be that this reflects referral bias on the part of family doctors. Similar symptoms may not be referred on in older people yet co-occurrence with other effects of ageing may mean these symptoms become more catastrophic. Prevalence is a function of age (Coles and Davis, 1983).

Management

The first principle of management is to approach hearing-impaired people sensitively, whether dealing with those who have pre- or post-lingual deafness. Communication is obviously made difficult and at the same time many professionals are not given enough training in this aspect of care. Especially with profound pre-lingually deaf people skilled communicators, who can use manual methods, are essential to assessment and treatment processes. With those who have acquired hearing loss it may be appropriate to provide amplifiers particularly, perhaps, in working with older patients. Aid provision is a first consideration if there is usable hearing, but not all can benefit (Thomas and Gilhome-Herbst, 1980).

There is no doubt that services for psychiatrically disordered deaf people are inadequate. Specialist services in the UK were first developed in 1964 for out-patients (in Manchester) and in 1968 for in-patients. Such clinics have remained rarities but their approach can be of value to those working with hearing-impaired people in other settings and have implications for the speech therapist. Denmark (1985) describes a specialist clinic taking referrals from all over Great Britain to evaluate whether there is a mental illness or problems experienced by the patient are actually due to communication difficulties. Of 250 referrals about half communicated manually, nearly one-fifth were non-communicative and the rest used oral or combined methods. In these subjects psychiatric diagnoses were made in 104, developmental disorders affecting communication were found in 48 and in 58 there were problems directly related to their hearing impairment – these findings are summarized in Table 3.1.

It is of fundamental importance to have professionals involved who have the ability to communicate manually as well as a knowledge of deafness. The assessment and treatment of mentally ill people with communication difficulty is very time consuming and difficult, as psychiatric interviews tend to be verbally based. Pyke and Littman (1982) describe a Canadian clinic and make similar points to those of Denmark. They found 25% of referrals had psychiatric problems 'solely due to deafness' and that family doctors tended to refer deaf people only when there was *major* mental illness compared with referrals of hearing people for psychiatric consultation. There were more cases of mentally handicapped individuals than would be expected in a normal population and one-quarter of their referrals were diagnosed psychotic.

Table 3.1 Diagnoses of 250 referrals to a psychiatric clinic for the deaf

Psychiatric Disorder		Developmental Disorder		Problem related to Deafness	
Schizophrenia	56	Mental handicap + other problem —	30	Behavioural	53
Neurosis/pers. disorder	26	Autism	7	Depression	3
Affective disorder	14	Central language disorder	6	Alcoholism	1
Organic	4	Other	5	Tinnitus	1
Schizo-affective	1				
Other	3				
Totals	104		48		58

It is clear, across national borders, that mental health services in all disciplines are not meeting the needs of the hearing-impaired population. Thacker (1988) reporting on the European Society of Mental Health and Deafness Congress drew attention to various delegates' comments on the inadequacies of provision, especially of long-term care. Many still 'remain in psychiatric hospitals and hospitals for the mentally impaired, living in total isolation because staff are unable to communicate with them effectively' (Denmark, 1985) and it appears deaf people on average are likely to stay much longer in psychiatric hospitals than hearing patients (Timmerman, 1988). Deaf adolescents are also very poorly catered for at present.

Management should not merely focus on direct intervention but – via a multidisciplinary approach – should be involved in preventative work before crises arise. This would involve counselling, education and social skills teaching, for example. Early diagnosis should be a further aim as intervention for hearing loss early on may decrease psychiatric symptoms (Eastwood et al., 1981). This wold apply to work with adults and children, often in the latter instance implying work with and through the family.

The psychiatric clinics described above use manual communicators, but there will be instances where interpreters are needed – for example, when psychiatrists or other workers are not fluent manual communicators. Care must be taken as there is a danger, particularly with mentally ill patients, of distortion, confusion and misunderstanding and the mere presence of a skilled interpreter does not mean communication can be left to him or her – the non-verbal cues given by the psychiatrist or other professional may assume even greater significance for the deaf person.

The role of the speech therapist

It has already been stated that the role of the speech therapist in general work with deaf populations is beyond the scope of this volume, but there is a need for speech therapists to be aware of their usefulness in working with mentally ill deaf or hearing-impaired individuals. Many of the techniques that may be employed will be discussed in Chapter 10, so only a brief outline of the approach needed will be offered here.

It is apparent that it is communication that is the crux of working in this field and the speech therapist's specialist knowledge can therefore be important in several ways. She can be crucial in guiding parents on how best to communicate with a deaf child during the formative years to reduce distancing and isolation and thus reduce psychosocial risks of behavioural and educational problems later in life. Advice on when manual methods should be employed may be offered alongside the opinions of other team members and teaching given in total communication skills.

The speech therapist is important within the psychiatric team partly in the role of teaching other professionals how best to communicate with deaf patients. Interaction is more tiring and slow, and deaf people may use different coping strategies. The preferred communication method for each individual must be determined. Non-verbal behaviours may be affected both by the hearing loss and any mental illness that coexists, so the therapist must educate others on non-verbal aspects of their own and the patient's behaviour. Advice can be offered on seating, proximity, language modification (slowing, avoiding complex structures or jargon, etc.) and manipulating the environment to avoid distractions and maximize communicative potential.

Psychiatric disorders may themselves reduce the communicative ability of a person, as has been stressed throughout this chapter, and attention must be given to this possibility rather than assuming the deafness is the cause. Assessment of language and communication skills may follow the principles outlined in the chapter on management, with precautions appropriate to the needs of deaf people in each age group. Work with individuals may take the form of direct intervention related to the hearing impairment or the psychiatric disorder, counselling and social skills training.

It is evident that the speech therapist working in specialist settings – in psychiatric practice, in the field of hearing impairment, or indeed in general adult/child work (as hearing loss and psychiatric symptoms are both so prevalent in communicatively impaired populations) – needs to have a good knowledge of the special rehabilitative needs of mentally ill deaf or hard-of-hearing people.

MENTAL HANDICAP AND PSYCHIATRY

Mental retardation, mental handicap and specific learning difficulty are all terms used to refer to 'sub-average general intellectual functioning which originates during the developmental period and is associated with impairment in adaptive behaviour' (Heber, 1961). It is not a unitary condition, but these labels act as blanket terms covering many different patterns of social, emotional, intellectual and physical problems and many degrees of severity (Purser, 1982).

Although, as always, there are problems in subgrouping or classifying on any one criterion, there does seem to be some justification in the frequently used severity gradings, in terms of predicting symptoms and rehabilitation needs (Tizard, 1966) so long as the arbitrary boundaries are recognized as fallible in individual cases. The usual distinctions made are between mild (IQ 50–70), moderate (35–49), severe (20–34) and profound (below 20). Approximately three-quarters of all those diagnosed as mentally handicapped fall into the mild group. The diagnosis of mental handicap, however, is not as clear cut as this may suggest as there is a continuum with normal intelligence and the boundaries are impossible to define solely on numerical criteria, as associated factors may mean two individuals with similar IQ levels function very differently. At times mental retardation may only be apparent later in life, as a result of social inadequacy and occasional instances of criminality. The relationship of mental handicap and criminal behaviour is poorly understood but there is some evidence of increased incidence of sex offences and arson, and Reid (1982) discusses possible reasons for these links.

Classification and diagnostic categories

Mental handicap is usually defined both in terms of social and intellectual functioning. ICD–9 classifies on the current level of functioning rather than on aetiology and stresses the need to use additional codes when, as often happens, psychiatric disturbances are also involved. While this system includes a separate axis for intellectual level, the DSM-III system subsumes mental retardation under its second axis of developmental and personality disorders.

Most discussions of psychiatric disorder in mental handicap agree that symptoms are modified by intellectual level and by brain damage. Certain symptoms may have little or no psychiatric significance in mentally handicapped people although in other groups they would be seen as highly relevant – for example, disorientation, echolalia, manneristic or repetitive movements. It is also crucial that psychiatrically disturbed behaviour is separated from underlying developmental delay, as an apparently deviant behaviour may be an immaturity, characteristic of a younger age group. Furthermore lack of verbal ability may render a person unable to describe or draw attention to symptoms and this can lead to great difficulty in establishing certain psychiatric diagnoses in severely retarded individuals. Some clinicians (e.g. Reid, 1982) feel it is 'difficult to conceive of psychiatric disturbance' in profoundly mentally handicapped people because they are so limited in their behaviour and reactions.

A further diagnostic factor to bear in mind, especially with those who have limited ability to express themselves, is that 'deviant' behaviour may in fact reflect a healthy response to stresses, such as bereavement or resettlement (Hallas *et al.*, 1978).

Despite these difficulties in diagnosis all mental illnesses found in a normal population can occur in mentally handicapped adults or children, both the major groups and less common conditions, like anorexia, which have nothing particularly distinctive in their presentation or treatment in a mentally handicapped population. It seems appropriate to offer brief comments on the former group – that is, the major mental illnesses, as they may differ in presentation in mentally handicapped people.

Hyperkinetic syndrome

There is some debate over the existence of hyperkinetic syndrome, which is reflected in wide discrepancies in prevalence between cultures – for instance, it is much more widely diagnosed in the USA than in the UK. It has been linked with minimal brain dysfunction but this term may mislead and there is no evidence of structural abnormalities in children thus diagnosed. Outcome varies: some settle to normal activity levels while in others hyperactivity persists or hypoactivity is seen. Consistency in approach is crucial, providing plenty of space seems to be beneficial, and drugs and/or behavioural techniques may be used. It may be that there is an underlying epilepsy, which should be suspected if the symptom is episodic in nature.

Early childhood autism

This has been discussed elsewhere in this volume and will not be given detailed attention here, other than to stress that the majority of autistic children are also of low intellectual level and must be managed accordingly.

Depression/mania

The prevalence of manic and/or depressive disorders in mental handicap has been put at between 12 and 35 in every 1000 (Reid, 1972; Corbett, 1979). Similar stresses as in normal populations can precipitate affective disorder (such as bereavement or childbirth) and similarly there may be a single or recurring episodes. Diagnosis may be difficult in severe intellectual impairment when observation of mood and behaviour, somatic or hysterical symptoms and family history become even more central because of the lack of verbal ability. Diagnosis is important, however, both because treatment is often successful (largely by medication) and because behaviours may otherwise not be set 'in the correct context of illness' (Reid, 1982) and thus responded to inappropriately. Suicide may be attempted by mildly mentally handicapped individuals (Gelder *et al.*, 1989; Reid, 1982).

Schizophrenia and paranoid psychoses

Diagnosis is difficult, as a degree of verbal fluency is needed and it is hard to know what weight to give to symptoms as mentally handicapped people show various behavioural 'quirks' anyway. The more intellectually impaired a person is the 'less the clinical features of mental disorder approximate to the clusters found in adult psychiatry' (Fraser, 1982). Symptoms may be qualitatively different – for example Gelder *et al.* (1986) suggest delusions and hallucinations are less elaborate. Treatment has vastly improved over the past twenty-five years with drugs and social care and diagnosis is vital to allow these benefits to schizophrenic mentally handicapped people. However, it does appear that there are increased side-effects of medication in this population which need to be considered. Deafness may play a causative role and is very common in the mentally handicapped population (Reid, 1982). A discussion of the possible link can be found earlier in this chapter.

Organic reaction types

There are well-established links between brain pathology and mental handicap, but progressive brain conditions may also occur – most notably dementia, which is becoming more prevalent in this group as life expectancy increases. Particular links between Alzheimer's disease and Down's syndrome exist. Clinical presentation is similar to normals, although onset may be earlier and progression more rapid (Heaton-Ward and Wiley, 1984) but below a certain intellectual level it is hard to establish a history of deterioration and thus to diagnose. Delirium may be more readily provoked in the mentally handicapped population but is otherwise not distinctive.

Neurotic, conduct and personality disorders

Reid (1982) states that it is hard to accept the validity of non-psychotic classifications in this population, but in order to plan treatment the categories are needed, and there is 'nothing unique in the symptoms'. Mentally handicapped people probably face more stress in life (e.g. educational failure, stigma, dependency, family disappointment) and this is reflected in a high incidence of neurotic disorder, often acted out behaviourally or hysterically as they cannot communicate verbally. Diagnosis in severe retardation is probably precluded. Treatment is by manipulation of the environment, family therapy, behavioural modification, limited use of drugs and explanation/support at the appropriate level.

Conduct disorders are common and may persist into personality disorder/psychopathy. As in other mental illnesses the problems so caused in terms of management may outweigh those due to the mental handicap itself. The focus of treatment is to match the individual better to their environment and consider the role of the family. Drugs and/or behaviour therapy may play a part. The distinction between neurotic conduct and personality disorder is far from clear, overlapping in presentation, course and precipitating factors (Reid, 1982).

Behavioural problems

Certain behaviours are associated with mental handicap and lead to severe management problems. Some clinicians feel there is a discrete subgroup or syndrome of multiple behavioural problems, which can be persistent and concentrated, with symptoms of aggression, restlessness, insomnia and self-injury. Other mentally handicapped people may show marked single aberrant behaviours, for example self-injury is seen particularly in some conditions (e.g. Lesch-Nyhan and Norrie's disease). Ritualistic, repetitive behaviour patterns are common and may indeed be communicative, thus having functional value. Sexual behaviour may be socially unacceptable and present management difficulties.

All psychiatric symptomatology in mentally handicapped people must be seen in the context of the whole person and the setting in which they are functioning.

The incidence of mental illness in mental handicap

The prevalence of mental handicap in under–20-year-olds is 3–4 in every 1000 population (Yule and Carr, 1980). Adult prevalences are harder to establish, particularly in the light of increased life expectancies for disabled people. Tizard (1964) points out the difference between true prevalence and what he describes as the administrative prevalence, which is those needing services.

Nearly all mentally handicapped individuals will have associated problems, for example, Fraser (1982) discusses the prevalence of psychiatric and communicative disorders. Heaton-Ward and Wiley (1984) mention autism, sensory defects, epilepsy, hyperkinetic syndrome, spasticity and superimposed psychiatric illness. All of these conditions will of course affect the management of the individual. Mentally handicapped people are very vulnerable to adverse social consequences of educational failure and social rejection.

As these comments suggest, overall the incidence of psychiatric illness is greatly increased in this population. Corbett (1979) found 47% of children and 46% of adults with severe mental retardation to have symptoms of mental illness, and this seems to be representative of the literature. Rutter *et al.* (1970) found psychiatric disorder to be up to four times more common in children with IQs two or more standard deviations below average.

Causes of mental illness in mental handicap

There are numerous causes of mental handicap, which can broadly be divided into genetic (e.g. Down's syndrome, phenylketonuria), infectious (e.g. maternal rubella), physical or chemical trauma, metabolic disorder (e.g. Lesch-Nyhan syndrome), brain damage and – although not primary in more severe levels – psychosocial or an environmental deprivation. Some prefer to divide causes into two broad groupings – organic and non-organic. There may, of course, be a mixture of causes.

Reid (1982) states that severe mental handicap will almost always involve significant brain pathology and that in mild cases there is often subtle pathology. This will affect various abilities, not just intellect, and seems, for example, to predispose to psychiatric disturbance and to seizures (Rutter *et al.*, 1970). Epilepsy is very common in mentally handicapped people – Reid *et al.* (1978) found over 30% of a hospitalized population had epilepsy.

The causes of mental illness may be directly linked therefore to the intellectual handicap, for instance as a mutual result of brain damage. Psychiatric disturbance may also stem from the environment as social adjustment is impaired and there is increased risk of social-educational deprivation or failure. It may also be that the psychiatric symptoms are secondary to the individual's primary disorder.

Management

It is crucial that any assessment or treatment considers the whole person and their social/physical environment. Observation is important as verbal interview is often difficult because of low levels of linguistic ability. Psychiatric diagnosis is important to enable appropriate treatment and to plan placement as it is often the psychiatric symptoms that make it unsuitable or difficult for an individual to remain at home, which explains the high prevalence of mental illness and of management difficulties in hospitalized patients.

Medical care will involve prescription and evaluation of medication and some psychotherapy input. This latter is very limited with the mentally retarded person but can support and encourage, perhaps particularly in a group setting, the mildly impaired. However, psychotherapy has a role with the family in many cases, to help them to adjust to the fact of having a handicapped child or adult in their midst. Parents experience great shock and grief often when the diagnosis is made and subsequently further difficulties arise in coping with the dependency of their child and the development of sexual maturity and a life outside the family.

Specialist therapies should also be available and psychologists have become increasingly involved in behaviour description and modification with this population. It is crucial that a multidisciplinary approach is adopted and that this applies whatever the setting, not just in hospital or residential care where it is admittedly easier to organize. This is not without problems and fragmentation of services is not uncommon and not helped by the division that exists in the UK and other countries between health and social services. The team should be involved not only in direct patient contact but also in prevention, early identification and intervention, domiciliary family support and in attempting to provide facilities to meet special needs – such as those of multiply handicapped people. The aim above all is to improve the quality of life of this population, while doing everything possible to reduce the incidence of mental handicap and of mental illness by preventative work.

Some educational systems are more supportive than others, some families need more assistance in order best to care for their handicapped relative, and – although usually outside the auspices of treatment plans – it may be that some cultures and societies enable these individuals to function more effectively (Barker, 1988).

Principles of management applied to the care of mentally handicapped people that have been particularly influential are those of normalization and personalization. The former refers to allowing the individual to function as normally as possible in and be accepted by society, and the latter to giving choices and decisions to the person. Reid (1982) cautions that these 'should not be allowed to assume the status of ideology, nor . . . be misused to deny a true appreciation of a retarded person's dependency needs and of their right to care and treatment'.

There is a need for full community support with educational, work and leisure facilities. Certainly such facilities have increased over recent years with the move away from medical models of care to a learning difficulties community-based approach. As Fraser (1982) indicates this has recognized the influence of environment and of the expectations of others upon individuals' performance. The aim now is to increase independence by providing necessary social, and in some cases residential, support. The resettlement of mentally handicapped people from 'subnormality' hospitals to the community has not proved easy, with resistance from professionals, families and sometimes the patients themselves. The resettlement of those who have superimposed mental illness is fraught with even more difficulties, and it is likely that more of this subgroup of the mentally handicapped population will continue to need residential care, as they present such particular management problems. If resettlement can be considered, intensive input is necessary to allow the transition from total institution to 'freedom', within the boundaries of ability and determined by medical and social needs.

The role of the speech therapist

Speech therapists have for some years been recognized as having an important role within the multidisciplinary care of mentally handicapped children and adults, in terms of assessing and treating communicative difficulties and feeding/swallowing problems. Therapists have been working in a variety of settings, ranging from hospitals to schools and clients' homes. While a full description of the speech therapist's role with mentally handicapped people is outside the scope of this text, this brief discussion is included in order to highlight the psychological/-psychiatric needs of this population.

Speech therapists have adopted the principles of care outlined above in the context of general management but, as the centrality of the ability to communicate in terms of quality of life is increasingly recognized, their role develops and expands. A range of communicative disorders is found in this population and there has been a considerable amount of research into language development in mentally retarded children. A review is offered by Rondal (1987), who highlights the value of speech therapy. Associated problems such as the risk of brain damage and the increased prevalence of deafness contribute to communicative handicap and there are high incidences of articulation, prosody and fluency disorders. At severe levels many will be non-verbal.

The speech therapist may be called upon to provide aids, to help individuals communicate needs and opinions, to increase social acceptability, to teach non-verbal communication when appropriate (e.g. Kiernan, 1977) and to promote the creation of an environment conducive to communication. This latter role extends to advising all disciplines as all need to be aware of and sensitive to communication in the patient/client and in themselves. Further discussion of the general role of the speech therapist will be left to others but in the context of this volume Reid's (1982) statement that the importance of speech therapy 'in the field of mental retardation, and individually in the treatment of associated psychiatric disorders, is of considerable, direct and practicable relevance' is a welcome recognition of the role with mentally ill people with learning difficulties.

However, not enough emphasis is placed upon the need to give attention to this impact of psychiatric disorder on intervention plans and there needs to be more research into how communicative abilities and needs are affected by psychiatric disorder existing with varying degrees of intellectual impairment. In many ways psychiatric care will be similar to that needed with other populations and comments within the sections in Chapter 2 on the role of the speech therapist in general psychiatric practice with children, adolescents, adults and elderly people will therefore be relevant, as will the later chapters on specific disorders and on management techniques.

ACQUIRED BRAIN DAMAGE AND PSYCHIATRY

'The domain of psychiatry encompasses a wide range of behavioural disorders associated with demonstrable neuroanatomical changes or neurophysiological derangements of the central nervous system' (Ludwig, 1980).

Although often psychiatric terms are not brought in to assist in the management of people with acquired brain damage, there is a growing body of opinion that feels this would be an important step forward and the following discussion will highlight the psychological/psychiatric needs of these patients – needs which will influence communicative processes and rehabilitation.

Causes and incidents of acquired brain damage

Brain damage may of course occur at any age and may be the result of a variety of causes. Focal damage may be due to cerebrovascular accident (CVA), to tumour or to penetrating head wounds (such as may result from gunshots), for example. Diffuse damage is seen in closed head injury and may result from disease processes affecting the central nervous system, such as Parkinson's disease, Huntington's chorea or Alzheimer's disease. Episodic brain pathology occurs in epilepsy. Acquired brain damage in childhood involves the added variable of developmental processes and there may be less distinction between diffuse and focal injury (Oddy, 1984).

Consideration of the incidence of focal, diffuse or episodic brain damage reveals some links between age and aetiology. CVA may occur at any age but incidence rises rapidly with age – Clifford Rose and Capildeo (1981) cite an annual incidence of 9 per 1000 aged 65–74, 20 aged 75–84 and 40 in the over-85-year-old group. Head injury tends to occur in younger age groups and the population is to some extent self-selecting in terms of pre-morbid activity patterns. Lewin (1970) estimated 7500 people in Britain each year have major head injury, that is with post-traumatic amnesia of more than 24 hours. Jennett (1982) cites 250 per 100 000 population are treated in hospital for head injury, of which 150 survive with significant disability.

In childhood causes tend to be more home accidents and some abuse, rather than accidents outside the home as in adults, when traffic, occupational or violence-related incidents are more common. In all cases whatever the precise nature of the damage the mental consequences will depend upon various factors, which Bond (1984) summarizes as: the mix of general and focal damage; secondary stress reactions; whether the brain is developing, mature or senescent; whether epilepsy occurs; and on pre- and post-traumatic social and personality characteristics.

Sequelae of acquired brain damage

Recovery, in degree and rate, varies between individuals and there are no fully reliable indicators of the level of functioning a person will eventually achieve. After closed head injury often there is a stage where the person is comatose, followed by a period of disorientation and post-traumatic amnesia – the length of which is often used as an indicator of severity. After this stage, with full consciousness, the main features of future disabilities emerge. Post-CVA similarly there may be a period of acute disorientation before full consciousness returns.

It is worth at this point briefly outlining some of the common sequelae of brain damage before specifically considering the psychiatric complications that may occur. Certain cognitive and mental impairments may confuse or mislead psychiatric diagnosis and thus rehabilitative planning and it is therefore important that therapists are aware of the diverse nature of difficulties and deficits with which the brain-damaged person may be left.

Cognitive sequelae

There may be residual deficits in memory, selective attention, information processing and speed, abstract thought and organization of thought. Rutter (1981), discussing children with brain damage, suggests intellectual defects are seen after diffuse or bilateral damage and are more pronounced after prolonged unconsciousness. Even after minor head injury or a mild CVA there may be evidence of cognitive slowing and resultant attentional deficits (van Zomeran *et al.*, 1984).

Communication deficits

Focal damage may result in aphasia (language disorder affecting comprehension and expression via auditory and visual modes); dyspraxia (a motor programming disorder affecting verbal output) or dysarthria (disturbed articulation due to muscular weakness or paralysis). These disorders may also be seen after closed head injury, when damage is diffuse, but persistent aphasia is thought in these cases to be rare (Newcombe, 1982) and dysarthria may then be 'the most serious permanent disorder of communication' (Thomsen, 1984). On long-term follow-up there are increasing reports of dysarthria and of persisting language problems (Brooks *et al.*, 1986) although often the latter are not truly aphasic in nature, but reflect underlying cognitive changes. There do seem to be some common sequelae in that verbal memory is impaired, naming disorders occur, subtle comprehension deficits are found and there is decreased fluency (Brooks, 1984), reading is slow and errorful and use of set phrases and incomplete sentences is common (Thomsen, 1984); however, such symptoms are not inevitable and each individual must be fully clinically assessed.

Initially after a closed head injury, with or without focal language impairment, there is a period when there is little or no desire to communicate, followed by a period of confused and disoriented language. Again this reflects the cognitive impairments suffered. Hagan (1984) discussed cognitive-language disorganization as the major communicative disability after any head trauma. This results from the disruption of attention, discrimination, sequential ordering, memory, categorization and integration of input. Individuals appear disorganized, stimulus bound, have reduced inhibition and decreased comprehension skills, and show irrelevant and confused expressive language marked by word-finding difficulty and inappropriate ordering of linguistic units.

Sensory and motor deficits

Focal or diffuse damage may lead to impairment of sensory functioning and perception and to physical handicap. These impairments have been given much more attention in clinical management in the past than have social, emotional and psychiatric disorders due to brain damage and will not be considered in detail here.

Personality and emotional changes

After apparently minor head injury or CVA there may be alterations in personality with, for example, increased irritability. Some changes will be discussed in relation to psychiatric disorder post-trauma, but it is worth stating that the emotional changes 'do not fit into the formal taxonomy of psychiatry' (Newcombe, 1982).

Personality changes are not uniform and mechanisms are likely to vary between individuals. Brooks and McKinlay (1983) suggest this will be due to the pattern of brain damage suffered, pre-morbid personality and their current social situation. There are few systematic studies but there appear to be a wide variety of altered features of behaviour and personality after brain damage and, in the case of head-injured people, these are reported by relatives more over the first year post-trauma and beyond, with increased threats of violence a particular development over time (Brooks *et al.*, 1986). Thomsen (1984) postulates that younger patients show more personality/emotional changes perhaps because 'the immature personality is particularly vulnerable'.

There has been a reluctance to accept self accounts of emotional change due to professionals' knowledge of well-documented cases of limited self-awareness and insight in brain-damaged people; however, Kinsella *et al.* (1988) suggest that self-report screening scales may be reliable. In the studies that have looked at emotional and personality change most have used the reports of relatives and evidence appears conclusive that it is these changes and psychiatric sequelae that result in increased burden on families, rather than sensory or physical disability (e.g. Thomsen, 1974; Bond, 1975).

McKinlay *et al.* (1981) found the most prevalent problems for families three months after closed head injury were the patient's slowness, tiredness and memory loss; after six months slowness, tiredness and irritability; and after one year irritability, impatience and tiredness. Changes that have been referred to in the literature include – in addition to these – apathy, silliness, sexual drive alterations, rigidity, anxiety and impaired social perceptiveness. Aggression is not uncommon and may be more readily released by alcohol than pre-morbidly (Bond,

1984). Personality changes seem to persist and there is usually associated cognitive impairment (Bond, 1984).

Social factors

Most studies have looked at the proportion of brain-damaged people who return to work to assess social recovery, but recently there has been an awareness that leisure activities are equally disrupted, regardless of physical handicaps. Social isolation is common and to patients themselves often appears the most devastating effect of their injury (Thomsen, 1974). In fact, excepting the most severely injured of working-age groups, work is resumed more quickly than are leisure and social activities. Return to work is furthermore a crude indicator of recovery because often people return only to some or to altered duties.

Social relationships within the family are affected often increasingly over time, as problems become more apparent. Parents appear to cope better than spouses of head-injured patients, although such a comparison is limited by age in CVA victims. Marital breakdown, isolation and educational/occupational difficulties continue even 10–15 years post-trauma (Thomsen, unpublished study).

In childhood too there are continued social problems, perhaps related to school failure, and family relationships seem most disrupted again some time after the damage in about 10% of cases (Klonoff and Paris, 1974). There are many stresses on parents and lack of discipline, over-protection and denial are common reactions (Oddy, 1984). Worsening reports of difficulties over time from parents and other relatives, regardless of the age of the brain-damaged individual, may reflect a decrease in the relatives' acceptance rather than objective changes in the handicapped person.

Psychiatric disorders in acquired brain damage

Organic brain syndromes

Certain behavioural patterns have been ascribed to focal cortical damage but may also be seen in diffuse damage that particularly affects certain brain areas, as in some closed head injuries. Frontal lobe damage can cause attentional and planning deficits, impulsivity and perseveration. There may be primitive reflexes. Typically patients are egocentric and irresponsible, the severity of behavioural disorder relating to the degree of returned insight (Bond, 1984). There may be clinically misleading signs of pseudo-depression or pseudo-psychopathy.

Temporal lobe damage may lead to memory and language deficits, epilepsy, hallucinations and occasionally affective or schizophrenic-like psychotic symptoms. Parietal lobe damage can disturb the body schema and cause motility disorder, while occipital damage may result in blindness, agnosias, illusions and hallucinations.

Ludwig (1980) points out that 'cortical lobe syndromes may often be misdiagnosed as functional psychiatric disorders, especially when there are no associated and obvious neurological deficits or localizing signs'. Psychiatric disorders linked thus include depression (in cases of frontal or temporal damage), hysterical reactions (parietal, occipital or temporal) and personality/social disorders (frontal or temporal).

Diffuse brain damage can lead to the so-called 'post-head trauma syndrome' characterized by a variety of psychiatric manifestations, and disease processes (as in Huntington's or Parkinson's disease) may also result in major psychiatric illness either as primary (i.e. disease caused) or secondary symptoms – depression, personality deterioration and compulsive thinking occur, for example.

Episodic brain pathology (epilepsy) may give rise to various controversial psychiatric syndromes – fugue, hysterical epilepsy, personality change, psychoses and others. However, the other side of the coin is that some signs of epilepsy may be mistaken for psychiatric symptomatology and this should be investigated if the latter present in stereotyped, time-limited episodes.

In summary organic brain syndromes can masquerade as functional psychiatric disorder, may be complications of other disorders (such as alcoholism) or of drug treatment, and may produce personality-behavioural disruptions which require psychiatric intervention.

Dementia

The label dementia is, and must be, used sparingly in cases of brain damage due to injury. It is worth mentioning, however, that there is a pseudo-dementia (Ganser syndrome) that may be seen. Specific attention is given to the problem of dementia in Chapter 8.

Depression

Depression may result after brain damage of any severity and Lishman (1978) suggests such feelings are common but usually transient, developing three to six months after insult when there is increased awareness of disability. Depression is thought to be a negative prognostic factor in terms of response to rehabilitation attempts. Kinsella *et al.* (1988) found the availability of a confidant was strongly related to the experience of depressive feelings.

A study of CVA patients by Ebrahim *et al.* (1987) looked at the incidence of depression and found a relationship with severity of the CVA but not with hemispheric laterality; however, the study excluded severely aphasic patients. Antidepressive medication is less often given to aphasic individuals (Lim and Ebrahim, 1983) perhaps because of the difficulties they present in terms of making any psychiatric diagnosis. Mood disturbance seems to contribute to longer hospital stays even with fairly minor functional disability.

It is likely that depression is more common after focal or diffuse damage than is realized or treated. Suicide is rare early on but Lishman (1978) noted a peak 15–19 years on in head injury cases. Mania occurs post-trauma occasionally and there seems to be a high incidence of epilepsy in these patients (Shukla *et al.*, 1987).

Psychoses

Paranoid ideas and delusions may occur as a transient symptom arising in the stage of disturbed consciousness. There have been reports of such a syndrome following prolonged intensive care/ventilation treatment. Lisham (1978) comments that persecution and marital infidelity figure prominently in post-trauma paranoia.

Schizophrenia-like psychoses increase in incidence after closed head injury, which appears related to the severity of brain injury. However, other factors must be involved as the incidence is still small (Davidson and Bagley, 1969). Thomsen (1984) describes early-onset and late-onset psychoses after blunt head trauma, with two of her eight cited cases having permanent problems. Diagnosis is often difficult and it may be necessary to undergo a trial period of medication.

Dissociative and behavioural disorders

It is thought by many that injury exaggerates pre-morbid traits but, interestingly, there have also been instances when previously objection-able behaviour has been moderated – for example, alcoholism. Anxiety and irritability are common and reactions tend to be more marked when encountering new situations or events. Wood (1984) describes dissociative disorders where, in order to keep control, there is a split from consciousness, stressing the devastating effect these have on rehabilitation attempts via behaviour modification. Some present with 'opposite' behaviour which is also difficult to cope with in therapy, as are obsessional/ritualistic behaviours. Behavioural problems may be a direct result of injury/damage or due to a psychological response to the situation.

Neuroses

A syndrome has been noted frequently after mild head injury and labelled 'compensation neurosis' (Lloyd, 1980). It occurs most often in men of lower socio-economic status and results in over-preoccupation with and exaggeration of symptoms. Outcome is favourable once litigation to do with the injury is resolved.

Psychiatric disorder in childhood head injury

The additional variables of development are important to consider in childhood-acquired brain damage. There have been few controlled studies but at the same time many references to psychiatric sequelae. Similar disorders occur as are seen in general child psychiatry (and thus the discussion in Chapter 2 will be relevant) but individual symptoms may differ, as Brown *et al.* (1981) point out, and disinhibition is rare in general clinics but does occur after severe head injury.

It is accepted that psychiatric disorder is more common after brain damage – Rutter (1981) found it to be twice as common as in non-brain-damaged children and James (1982) reports psychiatric signs in two-thirds of head-injured children (and neurological signs in under 10%). However, it is hard to explain the link. Mechanisms involved may include the severity of injury, the locus, the type of pathology, the age at injury (the debate continues as to hemispheric plasticity in the developing years), temperament and psychosocial factors. Children prone to accidents may have shown behavioural problems before injury which put them at risk.

There is no one stereotyped psychiatric syndrome seen after head injury, but there is a need for more study of post-brain damage *de novo* behaviours and signs. Some psychiatric disturbances may only appear years after the incident, perhaps as the child reaches a more demanding stage of development.

General management

Rehabilitation

The aim in rehabilitation is to attain each individual's potential level of functioning by relearning lost skills, developing compensatory abilities, learning to cope with residual deficits and restoring confidence. This involves utilizing 'the abilities of the patient in a structured way' (Muir Giles and Clark-Wilson, 1988) towards independence. In childhood the aim is not 'merely to return to the pre-morbid level but to place on the moving developmental stair' (James, 1982).

Little seems to be written about the positive factors in patients which aid rehabilitation – such as drive, orderliness, some retained cognitive abilities and some ability to discriminate the consequences of behaviour. Negative factors in planning rehabilitation include the existence of depression or of dissociative disorder, lack of awareness of disability persisting beyond six months post-incident, alcoholism and behavioural/psychiatric disorders.

Treatment has been based on clinical tests with an implicit assumption that deficits thus shown will affect a person's functioning. There are two main schools of thought in rehabilitation – cognitive and behavioural. The former is limited by the decreased initiative of patients which affects carry over, but it considers such abilities as memory and attention. Highly structured material is used, for example in developing visual imagery for memory work. Behavioural therapy uses learning theory to modify disordered behaviour and seems successful in quite severe cases given lengthy application and if carried over into social and work settings (Eames and Wood, 1985). Other models of rehabilitation have been stimulation and substitution. Recently the need for counselling has also been recognized, both for the affected individual and for families. Whatever approach is taken there is a pressing need for satisfactory evaluation of procedures and of relevant patient/therapist/situational factors. Such data are at present scanty but once obtained may be valuable, for example showing up when techniques prove to be too expensive in terms of time and effort for the benefits that result (Gloag, 1985).

Placement issues

The service to brain-damaged people has all too often been fragmented and placement has been a particular problem for children and young or middle-aged adults. Inappropriate placement may well have exacerbated problems – for example, Bond (1984) points out that discharge to more familiar surroundings can greatly reduce prolonged disturbed consciousness in children. Moving to general wards from intensive care is likely to result in more clues to orientation, if any behavioural problems are not too difficult for the ward to manage, and similarly involving known people in rehabilitation can aid orientation. Increased input with families can help them cope with the personality and behavioural changes that prove most handicapping in later months and years. Once the individual is medically stable it is advisable to transfer to a rehabilitation centre as soon as possible – although having said that there are few such centres available and children are especially poorly catered for.

Many go from hospital care to inactivity as a result of this, which engenders its own stresses and long-term psychiatric problems. 'Truly successful rehabilitation should have an impact on how the person spends his time' (Diller and Gordon, 1981) and this necessitates appropriate acute care, long-term accommodation/rehabilitation services and domiciliary follow-up, in order to consider the long-term emotional and other needs of these people and their families. These same needs exist for elderly brain-damaged individuals too, although aims will differ in some ways, for example in relation to employment.

Psychiatric intervention

Psychiatric diagnosis relies heavily on verbal material and in some cases patients will be unable to make use of this so that a trial period of drug therapy is indicated. Psychiatric intervention may consist of drug use or psychotherapy with families or individuals. Too often the psychiatric sequelae of brain damage are ignored by professionals, yet intervention is needed early on to reduce the incidence of psychiatric morbidity if this is possible (McKechnie, 1982). Results suggest intervention can reduce emotional stress and depression, for example. Psychiatric symptoms can, without doubt, sabotage rehabilitation and jeopardize the future quality of life for patients and their families.

In general little attention has been paid to the special needs of head-injured children and adults, and even CVA patients have suffered from a lack of broad aims in service and therapy planning beyond the merely physical. Oddy (1984) describes this as 'the challenge for all professions involved in the care of head-injured patients'. There is a need for multi-disciplinary involvement with the patient as a family and social being from the earliest point. All concerned need clear explanations and the opportunity to ask questions and be involved in decisions. Psychiatric teams should have a role in dealing with the often 'serious emotional and intellectual handicaps incurred' and sensitive consideration given to possible family reactions against psychiatric intervention (McKechnie, 1982).

A unified approach both in clinical team-work and at a high administrative level is necessary, to evaluate better the psychological needs of this population and how best they can be met in the short and the long term.

The role of the speech therapist

This discussion is not intended to cover the speech and language therapy that might be appropriate with this population, which is well covered by a variety of other texts (e.g. Hagan, 1984; Holland, 1984). The aim of this brief section is to stress the need for speech therapists to take account of the possibility of psychiatric disorder in people of any age who have acquired brain damage and appropriately adapt to their resultant needs in terms of planning assessment and rehabilitation. The evidence for long-term difficulties in communication, due to specific disorders or to impaired social-emotional skills, suggests a follow-up role is needed – in addition to involvement in the acute stages.

The need to consider cognitive deficits has long been accepted and Hagan (1984) and others recognize this in their approaches to assess-ment and therapy. Involvement may begin in the stage of deep coma and as soon as some degree of response occurs input will be functional (communication and feeding) and indirect. Manipulation of the environment and advice to staff and relatives can be crucial to support-ing through the initial stages but also prove valuable in preventing later emotional and psychiatric distress. The repeated links between mental health and communicative ability suggest this as a logical possibility but empirical research is necessary. A further role early on that may be crucial to reduce frustration is the consideration of simple alternative means of communication or of communication aids as supplements to speech.

In later stages social skills work may be valuable to improve conver-sational skills, sensitivity to listeners, use of environmental clues and so on. It is often useful to observe patients outside clinical settings (for instance at mealtimes or in group activities) as there may be functional communication difficulties that are not indicated by specific speech-language tests. Sarno (1984) for example found a third of closed head injury patients with coma have hidden linguistic deficits and, in addition, there may be social communication difficulties due not to the brain damage *per se* but to psychiatric disorder. Medication must also, of course, be considered. Problems may only become apparent when the person is confronting new situations and demands, which possibly should be taken into account during the rehabilitation period.

If there is a psychiatric disorder after diffuse or focal brain damage, in addition to specific speech and language work appropriate for the brain-damaged population, the chapter in this volume concerned with practical management issues will be relevant. Mazella Gordon and Wicks (1988) state 'the discrepancy between real and apparent ability has practical consequences for all aspects of rehabilitation, can be easily overlooked, and may lead to unrealistic expectations, resulting in feelings of helplessness and frustration'. The speech therapist can contribute greatly by ensuring all understand the limitations due to communicative disorders which stem either from the brain damage itself or from the secondary emotional and psychiatric sequelae and that they adapt accordingly.

FORENSIC PSYCHIATRY

Forensic psychiatry is a term that applies to all legal aspects of psychiatry, which includes civil law and laws regulating psychiatric practice, as well as that branch of psychiatry that deals with the assessment and treatment of mentally abnormal offenders. It is important to point out that the laws of different countries vary considerably and there are also differences between the legal and the psychiatric concepts of mental abnormality. Those working in clinical psychiatry must therefore work with the knowledge of two sets of laws – those relating to 'ordinary' psychiatric patients and those relating to mentally abnormal offenders. It is thought that social causes of crime are more important than psychological causes, but there is a group of offenders whose criminal behaviour is believed to be at least partly due to psychological factors.

The mentally abnormal offender is a criminal offender who suffers from a mental disorder and such people are a small minority of all offenders. Initial problems they present include whether they are fit to plead in court, whether treatment is necessary and if so where it should be provided – in the community, a psychiatric hospital, a special hospital, a regional secure unit or prison.

Special hospitals

Special hospitals consist of a secure perimeter wall and an 'air-lock' entrance system, so that all movements into and out of the hospital and patient movements within the hospital can be monitored. Full facilities for daily life, work, education, exercise, relaxation, socialization and treatment are provided. Special hospitals are staffed by nurses, psychiatrists, social workers, occupational therapists, educating staff, librarians, chaplains, physiotherapists, speech therapists, psychotherapists, administrative and clerical staff, catering and domestic staff.

The patients

In the UK approximately 74% of patients in secure hospitals suffer from mental illness, predominantly schizophrenia, and the remaining 26% from personality disorder (psychopathy). All patients are detained on a court order – in the UK the relevant legislation is section 37 of the Mental Health Act 1983 – and many will have a restriction order added (section 41). Less than 10% will be on treatment orders (section 3) and about 10% will have been transferred from prison (on a section 47–49) according to Faulk (1988). Offences include homicide, other violent acts, arson, sex offences and causing criminal damage.

The patient's stay is usually for five or more years; short stays are unusual unless the individual is sent to the hospital for assessment prior to sentence and then found unfit for treatment. Two of the special hospitals in the UK – Rampton and Ashworth – also take patients who are mentally handicapped with mild-moderate impairment (10%) and severe impairment (15%), but other hospitals do not cater for this population (e.g. at Broadmoor Hospital).

Treatment offered to these patients is similar to that in other psychiatric hospitals although considerable interest is focused on the patient's past, his offence and life around the time of the offence, his early life, successes and failures, relationships and knowledge and understanding of his mental illness. Treatment programmes are based on coping with daily living, understanding the past and looking towards the future to help to grieve for himself, then to grieve for the victim – which is to feel remorse. The offender needs to become acceptable and an accepted member of the community by stopping antisocial behaviour and developing social assets and a sense of responsibility.

Regional secure units

Regional secure units cater for those patients who are too difficult or dangerous to be dealt with in the community or in an open setting, but are not so disturbed as to require a special hospital. Most regions in Britain now have either an interim unit or their own regional unit, and they vary according to the security provided. As part of the rehabilitation of the individual is to enable them to return to the community patients will eventually have freedom to move unaccompanied outside the unit. The units are designed to be small enough for staff to manage easily – 50 beds is thought to be the maximum and less than this the ideal.

The patients

Most patients suffer from mental illness, predominantly schizophrenia, and the rest from personality disorder. In the UK patients are referred from National Health Service hospitals (25%), special hospitals (20%), courts and remand prisons (40–50%), community services (up to 10%) and ordinary prisons (1–2%) according to the figures given by Faulk (1988).

The length of stay varies from unit to unit, mostly between six to twelve months, with some units extending this to two years. The restricted patients will tend to stay the longest and some chronically ill people might have their length of stay determined by the difficulty of placing them back in the community. Treatment styles are usually based on a multidisciplinary approach and staffing levels are high, making it possible to organize individual programmes for each patient's needs. Types of treatment offered are similar to those in any psychiatric hospital.

Secure wards

Secure wards are wards within 'ordinary' psychiatric hospitals used to nurse patients who are disruptive or dangerous and who cannot be nursed on an ordinary psychiatric ward. Patients are admitted on the short term and once the acute disturbance is over they are returned to their former place. The staff offer supportive and individual attention and the length of stay may vary from a few days to a few weeks.

Psychiatric care in the penal system

The incidence of serious mental illness in prison seems to be the same as in the general population, that is 3–4% of both psychoses and affective disorders. Personality disorders are more prevalent (80%) as are alcoholism (50%), drug abuse (25%), epilepsy (1.5 times the normal rate) and mental handicap (possibly 14%) according to Faulk (1988). It is known that prisons contain large numbers of psychiatrically disturbed people – in a survey in the south-east of England, Gunn (1977) found 31% of prisoners to be psychiatrically disturbed. A medical service is provided in prison and the team consists of a prison medical officer who is assisted by hospital officers, some qualified psychiatric nurses and visiting psychiatrists. Treatment by medication and psychotherapy is offered.

The role of the speech therapist in a forensic setting

As previously stated patients in secure settings suffer from similar mental illnesses as patients in other settings apart from potential dangerousness. Good communication skills are seen as a precondition for successful participation in some of the therapeutic groups and so the speech therapist has a particular role in assessing and improving speech and language skills (Grounds *et al.*, 1987), and such practice may be seen, for example, in Broadmoor hospital, where one of the authors works. Treatment there is provided individually and in groups with the emphasis on communication – all treatment is with full cooperation of the nursing staff, who offer support to individual programmes and participate in group work.

Structured group work is multidisciplinary and includes social skills (shared at Broadmoor with the clinical psychology and nursing staff), communication skills and communication groups and dynamic psychotherapy (with a psychotherapist, psychiatrist and trained psychiatric nurses). Some structured groups are 'purpose built' to include particular personal needs of patients and deal with anger control, assertiveness training, interpersonal relationships, self-awareness and sex education.

The communicative needs of this population are added to by their traumatic history and the difficulties they face in coming to terms with this, some are unable to accept and understand their past and some may not even believe that it is indeed their own history! The opportunity to talk about the past is essential – to be able to describe the offence and talk about the time, events and relationships leading up to it will help the individual to put it into perspective whilst within a supportive environment. They can then take that history back into the community, perhaps to familiar places, and learn to live with it. To achieve this a particular language is needed, to describe events that may be too horrific for others to hear or for the person to discuss, to allow the individual to regain or develop insight about the offence and to accept responsibility, understand its significance and ultimately be strong enough to survive.

Having developed the ability to talk openly, freely and honestly for treatment purposes, the next stage of rehabilitation is to modify the use of language and communication around these events and so fit into society presenting acceptable codes of communicative behaviour. The ability to be able to adapt from one setting to another – perhaps an institutional setting to the community – and from one group of people to another demands sophisticated communication skills, which need to be learnt or relearnt as part of the rehabilitative process.

In forensic settings many patients are detained without limit of time and so the urgency to accomplish treatment aims before the patient is ready to move on is reduced. This is particularly important in the case of the personality-disordered patients who fill approximately one-third of the special hospital beds and eventually move on to regional secure units for further treatment. Treatment programmes can therefore be developed and expanded as needed, or adapted to a particular patient. For instance, two of the special hospitals in the UK (Rampton and Ashworth) have a mentally handicapped population which will need the traditional skills of the speech therapy service in addition to their needs in relation to their mental illness, any physical problems and other medical conditions. Care for the hearing impaired in forensic settings is important, in particular for the mentally handicapped who are often difficult to assess, and the speech therapist may be able to offer valuable assistance in diagnosing and supporting treatment with this group of patients.

Many patients in forensic settings have suffered long-term mental illness and institutionalization (either in psychiatric hospitals or prisons). Medication, although carefully monitored, can produce speech problems such as dysarthria. Some such speech disorders may be very severe and may be further exacerbated by acute psychotic symptoms as exhibited in the person's language.

Yet again the emphasis of treatment is through a team approach and language, speech, fluency, articulation and voice therapy will all be approached in a number of different ways – for instance, the therapist may offer individual and/or group therapy, social skills and general communication work, psychotherapy and many other types of structured educational and interpersonal programmes.

REFERENCES

Alpiner, J. G. (1978) *Handbook of Adult Rehabilitative Audiology*, Williams and Wilkins, Baltimore.

Ashley, J. (1973) *Journey into Silence*, Bodley Head, London.

Barker, P. (1988) *Basic Child Psychiatry*, 5th edn, Blackwell Scientific Publications, London.

Beethoven, L. van (1802) *Heiligenstadt Testament*, Hamburg Stadtbibliothek.

Bond, M. R. (1975) Assessment of the pscyhosocial outcome after severe head injury, in *Outcome of Severe Damage to the CNS*, CIBA Foundation Symposium, Amsterdam, **34**, 141–58.

Bond, M. (1984) The psychiatry of closed head injury, in *Closed Head Injury* (ed. N. Brooks), Oxford University Press, Oxford, pp. 148–78.

British Medical Journal (1977) *Deafness and Mental Health*, 22 Jan, 191.

Brooks, N. (1984) Cognitive deficits after head injury, in *Closed Head Injury* (ed. N. Brooks), Oxford University Press, Oxford, pp. 44–73.

Brooks, N., Campsie, L., Symington, C. *et al.* (1986) The five year outcome of severe blunt head injury: a relative's view. *Journal of Neurology, Neurosurgery and Psychiatry*, **49**, 764–70.

Brooks, D. N. and McKinlay, D. (1983) Personality and behavioural change after severe blunt head injury. *Journal of Neurology, Neurosurgery and Psychiatry*, **46**, 336–44.

Brown, G. W., Chadwick, O., Shaffer, D. *et al.* (1981) A prospective study of children with head injury. *Psychological Medicine*, **11**, 63–78.

Clifford Rose, F. and Capildeo, R. (1981) *Stroke – The Facts!* Oxford University Press, Oxford.

Coles, R. R. A. and Davis, A. C. (1983) *Tinnitus and Ageing*, paper to BSA meeting/Geriatric Audiology, November.

Cooper, A. F. (1976) Deafness and psychiatric illness. *British Journal of Psychiatry*, **129**, 216–26.

Corbett, J. A. (1979) Psychiatric morbidity and mental retardation, in *Psychiatric Illness and Mental Handicap* (eds F. E. James and R. P. Smith), Gaskell Press, London.

Davidson, K. and Bagley, C. R. (1969) Schizophrenia like psychoses associated with organic disorders of the CNS, in *Current Problems in Neuropsychiatry* (ed. R. N. Herrington), *British Journal of Psychiatry* Publ. no. 4, pp. 113–84.

Davis, A. C. (1983) Hearing disorders in the population in *Hearing Science and Hearing Disorders* (eds M. E. Lutman and M. P. Haggard), Academic Press, London.

Denmark, J. C. (1985) A study of 250 patients referred to a department of psychiatry for the deaf. *British Journal of Psychiatry*, **146**, 282–6.

Diller, L. and Gordon, W. (1981) Intervention for cognitive deficits in brain injured adults. *Journal of Consultative Clinical Psychology*, **49**, 822–34.

Eames, P. and Wood, R. (1985) Rehabilitation after severe head injury. *Journal of Neurology, Neurosurgery and Psychiatry*, **48**, 613–19.

Eastwood, M. R., Corbin, S. and Reed, M. (1981) Hearing impairment and paraphrenia. *Journal of Otolaryngology*, **10** (4), 306–8.

Eastwood, M. R., Corbin, S. L., Reed, M. *et al.* (1986) Acquired hearing loss and psychiatric illness: an estimate of prevalence and psychomorbidity in a geriatric setting. *British Journal of Psychiatry*, **147**, 552–6.

Ebrahim, S., Barer, D. and Nouri, F. (1987) Affective illness after stroke. *British Journal of Psychiatry*, **151**, 52–6.

Faulk, M. (1988) *Basic Forensic Psychiatry*, Blackwell Scientific Publications, London.

Frankenburg, F. R., Sloman, L. and Perry, A. (1985) Issues in the therapy of hearing children with deaf parents. *Canadian Journal of Psychiatry*, **30**, March, 98–102.

Fraser, W. I. (1982) Proper settings for the mentally handicapped in *Rehabilitation in Psychiatric Practice* (ed. R. G. McCreadie), Pitman, London, pp. 243–62.

Gelder, M., Gath, D. and Mayou, R. (1986) *Oxford Textbook of Psychiatry*, Oxford University Press, Oxford.

Gelder, M., Gath, D. and Mayou, R. (1989) *Oxford Textbook of Psychiatry*, 2nd edn, Oxford University Press, Oxford.

Gilhome-Herbst, K. and Humphrey, C. (1980) Hearing impairment and mental state in the elderly living at home. *British Medical Journal*, **281**, 903–5.

Gloag, D. (1985) Rehabilitation after head injury. *British Medical Journal*, **290**, 913–16.

Gravell, R. (1988) *Communication Problems in Elderly People: Practical Approaches to Management*, Croom Helm, London.

Grounds, A. T., Quayle, M. T., France, J. *et al.* (1987) A Unit for 'psychopathic disorder' patients in Broadmoor Hospital. *Medical Science and the Law*, **27** (1), 21–31.

Gunn, J. (1977) Criminal behaviour and mental disorders. *British Journal of Psychiatry*, **130**, 317–29.

Hagan, C. (1984) Language disorders in head trauma, in *Language Disorders in Adults: Recent Advances* (ed. A. Holland), College Hill, San Diego, pp. 245–82.

Hallas, C. H., Fraser, W. I. and MacGillivray, R. C. (1978) *The Care and Training of Mentally Handicapped*, 6th edn, Wright, Bristol.

Harrop-Griffiths, J., Katon, W., Dobie, R. *et al.* (1987) Chronic tinnitus: associations with psychiatric diagnoses. *Journal of Psychosomatic Research*, **31** (5), 613–21.

Harry, B. (1986) Interview, diagnostic and legal aspects in the forensic assessments of deaf persons. *Bulletin of the American Academy of Psychiatry and Law*, **14** (2), 147–62.

Harry, B. and Farazza, A. R. (1984) Brief reactive psychosis in a deaf man. *American Journal Psychiatry*, **141** (7), 898–9.

Hawthorn, M. R., O'Connor, S., Britten, S. R. and Webber, P. (1987) The management of a population of tinnitus sufferers in a specialised clinic. Parts I-III. *Journal of Laryngology and Otology*, **101**, 784–99.

Heaton-Ward, W. A. and Wiley, Y. (1984) *Mental Handicap*, Wright, Bristol.

Hebb. D. O., Heath, E. A. and Stuart, E. A. (1954) Experimental deafness. *Canadian Journal of Psychology*, **8**, 152–6.

Heber, R. (1961) A manual on the terminology and classification in mental retardation, 2nd edn. *American Journal of Mental Deficiency*, monograph.

Holland, A. (1984) *Language Disorders in Adults: Recent Advances*, College Hill, San Diego.

James, D. (1982) Chronically disabled children and their families, in *Rehabilitation in Psychiatric Practice*, (ed. R. G. McCreadie), Pitman, London, pp. 215–39.

Jennett, B. (1982) Research aspects of rehabilitation after acute brain damage in adults. *Lancet*, **ii**, 1034–6.

Kiernan, C. (1977) Alternatives to speech: a review of research on manual and other forms of communication with the mentally handicapped and other non-communicating populations. *British Journal of Mental Subnormality*, **23**, 6–28.

Kinsella, G., Moran, C., Ford, B. and Ponsford, J. (1988) Emotional disorder and its assessment within the severe head injured population. *Psychological Medicine*, **18**, 57–63.

Klonoff, H. and Paris, R. (1974) Immediate, short term and residual effects of acute head injuries in children, in *Clinical Neuropsychology: Current Status and Applications* (eds R. M. Reitan and L. A. Davison), Wiley, New York, pp. 179–210.

Knapp, P. H. (1948) Emotional aspects of hearing loss. *Psychosomatic Medicine*, **10**, 203–22.

Kugler, B. T., Caudrey, D. J. and Gruzelier, J. H. (1982) Bilateral auditory acuity of schizophrenic patients. *Psychological Medicine*, **12**, 775–81.
Lewin, W. (1970) Rehabilitation needs of the brain injured patient. *Proceedings of the Royal Society of Medicine*, **63**, 28–32.
Lim, L. M. and Ebrahim. S. (1983) Depression after stroke: a hospital treatment survey. *Postgraduate Medical Journal*, **59**, 489–91.
Lishman, W. A. (1978) *the Psychological Consequences of Cerebral Disorder*, Blackwell Scientific Publications, London.
Lloyd, J. H. (1980) Compensation neurosis. *Australian Family Physician*, **9**.
Ludwig, A. M. (1980) *Principles of Clinical Psychiatry*, Free Press/Macmillan, London.
Mahapatra, S. (1974) Psychiatric and psychosomatic illness in the deaf. *British Journal Psychiatry*, **125**, 450–1.
Mazzella Gordon, C. and Wicks, K. L. (1988) Treating communication disorders in the brain injured adult, in *Rehabilitation of the Severely Brain Injured Adult: A Practical Approach* (eds I. Fussey and G. Muir Giles), Croom Helm, London, pp. 116–29.
McKechnie, A. A. (1982) Head injury – its psychological sequelae and compensation neurosis in *Rehabilitation in Psychiatric Practice* (ed. R. G. McCreadie), Pitman, London.
McKinlay, W. W., Brooks, D. N., Bond, M. R. *et al.* (1981) The short term outcome of severe blunt head injury. *Journal of Neurology, Neurosurgery and Psychiatry*, **44**, 527–33.
MRC Institute of Hearing Research (1985) Epidemiology of tinnitus. *CIBA Foundation Symposium*, 16–34.
Moore, N. C. (1981) Is paranoid illness associated with sensory defects in the elderly? *Journal Psychosomatic Research*, **25** (2), 69–74.
Muir Giles, G. and Clark-Wilson, J. (1988) Functional skills training, in *Rehabilitation of the Severely Brain Injured Adult: A Practical Approach* (eds I. Fussey and G. Muir Giles), Croom Helm, London, pp. 69–101.
Newcombe, F. (1982) The psychological consequences of closed head injury: assessment and rehabilitation. *Injury*, **14**, 111–36.
Norris, M. L. and Cunningham, D. R. (1981) Social impact of hearing loss in the aged. *Journal of Gerontology*, **36** (6), 727–9.
Oddy, M. (1984) Head injury during childhood: the psychological implications, in *Closed Head Injury* (ed. N. Brooks), Oxford University Press, Oxford, pp. 179–94.
Parker, A. (1983) Speech conservation, in *Rehabilitation and Acquired Deafness* (ed. W. J. Watts), Croom Helm, London, pp. 234–50.
Post, F. (1966) *Persistent Persecutory States of the Elderly*, Pergamon, Oxford.
Purser, H. (1982) Clinical child psychology, in *Psychology for Speech Therapists* (ed. H. Purser), the British Psychological Society/Macmillan Press, London, p. 101–40.
Pyke, J. M. and Litman, S. K. (1982) A psychiatric clinic for the deaf. *Canadian Journal of Psychiatry*, **27**, 384–9.
Ramsdell, D. A. (1962) The psychology of the hard of hearing and deafened adult, in *Hearing and Deafness* (eds H. Davis and S. R. Silverman), Holt, Rinehart and Winston, New York.
Reid,A. H. (1972) Psychoses in adult mental defectives. *British Journal of Psychiatry*, **120**, 205–18.

Reid, A. H. (1982) *The Psychiatry of Mental Handicap*, Blackwell Scientific Publications, Oxford.

Reid, A. H., Ballinger, B. R. and Heather, B. B. (1978) Behavioural syndromes in a sample of 100 severely and profoundly retarded adults. *Psychological medicine*, **8**, 399–412.

Rondal, J. A. (1987) Language development and mental retardation, in *Language Dvelopment and Disorders* (eds W. Yule and M. Rutter), MacKeith Press, London, pp. 248–61.

Roth, M. and McClelland, H. A. (1971) Vestnik Academicheskith Nauk. *SSSR Meditsina*, **5**, 77.

Rutter, M. (1981) Psychological sequelae of brain damage in children. *American Journal of Psychiatry*, **138** (12), 1533–44.

Rutter, M., Tizard, J. and Whitmore, K. (1970) *Education, Health and Behaviour*, Longman, London.

Sarno, M. T. (1984) Verbal impairment after closed head injury. *Journal Nervous and Mental Diseases*, **172**, 475–9.

Shukla, S., Cook, B. L., Mukherjee, S. *et al.* (1987) Mania following head trauma. *American Journal of Psychiatry*, **144** (1), 93–5.

Thacker, A. (1988) European study will probe psychiatric problems of deaf. *Therapy Weekly*, 8 December, 3.

Thomas, A. J. (1981) Acquired deafness and mental health. *British Journal of Medical Psychology*, **54**, 219–29.

Thomas, A. J. and Gilhome-Herbst, K. R. (1980) Social and psychological implications of acquired deafness for adults of employment age. *British Journal of Audiology*, **14**, 76–85.

Thomsen, I. V. (1974) The patient with severe head injury and his family. *Scandinavian Journal of Rehabilitative Medicine*, **6**, 180–3.

Thomsen, I. V. (1984) Late outcome of very severe blunt head trauma. *Journal of Neurology, Neurosurgery and Psychiatry*, **47**, 260–8.

Timmerman, L. (1988) Paper presented at *European Society for Mental Health and Deafness Congress*, Rotterdam.

Tizard, J. (1964) *Community Services for the Mentally Handicapped*, Oxford University Press, Oxford.

Tizard, J. (1966) Mental subnormality and child psychiatry. *Journal of Child Psychology and Psychiatry*, **7**, 1–15.

van Zomeran, A. H., Brouwer, W. H. and Deehan, B. G. (1984) Attentional deficits, in *Closed Head Injury* (ed. N. Brooks), Oxford University Press, Oxford, pp. 74–107.

Vernon, I. M., Griffin, D. H. and Yoken, C. (1981) Hearing loss. *Journal of Family Practice*, **12** (6), 1152–8.

Wood, R. L. (1984) Behaviour disorders following severe brain injury, in *Closed Head Injury* (ed. N. Brooks), Oxford Univeristy Press, Oxford, pp. 195–219.

Yule, W. and Carr, J. (1980) *Behaviour Modification for the Mentally Handicapped*, Croom Helm, London.

4

Neurotic disorders

Jenny France

'Neurotic disorders' is a global term used to cover minor psychiatric conditions such as anxiety, depression, obsessional and phobic neuroses. They are mental disorders without an organic basis and where the patient does not lose touch with reality. When the term neurotic disorders was first introduced, in the middle of the eighteenth century, it was used to define disorders of sense and motion caused by a 'general affliction of the nervous system'. It covered a wide range of conditions such as hysteria, hypochondriasis, melancholia, palpitations, epilepsy, mania, chorea, astheima and diabetes. By the end of the nineteenth century, the concept of neurosis had been refined to mean psychiatric disorders which did not include either mania or psychotic states.

Freeman (1988) states that Freud introduced the term psychoneurosis, which he used to mean three specific syndromes: anxiety-hysteria (phobic anxiety); obsessive-compulsive neurosis; and hysteria proper. Freud (1894a) saw psychoneurosis as resulting from unconscious conflicts and saw these conflicts leading to unconscious perception of anticipated danger which evokes defence mechanisms that become manifest as personality disturbances or neurotic symptoms or both. Defence mechanisms are concerned with everyday thoughts and actions and are used by people to protect themselves against the disorganizing effect of overwhelming anxiety and include regression (resorting to behaviours learned at an earlier stage of development) or denial when by an unconscious distortion a problem is no longer seen to be important. Freud went on to distinguish psychoneuroses from the 'actual' neuroses which were neurasthenia and anxiety neurosis. He used the term neurosis in two ways, firstly to indicate an aetiological process – the unconscious conflict arousing anxiety and leading to maladaptive use of defence mechanisms that result in symptom formation – and secondly as a descriptive term to indicate a painful symptom in one individual who is fully in touch with reality (Freeman, 1988).

Today the term covers all forms of non-psychotic and non-organic disorders and there is now even a move to abandon the category of neurosis, which has been almost accomplished by the DSM-III-R. The ICD–10 is likely to retain the term 'neurosis' but only to cover a whole group of syndromes, and individual syndromes are to be referred to as disorders. The DSM-III-R states that the features of this group of disorders are symptoms of anxiety and avoidance behaviour, and include Panic Disorder, Phobic Disorders and Obsessive–Compulsive Disorder (1987).

The ICD–9 defines neurotic disorders as 'Mental disorders without any demonstrable organic basis in which the patient may have considerable insight and has unimpaired reality testing in that he usually does not confuse his morbid subjective experiences and fantasies with external reality. Behaviour may be greatly affected, although usually remains within socially acceptable limits, but personality is not disorganized. The principal manifestations include excessive anxiety, hysterical symptoms, phobias, obsessions and compulsive symptoms and depression'. (1975). Table 4.1 demonstrates the similarities between the two classifications.

When comparing childhood behaviour with adult neurotic disorders, Rutter (1972) states that most neurotic children become normal adults and most neurotic adults develop their neurotic disorder only in adult life; females are the more likely sufferers, whereas with children there are likely to be more boys who suffer and the ratio of predominance changes from boys to girls during adolescence. Very little is known, as yet, about childhood behaviours and personality traits that may be associated with adult neurotic disorders.

Neurotic disorders can be thought of as exaggerated forms of normal reactions to stressful events. Interesting and important questions are why some people develop a neurotic disorder when others do not and why more women are affected than men? Neurotic disorders do not cause death, but those suffering from neuroses tend to die prematurely – suicide, alcoholism and drug abuse might account for some. Hospitalized neurotics are more at risk than others (Freeman, 1988).

INCIDENCE OF NEUROTIC DISORDERS

Neurotic disorders are considered minor psychiatric disorders and only the most severe of these disorders are referred to a psychiatrist for treatment. Fewer still are admitted to hospital, the majority of these patients being treated by their general practitioner. It is worth stating here that a few neurotic disorders are or can be severe and disabling and some show poor response to treatment.

Table 4.1 Classification of neurotic disorders in ICD–9 and DSM–III–R

ICD–9	DSM–III–R
Anxiety state	Panic disorder Generalized anxiety disorder
Hysteria	Conversion disorder Psychogenic disorder Psychogenic fugue Multiple personality Atypical dissociative disorder Facticious disorder with physical symptoms
Phobic state	Phobic state Agrophobia without panic attacks Agrophobia with panic attacks Social phobia Simple phobia
Obsessive compulsive disorder	Obsessive–compulsive disorder
Neurotic depression	Dysthymic disorder (depressive neurosis)
Neurasthenia	Chronic facticious disorder
Depersonalization syndrome	Depersonalization disorder
Hypochondriasis	Hypochondriasis, a typical somatoform
Other	Other disorder Somatization disorder

Sources: DSM–III–R (1987) *Diagnostic and Statistical Manual of Mental Disorders*, 3rd edn – Revised, American Psychiatric Association, Washington, DC; International Classification of Diseases (1975) *Manual of the International Statistical Classification of Diseases, Injuries and Causes of Death*, Vol. 1, World Health Organization, Geneva, 1977

About 63% of all psychiatric cases seen by a general practitioner will be neurotic disorders, and only about 4% of other psychiatric cases will present with psychoses and character disorders. The largest percentage of patients are women (Shepherd *et al.*, 1966). A study of those patients treated by their general practitioner found that 24% improved, 52% showed a variable course through the year and 25% a chronic course (Mann *et al.*, 1981). A good outcome was associated primarily with the patient having a stable supportive family life, being young and male and without a physical illness and not receiving psychotropic medication. The chronic course was associated with the patient being older, having more psychological disturbances at onset, concomitant physical illness and recurring medication (Freeman, 1988). In some studies it was found that depression formed the greater part of the psychiatric morbidity.

Social measures and severity of illness rather than type of neurotic disorder or personality assessment appeared to be the most useful means of predicting outcome. A study of psychiatric out-patients by Huxley *et al.* (1979) showed that the initial severity of neurotic illness rather than any particular diagnosis was the best predictor of the eventual outcome of the neurosis.

Neurotic disorders can be considered at three levels: individual symptoms which may be experienced by normal people from time to time and are common in the general public; the undifferentiated neurotic syndrome (sometimes called minor emotional disorder), which is when a variety of neurotic symptoms occur together without any one predominating – these people are usually seen in general practice and frequency shows a wide variation; and specific neurotic syndromes when one type of symptom predominates. These people are usually seen in psychiatric practice and estimates of prevalence vary considerably (Gelder *et al.*, 1986). It is known that individual neurotic symptoms are very common in the general population. The frequency of undifferentiated neurotic disorders shows wide variation and probably this category forms about two-thirds of all the psychiatric cases seen in general practice, and the most frequent symptoms are anxiety, depression, irritability, insomnia and fatigue (Hibbert, 1988).

In individual neurotic syndromes, anxiety neuroses and mild depressive states are more common than hysteria or obsessional neuroses. Neurotic conditions vary from brief reactions to stress to chronic disorders, and out of a total population of 197 251 patients admitted or readmitted to hospital in England during 1986 15 269 people, (4978 males and 10 291 females) were suffering from neurotic disorders (first-time admissions are very many fewer than readmission totals) (DHSS, 1986). In undifferentiated neuroses, Hibbert (1988) found frequencies of anxiety and worry 93%, despondency and sadness 81%, fatigue 81%, somatic symptoms (of anxiety) 59%, sleep disturbance 57%, irritability 43% and obsessions and compulsions 22%.

DESCRIPTION OF NEUROTIC DISORDERS

Anxiety disorders

Anxiety disorders are the most common form of neurotic disorder in developed countries. They are found predominantly in young adults and sex distribution in hospital is equal, whereas in general practice two-thirds of the patients are women (Thorley, 1986). There are acute and chronic anxiety states. The acute states have a sudden onset occurring perhaps as a reaction to severe external stress, they tend to run a short course and have a good prognosis, resolving completely. Chronic disorders run a prolonged course and may not be associated with stressful events; these people often worry and have high anxiety traits (traits are habitual tendencies towards certain behaviours, for example, worrying). Factors that determine poor outcome of anxiety disorders are increasing age, long duration of illness and lower socio-economic class (Freeman, 1988). Those people suffering from anxiety disorders present with a number of symptoms which are centred around anxiety, of which the cause is only partly understood. They may present as attacks of anxiety or panic which can last for minutes, hours or days – or become chronic. The general symptoms might include apprehension, poor concentration, fear of losing control, and fears of impending disaster or disease. Irritability, depersonalization, dizziness, faintness, sweating, tremor, chest pain, palpitations and respiratory distress might also be present (Lader and Marks, 1971), with the addition of worrying thoughts of maladaptive cognitions. The appearance of the person is said to be characteristic: a tense, pale, strained-looking face, furrowed brow, tense posture, restlessness and sweating. Physical symptoms include a dry mouth, difficulty swallowing and respiratory symptoms of difficulty inhaling or overbreathing. These symptoms may be related to general muscular tension. Sleep might be disturbed with unpleasant dreams.

Anxiety might cause the sufferer a need to escape difficult situations and avoid those he fears, thereby creating further difficulties when faced with similar situations in the future (avoidance behaviour). It is important to point out that anxiety symptoms occur in all psychiatric illnesses. In some illnesses there might be difficulty in diagnosis as anxiety is a common symptom of depressive illness (Gelder *et al.*, 1986). Also those suffering anxiety often experience depressive symptoms. In fact, some of the less severe forms of depressive disorders have features that meet the criteria for neurotic disorders, as they include prominent anxiety symptoms.

Anxiety disorders in children and adolescents

Anxiety disorders in children and adolescents can arise from fears related to basic needs for survival, separation anxiety, being abandoned or sent away and fear associated with loss of self-esteem (Wolff, 1988). Wolff goes on to state that children up to 7 or 8 are particularly prone to irrational anxieties due to their cognitive immaturity. Like adults they use defence mechanisms to protect themselves.

Aetiology of anxiety

Genetics

Symptoms of anxiety are found to be more frequent in relations of patients with anxiety neuroses than in the general population, although this could understandably be the result of upbringing rather than inheritance. Twin studies provided evidence to suggest that anxiety neuroses might have a genetic cause (Gelder *et al.*, 1986).

Psychoanalytic theories

These theories state that anxiety is experienced when the ego is over-whelmed by excitation. Freud (1894b) thought that there were three possible sources: the outside world – realistic anxiety; the id – neurotic anxiety; and the superego – moral anxiety. Another theory is that of anxiety experienced during birth – the child is thought to be over-whelmed at the moment of separation from its mother (Gelder *et al.*, 1986).

Learning theory

If for example a person becomes frightened by an experience or sensation, or experiences frightening sensations in particular circumstances, anxiety may be subsequently provoked repeatedly by these physical symptoms or in these circumstances. Patients with severe anxiety give an account of such learning experiences, while those with milder forms do not (Hibbert, 1988).

Panic disorder

Panic disorder is given separate status by DSM-III-R (see Table 4.1) but not by ICD-9; it is thought that ICD-10 will include a category of panic disorder subtitled episodic anxiety.

Panic attacks are recurrent attacks of severe anxiety which is not restricted to any particular situation or set of circumstances and are therefore unpredictable (Freeman, 1988). The symptoms are similar to, although perhaps more exaggerated than, those in general anxiety – the sudden onset of palpitations, sweating and feelings of unreality, and there is almost always a secondary fear of either dying, losing control or going mad. These attacks might last for minutes or longer.

Both DSM-III-R and ICD-10 require the occurrence of at least three attacks within a three-week period in circumstances where there is no objective danger, for a diagnosis. Panic attacks are further complicated by fear of loss of control and helplessness, thereby resulting in the patient becoming reluctant to be alone or in public places away from home and so panic disorder may well result in the development of phobias. Freeman (1988) states that 3.7% of the general population meet the criteria of panic disorder and 11% of the population have experienced panic attacks at some time. There is evidence to suggest that some of the physical symptoms of panic attacks might well be attributed to hyperventilation (Beck and Emery, 1985).

Phobic disorder

Phobic anxiety is similar to other types of anxiety and varies in severity from mild fear to terror. Everyone experiences normal fears, both children and adults alike, but these fears do not lead to total avoidance of feared objects, places and situations. It is when these fears become severe enough to handicap a person in his daily life that they can be considered phobias. Phobias might take the form of fear of certain rodents, insects or animals, heights, flying, the dark and open or closed spaces.

Animal phobias

Animal phobias are said to be the rarest – they develop in childhood and lose their severity towards adulthood. Most sufferers are women although phobias experienced during childhood occur equally in the sexes (Freeman, 1988).

Agoraphobia

Agoraphobia has many similarities to general anxiety but there is a predominant fear of open or closed spaces, social situations, crowds, and in particular travelling on buses or trains. 75% of the sufferers are women and the symptoms develop around the late teens until the mid-thirties. Accompanying symptoms are panic attacks, depression and dizziness (Freeman, 1988).

Social phobias

Social phobias are fears of meeting people or of eating, drinking, blushing or behaving oddly in public. It is a fear of appearing ridiculous to others and there are few associated symptoms. Men and women suffer social phobias equally and the onset is in the teens or early adulthood and seldom develops after the age of 30 (Freeman, 1988).

Phobic disorders in children and adolescents

Phobic children are said to function happily except in specific situations; for example, they may be afraid of particular objects or situations, such as a fear of open spaces, school, snakes or mice, but if they avoid these fears they will be symptom free. The most severe cases are usually of minor prognostic importance and are not of a sufficient degree to affect much of the child's functioning (Evans, 1982).

Aetiology of phobias

Infants are not born with fears but acquire them throughout childhood and little is yet known as to why some of these childhood fears become fixed as phobias and persist into adulthood.

Obsessive–compulsive disorders

Obsessional disorders are characterized by obsessional thinking and compulsive behaviour, accompanied by anxiety, depression and depersonalization, and can be very disabling. The patient suffers from obsessional thoughts – these are words, ideas, beliefs and images that the patient recognizes as his own and which intrude forcibly into his mind. The thoughts might take the form of single words, phrases or rhymes (Gelder *et al.*, 1986). As they are usually unpleasant the patient attempts to exclude them but resistance of the compulsion is variable. These recurring ideas can prevent logical thought and might well be accompanied by ritualistic behaviour which includes mental activities (for example, repeating words and phrases, and counting), as well as repeating behaviours such as hand washing, which might arise from obsessive thoughts of contamination. Anxiety is a common component of obsessional disorders and may increase or decrease following the rituals. Obsessive–compulsive disorders are less common than anxiety disorders and prevalence varies from about 1.5% to 3% of adult psychiatric patients, of which 0.29% and 0.42% in England and Scotland will be admitted to hospital (Thorley, 1986). Men and women are equally affected.

Obsessive–compulsive disorders in children and adolescents

Obsessive–compulsive disorders in children and adolescents are characterized by the presence of obsessive thoughts and compulsive actions or combinations of both. It is thought that children have much greater difficulty in tolerating the inherent contradictions between loving and concern and feelings of hate and they usually attempt to distance themselves and their feelings in the area in which they feel ill at ease (Evans, 1982). Obsessive-compulsive disorders are considered the most complicated of the neurotic disorders and this condition does not usually occur until children are well developed. It has also been found that children functioned normally before the illness, that there was often evidence of parental disturbance and in some cases there might be excessive ambivalence and markedly open aggressive feelings towards one or both parents (Evans, 1982).

Aetiology of obsessive–compulsive disorders

It is the frequency, intensity and persistence of the symptoms that divide those suffering from a neurosis and the normal population, who also experience intrusive thoughts which might be sexual or aggressive and increase with stress, but these do not persist and occur very occasionally (Rachman and Hodgson, 1980). It is thought that obsessional personality traits can be accounted for by genetic influences and it was found that 5–7% of the parents of obsessive neurotics are also sufferers. There is no evidence to suggest that diseases of the central nervous system are responsible for obsessional disorders, or that obsessional mothers transmit symptoms to their children by imitative learning – these children are considered more at risk of non-specific neurotic symptoms, not obsessive symptoms (Gelder *et al.*, 1986).

Psychoanalytic theories based on Freud (1895) suggest that symptoms result from repressed impulses of aggression or of a sexual nature; the regression to the stage of anal development might be considered consistent with the patient's frequent concern over excretory functions and dirt. Although this is a theory it is not considered convincing to all. The learning theory is also not convincing as anxiety can either increase or decrease after rituals.

Prognosis is worse with increasing severity of symptoms and continuing stress but about two-thirds of cases will improve by the end of a year; other cases fluctuate, with periods of remission lasting from months to years.

Hysteria

It appears that hysteria is not a unitary illness but more likely to be a group of syndromes. It is known that psychiatrists have difficulty agreeing on what the terms 'hysteria' and 'hysterical' convey (Freeman, 1988) and that the DSM-III-R and the draft of the ICD–10 have abandoned the term 'hysteria' because of its confused and vague meanings. Disassociation – the disturbance or alteration in the normally integrative functions of identity, memory, or consciousness (DSM-III-R) – is a common property of all individuals, but a propensity to disassociate may be the hallmark of hysteria (Thorley, 1986). Disassociative states include disorders of memory, consciousness and intellect, whereas conversion symptoms are divided into mental and physical symptoms. The mental symptoms include amnesia, fugue and behaviour like that of major mental illness and 'multiple personality'. Physical symptoms include paralysis, fits, aphonia, blindness, deafness, anaesthesia, disorder of gait and abdominal pain. Gelder *et al.* (1986) report that the symptoms of hysteria usually confer some advantage on the patient. Hysteria produces symptoms and signs of disease when it occurs in the absence of physical pathology, the symptoms are produced unconsciously and they are not caused by overactivity of the sympathetic nervous system. Hysteria therefore gives rise to many errors of diagnosis but hysterical symptoms are common and hysterical neurosis is not (Gelder *et al.*, 1986).

The variety of symptoms is enormous and patients suffering from hysteria often show less than the expected amount of distress. The motor symptoms of hysteria are not accompanied by the expected signs of genuine physical illness; for example, changes in reflex are not present, muscle wasting is not observed, and symptoms tend to reduce when there is distraction and increase with attention.

Hysterical aphonia or conversion aphonia may manifest as whispering, muteness or unusual dysphonias and these conversion reactions permit people to avoid awareness of stress or emotional conflict that might be so severe that avoidance behaviours are developed to counteract stressful situations (Stemple, 1984). Sensory symptoms which include anaesthesia, paraesthesia, hyperaesthesia and pain are distinguished from organic disease by a distribution that does not conform to the known innervation of the part and by their response to suggestion. Mental symptoms include amnesia, fugue, hysterical pseudomentia, somnambulism and multiple personality. In an hysterical fugue the patient loses his memory and also wanders away from his usual surroundings and when found will deny memory of his whereabouts and knowledge of his personal identity.

Gelder *et al.* (1986) describe the difficulties of differential diagnosis and states that hysteria can be mistaken in three ways. First, the symptoms may be those of physical disease that has not yet been detected; secondly, undiscovered brain disease may in some unknown way 'release' hysterical symptoms; and, thirdly, physical disease may provide a non-specific stimulus to hysterical elaboration of symptoms by a patient of histrionic personality. It is stressed that the greatest difficulty arises in distinguishing hysteria from organic disease of the central nervous system. Four points have been identified to help minimize misdiagnosis (Gelder *et al*, 1986); these are age, stress, secondary gain and indifference. Age is a good guide as hysteria seldom appears after the age of 40. Hysteria is found to be provoked by stress. An important feature of hysteria is that it is characterized by a sudden onset of symptoms in clear relation to stress. The course is often a short duration and although at times incapacitating whilst it lasts it seldom leaves permanent disability. It is known that hysteria is more common in women than men and that it varies widely from culture to culture (Thorley, 1986).

Hysteria in children and adolescents

Hysteria in children and adolescents is thought to occur when the child is unable to tolerate anxiety engendered by some experience of expectations and sees no successful solution. Hysteria enables the child to avoid panic and disintegration and it is usually of brief duration (days or weeks) although it can be of prolonged nature. It is considered to be unusual in children and adolescents and occurs in either sex but is more common in females (Evans, 1982).

Aetiology of hysteria

Hysteria has been recognized as a condition since ancient times but has only relatively recently been associated with strong emotions, possibly associated with people who have a predisposition to hysteria (Gelder *et al.*, 1986). Genetic studies have been unable to prove that there is any genetic activity in hysteria although organic disease is sometimes associated with hysteria. Psychoanalytic theories follow Freud's (1894a) early work on hysteria and the assumption made by contemporary analysts is that the conversion symptoms possess specific psychic content and may be a precise symbolic representation communicating some otherwise hidden or unexpressed intra-psychic conflict. Freud's theory is that conversion stems from mental energy that is converted into certain physical symptoms. Thorley (1986) states that it is a distinctive feature of a bodily state for a personal problem.

AETIOLOGY OF NEUROTIC DISORDERS

The aetiology of neurotic disorders is still not clearly understood but it is thought that major happenings in a person's life, especially stressful events and losses, could predispose towards neurotic illnesses. Everyone uses defence mechanisms to limit and constrict awareness so that threatening cues from either the inner or outer environment can be excluded. Psychological theory maintains that excessive use of these mechanisms leads to eventual neurotic breakdown (Freeman, 1988).

Brown and Harris's (1978) work on depressed women states that three factors operate: vulnerability factors, long-term difficulties and provoking agents. There is still a question mark about whether life events do in fact precipitate the decision to seek medical help. It is thought that minor life events only play a small part and that major events or multiple events may provoke a neurotic illness in a previously stable person.

Social relationships

Evidence has been produced to suggest that lack of social relationships is associated with neurotic illness, and the former usually produces the latter. Those people who view their social relationships as inadequate have an increased risk of developing neurotic symptoms under conditions of adversity. Symptoms can also emerge in those who consider themselves deficient in care, support or concern from those around them. It is thought that neurotic symptoms can be seen as care-eliciting behaviour (Freeman, 1988). The capacity to withstand stress and its converse, the predisposition to neurotic disorders, arise partly from inheritance and partly from upbringing. There is a fair degree of agreement that the most important period is *not* limited to early childhood and that relatives outside the family are as influential as those within the family.

Family

There is a suggestion that neurotic individuals seek each other out and mate selectively and studies show that neurotic illness in one partner creates stress under which one spouse breaks down. Males have sick wives more often than females have sick husbands and marriage appears to be a protective factor for men and a vulnerability factor for women (Freeman, 1988).

Genetic factors

There is little evidence for a true genetic component in neurotic disorders, but over the last few years there has been some evidence to suggest there might be familial or probably genetic components linked to panic disorder and possibly to agoraphobia (Freeman, 1988).

Physical illness and organic pathology

Both of these conditions are thought to influence neurotic symptomatology (Thorley, 1986).

Employment factors

Many studies measuring anxiety and depression in unemployed people have shown deficit compared with the employed. It has been found that unemployed teenagers are twice as likely to suffer minor psychiatric disorders as those with jobs. Evidence has also been gathered to suggest that spouses of the unemployed become mentally ill and children develop conduct and behaviour disorders (Thorley, 1986).

Sociological aspects

It is difficult to know where the psychiatrist or physician should draw the line between neurotic disorders and the concepts of the sick role and illness behaviour. It is suggested that they need to look beyond the behaviour or symptoms and any underlying pathology to examine the psychological gains and advantages that the patient accrues from their prolongation (Pilowsky, 1978).

COMMUNICATION AND SPEECH PROBLEMS

The variety of communication and speech problems associated with neurotic disorders encompasses every aspect of speech, language and communication. There are those speech disorders which accompany neurotic disorders, those which result from neurotic disorders, and there are the communication problems that result from social inadequacy and perhaps exacerbate a neurotic disorder. The dividing line between these three categories is at times difficult to define and can be likened to the old question of 'which comes first – the chicken or the egg?' Does social incompetence produce failure, avoidance, anxiety, phobias, or is it that anxiety results in incompetent social functioning and inadequate communication? Stemple (1984) is of the opinion that by the time these patients are referred to a speech therapist/pathologist they are truly seeking relief from the disorder and are subconsciously ready for a change. He goes on to state that some patients may continue to receive secondary gains from the disorder and resist therapeutic modifications, but the majority will respond quickly to direct voice therapy. Needless to say it is always essential to establish that there is no organic pathology before proceeding with therapy. Few stutterers are socially at ease; the majority suffer from anxiety, particularly in speech situations, and in their negative attitudes produce avoidance strategies in relation to communication (Dalton, 1983).

In the case of anxiety it is known that anxious patients may show their anxiety in rapid and breathy speech, and have a tense posture and jerky and poorly controlled gestures. They are often over-sensitive to the reactions of others, fear that they are saying or doing the wrong thing and dread being the centre of attention. Some develop phobias to specific social situations (Trower *et al.*, 1978).

A shy person may lack adequate social skills, fear negative evaluation, lack self-confidence, have low self-esteem, or experience anxiety, or may have any combination of these problems. As in the case of reticence, the problem of shyness produces avoidance of communication situations. Communication avoidance is assumed to be a type of performance anxiety in which the person experiences anxiety when anticipating or engaging in communication with other people. Some people cannot communicate well, and because of this the quality of their lives is affected. They avoid communication because they believe they will lose more by talking than by remaining silent, as communication causes them pain and provides little pleasure, so gradually avoidance of communication becomes a way of life. The individual adapts to a pattern of avoidance behaviour and acquires a personality based on avoidance of communication. Such people do not comprehend the possibility of pleasure from human interaction (Phillips, 1984). The results of such behaviour suggests that this will affect the patient's feelings towards others and he might appear annoying, cold, destructive, bad-tempered, isolated or inept and so will be unrewarding to others. These impressions are conveyed by speech and non-verbal signals, using little eye contact, seldom smiling and using few gestures. Those who survive their anxiety and attempt to come to terms with it can also experience vocal disorders resulting from chronic anxiety.

It is learned from a number of sources that the voice is considered to be a 'sensitive reflector of emotional states and that speech is not always used solely for the communication of meanings but may also constitute the expression of feelings' (Brody, 1943). Moses (1954) was convinced that both neurotic disorders and psychoses manifested abnormalities of voice (and that through voice neurotic patterns can be discovered) and also thought that content and meaning of speech were useful differentiators between neurotic disorders, schizophrenia and personality disorders. Moses was able to differentiate between the neurotic and schizophrenic patient by their vocal expression! This demonstrates the need to listen as broadly as possible and attribute vocal styles to voice pathology, emotional states and mental disorders as well as making use of language as a major indicator of pathology.

Voice disorders may result from short-term anxiety and stress and are thought to occur in those who have a predisposition to be tense and anxious. As previously mentioned hysterical voice disorders producing both aphonia and dysphonia present with the dual treatment problems of treating the voice and treating the patient. Green (1975) states that the recovery of the voice is not the sole aim of treatment. Therapy must aim at removing or alleviating the causes and obtaining better adjustment to the difficulties by gaining some insight into the connection between the vocal symptoms and the precipitating factors. Voice disorders also occur in obsessional states and compulsive idiosyncratic speech mannerisms might also be evident.

Language use can also be involved as the patient's rituals might be continuous checking with others that he is not offending or disturbing them by repeating words and phrases which can interrupt the flow of conversation. As the predictability of the subject matter and repetitions will often drive others away, this behaviour is a real test of tolerance. Speech generally, but articulation in particular, can be affected by some of the medication prescribed – a dry mouth producing reduced salivation will hinder clear articulation, and if head posture is down both volume and clarity of speech is affected.

ASSESSMENT, MANAGEMENT AND TREATMENT

Initially assessments should ensure that the patient does not suffer from a physical disease, depressive disorder, schizophrenia or dementia. To exclude the probability of organic disease, a full medical history and examination should be part of the investigations. Often the age of the patient and duration and type of symptoms will act as a guide to diagnosis. Once organic disease, affective disorder, schizophrenia and dementia are excluded, the severity of the neurotic symptoms will determine treatment needs based on how long they have been present and whether the cause of the stress is likely to persist. The patient's personality also needs to be taken into account.

Overall, management needs to include measures to reduce symptoms, steps to help the patient solve the problems of his life and treatment to help the patient improve his relationships. (Further details on management will be found later in this chapter and in Chapter 10.)

Referral

Many of these patients will be seen by their general practitioner and treated or referred on to clinical psychologists or speech therapists or if severely impaired to the out-patient clinic and the psychiatrist. The psychiatrist, in turn, might supervise treatment, refer to other agencies, or if the problem is severe and persistent might commit the patient to hospital or, as is more likely, to a specialized unit for these disorders. It is therefore possible for a speech therapist to see and treat patients suffering from these disorders, particularly hysterical aphonia, in a community speech therapy clinic after direct referral from the patient's general practitioner; psychiatrists might make direct referrals to speech therapy hospital out-patient clinics and most of these cases will be referred with some form of speech pathology as a presenting symptom; hospital in-patients might be referred from within the multidisciplinary team, but as these patients usually have a short stay any treatment started in hospital will need to be continued in out-patient clinics eventually.

Treatment of anxiety states

Treatment can begin by offering support and in some cases this alone is enough. In other cases, counselling, psychotherapy and in addition social work assistance might be helpful. Patients should be encouraged to feel responsible for and carry out treatment procedures themselves and for actively attempting to solve their problems in life. In addition efforts should be made to help patients to rebuild their self-confidence and self-esteem (Hibbert, 1988). Drugs are possibly used more widely than is necessary and should perhaps be avoided unless other methods of treatment fail. Although drugs relieve symptoms, they might encourage dependence.

Drugs for anxiety states

The drugs prescribed for severe anxiety states (see Appendix 4.1) are benzodiazepines, which are centrally and long-acting drugs and considered more suitable than hypnotic agents. Benzodiazepines act on the brain stem and can therefore produce drowsiness, increase the seizure threshold and thus act as an anticonvulsant. They depress activity in

107

the limbic system and so recent memory may be impaired. The toxic effects of diazepines may increase anxiety and produce hostility, and confusion in elderly people. Other occasional side-effects are confusion and dry mouth. Benzodiazepines depress spinal reflexes but do not produce dysarthria except in toxic dosage and when abused with other drugs (Maguire, 1986). Barbiturates are used less now than previously because of their tendency to produce dependency.

Behaviour and cognitive therapy

Anxiety management training consists of three groups of elements: the explanation of the nature of anxiety and the rationale of treatment to the patient; the control of symptoms using relaxation, distraction, exercise, restructuring of thoughts and panic management; and thirdly avoidance controls of exposure and confidence rebuilding by encouraging positive activities (France and Robson, 1986). Gelder (1988) gives some detail of treating the maladaptive cognitions by using 'thought stopping', which is a sudden distraction used to interrupt a sequence of repetitive anxious thoughts. 'Self talk' is used to replace frightening thoughts by reassuring ones, and finally 'cognitive restructuring' may be used, which is making the thoughts less frequent by altering the belief structure from which they arise. It is thought that relaxation training can be as effective as drugs in reducing anxiety of a mild or moderate degree but is likely to be more effective within an anxiety management package.

Treatment of phobias, obsessive–compulsive disorders and hysteria

As phobias are sometimes secondary to depressive disorders, it is considered important to treat the primary condition. Anxiolytic drugs may produce some relief and in order to reduce avoidance behaviour one of the many forms of behavioural therapy methods might be employed (Gelder *et al.*, 1986).

Treatment of obsessive-compulsive disorders often needs to consider an accompanying depression as well, and if the depression is treated effectively improvement is likely in the obsessive symptoms. As obsessionals often involve their families in their rituals, family members need to be interviewed and perhaps involved in the treatment. Anxiolytic drugs will once again give symptom relief and help the depression but should not be relied upon in the long term. Behaviour therapy again can help these patients although is considered less effective for treating obsessive thoughts. Other forms of psychotherapy are seldom considered helpful.

Hysteria often responds to support and counselling; it is important to explain to the patient that the disability is not physical and to provide some details of what is actually happening to produce the symptoms. Direct the attention away from the symptoms and towards the problems that have provoked them. It is essential that all those involved with the patient should adopt a consistent approach to the patient (Gelder *et al.*, 1986).

Hypnosis has been proved to be successful in some cases of hysteria and some patients respond well to psychotherapy. Behaviour therapy has a limited value and medication is thought to have no part to play. Most of these patients do well with simple treatment, unless there is a strong motivation to remain ill, and all patients should be followed carefully for long enough to exclude organic disease as a cause of their problems (Gelder *et al.*, 1986).

Speech therapists are becoming more involved with rehabilitation programmes for the mentally ill in many different settings (Rustin and Kuhr, 1989), and as many of this client group are now in the process of being settled in the community, research as to how best to provide adequate and appropriate management is ongoing.

Overall the largest area in need of help from the speech therapist is that of social and communication inadequacy and support. Treatment for some specialized speech performance such as public speaking in various social settings can be included in the social skills package. More detail on treatment for these disorders will be found in Chapter 10.

REFERENCES

Beck, A. T. and Emery, G. (1985) *Anxiety Disorders and Phobias*, Basic Books, New York.

Brody, M. W. (1943) Neurotic manifestations of the voice. *Psychoanalytic Quarterly*, **12**, 371–80.

Brown, G. and Harris, T. (1978) *Social Origins of Depression*, Tavistock Publications, London.

Dalton, P. (1983) Psychological approaches to the treatment of stuttering in *Approaches to the Treatment of Stuttering*, (ed. P. Dalton), Croom Helm, London.

DHSS, Mental Health Statistics for England (1986). *Mental Illness Hospitals and Units in England: Diagnostic Data*, Booklet 12, a publication of the government statistical service.

DSM-III-R (1987) *Diagnostic and Statistical Manual of Mental Disorders*, 3rd edn – revised, American Psychiatric Association, Washington, DC.

Evans, J. (1982) *Adolescent and Pre-Adolescent Psychiatry*. Academic Press, London/Grune and Stratton, New York.

France, R. and Robson, M. (1986) *Behaviour Therapy in Primary Care*. Croom Helm, London.

Freeman, C. P. (1988) Neurotic disorders, in *Companion Guide to Psychiatric Studies*, 4th edn (eds R. E. Kendell and A. K. Zealley), Churchill Livingstone, Edinburgh, pp. 374–406.

Freud, S. (1894a) The aetiology of hysteria, in *Early Papers*, Vol. 1 (ed. S. Freud), Hogarth Press, London, 1924.

Freud, S. (1894b) *On the Grounds for Detaching a Particular Syndrome from Neurasthenia under the Description Anxiety Neurosis* (standard edition) Vol. 3, Hogarth Press, London, 1962.

Freud, S. (1895) Obsessions and phobias, their physical mechanisms and their aetiology, in *The Standard Edition of the Complete Psychological Works*, Vol. 3 (ed. J. Strachey), Hogarth Press, London.

Gelder, M. (1988) The treatment of anxiety and depressive disorders without drugs in *Perspectives in Psychiatry*, (eds P. Hall and P. Stonier), Wiley, Chichester, pp. 59–69

Gelder, M., Gath, D. and Mayou, R. (1986) *Oxford Textbook of Psychiatry*, Oxford University Press, Oxford.

Green, M. C. L. (1975) *Voice and its Disorders*, Pitman Medical, London.

Hibbert, G. A. (1988) The neuroses, in *Essential Psychiatry* (ed. N. Rose), Blackwell Scientific Publications, Oxford, pp. 74–83.

Huxley, P. J., Goldberg, D. P., Maguire, P. and Kincey, V. (1979) The prediction of the course of minor psychiatric disorders. *British Journal of Psychiatry*, 135–535.

International Classification of Diseases (1975) *Manual of the International Statistical Classification of Diseases, Injuries and Causes of Death*, Vol. 1, World health Organization, Geneva, 1977.

Lader, M. H. and Marks, I. M. (1971) *Clinical Anxiety*, Heinemann, London.

Maguire, T. (1986) *Pharmacological Effects in Speech and Language*, paper presented at Speech Therapy Special Interest Group, Broadmoor Hospital.

Mann, A. H., Jenkins, R. and Belsey, E. (1981) A twelve month outcome of patients with neurotic illness in general practice. *Psychological Medicine* **11** (3), 535–50.

Moses, P. (1954) *The Voice of Neurosis*, Grune and Stratton, New York.

Phillips, G. (1984) A perspective on social withdrawal, in *Avoiding Communication: Shyness, Reticence and Communication Apprehension* (eds J. A. Daly and J. C. McCroskey), Sage Publications, Beverley Hills, pp. 51–66.

Pilowsky, I. (1978) A general classification of abnormal illness behaviours. *British Journal of Medical Psychology*, **51**, 131–7.

Rachman, S. and Hodgson, R. S. (1980) *Obsessions and Compulsions*, Prentice-Hall, Englewood Cliffs, New Jersey.

Rustin, L. and Kuhr, A. (1989) *Social Skills and the Speech Impaired*, Taylor and Francis, London.

Rutter, M. L. (1972) Relationships between child and adult psychiatric disorders. *Acta Psychiatrica Scandinavica*, **48**, 3–21.

Shepherd, M., Cooper, B., Brown, H. C. and Kalton, C. W. (1966) *Psychiatric Illness in General Practice*, Oxford University Press, Oxford.

Stemple, J. C. (1984) *Clinical Voice Pathology Theory and Management*, Charles E. Merrill, Oxford.

Thorley, A. (1986) Neurosis in personality disorder, in *Essentials of Postgraduate Psychiatry*, 2nd edn (eds P. Hill, R. Murray and A. Thorley), Grune and Stratton, New York, pp. 195–259.

Trower, P., Bryant, B. and Argyle, M. (1978) *Social Skills and Mental Health*, Methuen, London.

Wolff, S. (1988) Psychiatric disorders in children in *Companion to Psychiatric Studies*, 4th edn (eds R. E. Kendell and A. K. Zealley), Churchill Livingstone, Edinburgh, pp. 505–34.

APPENDIX 4.1: DRUGS USED IN TREATING NEUROTIC DISORDERS

Antianxiety/sedatives (anxiolytics)	Non-proprietary name	Proprietary names	Mode of action	Adverse effects
(a) Benzodiazepines	Diazepam Oxazepam Lorazepam	Valium Serenid Ativan	Acts on brain stem Depresses limbic system	Drowsiness and dry mouth Loss of memory Confusion in elderly HABITUATION
(b) β-Adrenoreceptor blockers	Propranolol	Inderal	Peripheral action reducing tremor, palpitations and altering somatic symptoms Little central action	Sleep disturbance Brochospasm, etc.
(c) Sedatives	Chloral betaine Chloral hydrate Triclofos sodium	Welldorm Noctec	Central	Headache Excitement Delirium
Benzodiazepines (see above)	Nitrazepam Temazepam Triazolam	Mogadon Normison Halcion	see above (Benzodiazepines)	see above
(d) Buspirone	Buspirone	Buspar	Distinct from benzodiazepines ? Less sedative and addictive	Dizziness, headache, fatigue, dry mouth

5

Psychoses

Jenny France

The pyschoses are considered to be the major mental illnesses and include features such as incoherent speech, bizarre and idiosyncratic beliefs and purposeless or unpredictable or violent behaviour with apparent absence of concern for one's own safety and comfort (Roth and Kroll, 1986). The psychotic illnesses include organic psychoses, drug psychoses, the major affective (mood) disorders, schizophrenia and paranoid states.

The DSM-III-R (1987) classifies the disorders into organic mental disorders, psychoactive substance abuse disorders, schizophrenia, delusional (paranoid) disorders, psychotic disorders not elsewhere classified and finally mood disorders. The ICD–9 (1975) has two groups – the organic psychotic conditions and other psychoses – and gives an overall definition of psychoses as 'mental disorders in which impairment of mental function has developed to a degree that interferes grossly with insight, ability to meet some ordinary demands of life or maintain adequate contact with reality. It is not an exact or well-defined term. Mental retardation is excluded.'

The organic psychoses feature impairment of memory, orientation, comprehension, calculation, learning capacity and judgement, with the addition of alteration of mood, disturbance of behaviour and personality and impairment of volition. Acute disorders with a short course are referred to as delirium, and dementia runs a chronic course. They come under the heading of senile and pre-senile organic psychotic conditions, and this whole area will be dealt with in Chapter 8. Alcoholic psychoses include delirium tremens, Korsakov's psychosis, other alcoholic dementia and/or hallucinations and alcoholic jealousy.

Drug psychoses as a result of substance abuse (for example, barbiturates) produce withdrawal syndrome, paranoid and/or hallucinatory states induced by drugs (delusional disorder) and pathological drug intoxication. The transient organic psychotic conditions are acute confusional state (delirium) and subacute confusional state.

The schizophrenic disorders are the most prevalent of the psychoses; the affective disorders include the major affective disorders such as the manic-depressive psychoses, paranoid states (disorders), and other non-organic psychoses complete the list. These are illnesses where at their most severe patients' behaviour is far from everyday life; they live in a world of their own and fantasy may seem fact to them. Glimpses of their world show that they answer voices that others cannot hear or suffer torment and punishments that are not understood by others. They have severe problems relating to their environment and other people, contact with reality is poor and they lack insight. It is the disorganization of their minds that is their illness, and many patients refuse to believe they suffer from this illness. If eventually they develop insight into their predicament the resulting horror, in some cases, can be overwhelming.

The size of the problem that psychotic illnesses present to the health services is represented by the number of admissions and readmission to hospital during 1986. Schizophrenia and paranoid illness took up 29 419 beds, the affective psychoses 24 633, senile and pre-senile dementias 20 858, alcoholic psychoses 775, other psychoses including drug-induced psychoses 17 992, with a final total of 93 677 (DHSS, 1986).

Throughout this chapter when referring to psychotic symptoms certain terms will be used relating to many of the disorders, and so before discussing specific disorders more detail of this terminology will be given.

DESCRIPTION OF PSYCHOTIC SYMPTOMS

Gelder *et al.* (1986) divide the symptoms and signs into disorders of perception, thinking, emotion, motor symptoms, disorders of body image, memory, consciousness and insight and the mechanisms of defence.

Perceptions of imagery

Perceptions can alter in intensity and quality. In mania perceptions often seem very intense whereas in depression sounds and colours may seem less intense. In schizophrenia, changes in quality occur and sensations sometimes appear distorted and unpleasant.

The most important abnormality of perception in psychiatry is hallucinations, which are perceptions occurring in the absence of a stimulus which the patient takes to be real. Hallucinations come in many forms – auditory, visual, gustatory, tactile or somatic – and they may be simple or complex. For example, simple auditory hallucinations would include indistinct sounds or mutterings whereas those that are complex might be voices speaking clearly and sometimes a recognizable voice of a relative or friend. These voices may appear to speak words, phrases or sentences and some voices even anticipate what the patient thinks, or speaks his own thoughts as he thinks them.

Pseudo-hallucinations are similar to true hallucinations but lack the full qualities of true perceptions. A patient might hear a voice in his head and this would be a pseudo-hallucination. Illusions are deceptions of the sense where the sufferer misperceives things they see or hear.

Hallucinations may occur in all kinds of psychoses but are not necessarily an aid to diagnosis as healthy people experience hallucinations too. However, the form and content of auditory hallucinations can help diagnosis; for instance, voices heard talking to or about the patient and voices which appear to be talking to each other referring to the patient in the third person are called third-person hallucinations and are associated with schizophrenia. Voices with derogatory content suggest depressive psychosis, especially when the patient accepts the unjustified, whereas a schizophrenic patient is more likely to resent them. Visual hallucinations are not as helpful towards diagnosis but hallucinations of taste and smell, which are less frequent, may occur in schizophrenia or severe depressive disorders. Tactile and somatic hallucinations also occasionally occur in schizophrenia.

Disorders of thinking

The main way of recognizing disorders of thinking is through the patient's speech and writing. There are four divisions: stream, connection, possession and content of thought. There will be further discussion of disorders of thinking later in this chapter.

The stream of thought is how fast one thought follows another, and can be slowed as in depression or accelerated as in hypomania, where it might take the form of pressure of thought, in which the thoughts follow the same topic, or flight of ideas where the topic changes rapidly.

Disorders of connections between thoughts are seen in schizophrenia, hypomania and organic disorders. Thought block is the stopping of a line of thought and occurs in an extreme form in schizophrenia, together with schizophrenic thought disorder, for example, knight's move in thought – moving from one thought to another without any logical sequence. There may be a loosening of the associations between thoughts in schizophrenia and this may be combined with interpenetration of themes, where there are two or more subjects woven ran-

115

domly into the patient's speech, and with overinclusiveness, which is a tendency to excessive generalization. Concrete thinking is another phenomenon which is an acquired inability to think in abstract terms. Schizophrenic patients also produce neologisms (new words) and metonyms (approximately correct use of real words and phrases). The overall effect is likely to bemuse the listener. At its worst, schizophrenic speech may become completely unintelligible – this is called word 'salad' or verbigeration. Neologisms and metonyms also occur in hypomania but here the flight of ideas has some logical connection between thoughts. Organically impaired patients show perseveration, which is a repetitive activity in which there is an inability to stop one thing and move on to the next, and it is a diagnostically useful organic symptom.

Disorders of possession of thought occur in schizophrenia and include thought insertion. The patient experiences the thoughts in their head as those of some other person or agency or thoughts put there by somebody else. Thought withdrawal is the experience of one's thoughts being taken out of one's head. Thought broadcasting is an extension of thought withdrawal in which the patient experiences their thoughts travelling out of their head and other people having access to them.

Delusions, which are abnormal beliefs, are the most important part of the abnormalities of thought content. They are false beliefs which are firmly held and are not susceptible to the ordinary processes of reasoning and appeal to evidence, and are culturally atypical or out of step with the beliefs conventionally held among people of the same culture and ethnic background of the patient (Fulford, 1988). The most important kinds of delusions are persecutory or paranoid delusions and these reflect a distorted relationship between patient and the world about them; they are persecutory, self-referential and grandiose. Other delusions include hypochondriacal delusions, which are concerned with illness; religious delusions; jealousy, which is more common among men; guilt and worthlessness, which are usually found in depressive illnesses; and nihilism, which includes pessimistic ideas about death or impending doom and is usually associated with degrees of depressive mood change. Delusions of grandeur occur in mania and schizophrenia and are beliefs of exaggerated self-importance. Delusions of reference are ideas that objects, events or people have a personal significance for the patient. Delusions of control are delusions where the patient believes that his actions, impulses or thoughts are controlled by an outside agency.

Disorders of emotion

Changes of emotion are found in all kinds of psychiatric disorders, particularly in the affective disorders (depression and elation) and anxiety states. They are also common in organic psychoses and schizophrenia.

Depersonalization and derealization are feelings of unreality which are difficult to describe and said to be unpleasant. These feelings are often accompanied by morbid experiences and include changes in the experience of time and body image (such as a feeling that a limb has altered and is deformed), and feelings of being outside one's own body and observing one's activities from above. There are various theories about the causes of depersonalization and derealization but no satisfactory explanation has been found.

Motor symptoms

These include abnormalities of social behaviour, facial expression and posture, and are common in all mental illnesses. Motor symptoms are obscure among schizophrenic patients and include mannerisms such as making the sign of the cross as a greeting. Stereotypes are repeated movements such as rocking, posturing, adopting and maintaining unusual body postures and echopraxia (the imitation of movements of others).

Disorders of the body image

Abnormalities of body image occur and little is known about the cause. They arise in neurological as well as psychiatric disorders and they might include, for example, continuous awareness of parts of the body that have been lost or feelings that a limb is enlarging, becoming smaller or distorted.

Disorders of memory

Disorders of memory might include amnesia (the failure of memory) or short-, medium- and long-term memory disorders, where registration, retention, recall and recognition are impaired. Other aspects of impaired memory include *déjà vu*, when a patient describes a situation or event as having been encountered before, and *jamais vu*, the reverse situation, when the patient fails to recognize a situation or event encountered before (Gelder *et al.*, 1986).

Disorders of consciousness

Consciousness is awareness of one's environment and in acute organic disorders confusion, partial impairment of consciousness, illusions, hallucinations, delusion and mood change may be experienced.

Insight

Insight is described as being the awareness of one's own mental condition. It is thought that loss of insight distinguishes psychoses from neuroses and that neurotic patients retain insight while psychotic patients lose it. As this is variable it is not therefore a reliable way of distinguishing between the two. Diagnosis may be as a result of four questions: is the patient aware of phenomena that other people have observed (for example, the patient's overactivity or elation), does he recognize that these phenomena are abnormal, if he recognizes this does he consider they are caused by mental illness, and if he accepts that he is ill, does he think he needs treatment? (Gelder *et al.*, 1986).

The mechanisms of defence

Mechanisms of defence are processes that may help to explain certain kinds of experience or behaviour; they are automatic and unconscious and are said to have been used to account for the psychopathology of everyday life and to explain the aetiology of mental disorders (Freud, 1936). Defence mechanisms include repression, the exclusion from awareness of impulses, emotions and memories that would distress if allowed to enter the conscious; denial, when a person behaves as though unaware of something which he may reasonably be expected to know; and projection – the unconscious attribution to another person of thoughts or feelings and so rendering them more acceptable. Regression is the unconscious adoption of behaviour more appropriate to an earlier stage of development; reaction formation is the unconscious adoption of behaviour opposed to that which would reflect true feelings and intentions; displacement, transferring emotion from a situation or object to another which will give less distress; rationalization, the unconscious provision of a false but acceptable explanation for behaviour which has other less acceptable origins; sublimation is the unconscious diversion of unacceptable impulses into acceptable outlets; and finally, identification, the unconscious process of taking on some activities or characteristics of another person, perhaps to reduce the pain of separation or loss (Gelder *et al.*, 1986).

ORGANIC DISORDERS

Organic mental disorders are a class of disorders of mental functioning and behaviour caused by permanent damage to the brain, or by temporary dysfunction of the brain, or by both of these factors, the results of which can impair cognitive functions, emotions and motivation of behaviour. As has been stated, delirium and dementia are associated with cerebral pathology; delirium tends to be transient and dementia prolonged or chronic. In the most severe cases, psychotic symptoms may occur.

There is a wide variety of emotional, behavioural and motivational abnormalities associated with organic mental disorder and it is difficult to know whether the symptoms are the direct result of the damage to the brain or are essential features of these disorders. Severe emotional disturbance may accompany cognitive impairment. Anxiety, depression, irritability and shame of varying degrees of intensity may be present.

Organic mental disorders may occur at any age. Delirium is most apt to occur at the extremes of the life cycle and dementia is most common in elderly people (Kaplan and Sadock, 1985).

Organic psychotic conditions and the term 'dementia' include organic psychosis, as described under the main heading of the ICD–9 classification (see Table 5.1) and are of a chronic or progressive nature, which if untreated are usually irreversible and terminal. The term 'delirium' includes organic psychoses with a short course in which the above factors are overshadowed by clouded consciousness, confusion, disorientation, delusions, illusions and often vivid hallucinations (Gelder *et al.*, 1986).

Table 5.1 Organic psychotic conditions, ICD–9 Classification 1975

Senile and pre-senile organic psychotic conditions
Alcoholic psychoses
Drug psychoses
Transient organic psychotic conditions
Other organic psychotic conditions

Organic hallucinosis

Organic hallucinosis is a mental disorder in which recurrent or persistent hallucinations are the predominant or only symptom, and is attributed to a clearly defined organic factor (see Table 5.2). It is considered uncommon but most likely to be encountered in a setting of chronic

Table 5.2 Factors causing organic hallucinosis

Substance abuse	Alcohol Hallucinogens: LSD Mescaline Morning glory seed Cocaine
Drug toxicity	e.g. Levodopa Ephedrine Propanolol Methylphenidate
Space-occupying lesions of the brain	Neoplasm Aneurysm Abscess
Other factors	Migraine Huntington's chorea Cerebrovascular disease Hypothyroidism Disease of the sense organs

Based on Z. J. Lipowski (1985) in *Modern Synopsis of Comprehensive Textbook of Psychiatry/IV*, 4th edn (eds H. I. Kaplan and B. J. Sadock), Williams and Wilkins, Baltimore

alcoholism or hallucinogen abuse, or perhaps as a toxic side-effect of some drugs. The onset is usually acute and the duration may last for days or weeks. In a few patients, hallucinosis becomes chronic and schizophrenic features may appear. Diagnosis relies upon the patient's history and psychotic examination and absence of delirium, dementia, organic delusional syndrome and organic affective syndrome. Visual hallucinosis might be caused by cerebral lesions and hallucinogen abuse (Kaplan and Sadock, 1985). Treatment due to the usual temporary nature of the disorder may be simply reassurance but psychotherapy might be necessary and hospitalization will be advisable in some more severe cases.

Organic delusions syndrome

This mental disorder is characterized by a predominance of delusions and is attributed to an organic factor. It might be caused by a variety of chemical substances, or cerebral and systemic diseases. Kaplan and Sadock (1985) note that there might be an association between amphetamine intoxication and paranoid psychosis and between lesions involving the limbic system and schizophreniform psychosis. The delusions may vary and be either persecutory or delusions of jealousy and may also be accompanied by hallucinations; other schizophrenic disorders may also be present (see Table 5.3). The prognosis will depend on the underlying cause and/or the duration, which may vary, with a few becoming chronic. Treatment will once again depend on the cause and then it usually follows treatment applicable to schizophrenic and paranoid disorders.

Table 5.3 Conditions associated with organic affective (mood) syndrome

Drugs	Riserpine, corticosteroids, levodopa, oral contraceptives, amphetamines, hallucinogens
Endocrine diseases	Addison's disease, hyperparathyroidism
Infectious diseases	Influenza, infectious hepatitis, viral pneumonia
Pernicious anaemia Brain tumour Parkinsonism Carcinoma of the pancreas	

Based on Z. J. Lipowski (1985) *Modern Synopsis of Comprehensive Textbook of Psychiatry/IV*, 4th edn (eds H. I. Kaplan and B. J. Sadock), Williams and Wilkins, Baltimore

Organic affective syndrome

The essential feature of organic affective syndrome is a prominent and persistent depressed, elevated or expansive mood, resembling either a manic episode or a major depressive episode that is due to a specific organic factor. The syndrome is usually caused by toxic or metabolic factors and may vary in severity from mild to severe or psychotic, and delusions and hallucinations may be present. The course may vary depending upon the cause and may even last after treatment for the underlying cause has been successful. Treatment will need to be for the physical and affective symptoms and some cases will need the addition of psychotherapy (Kaplan and Sadock, 1985).

Substance-induced organic mental disorders

Organic mental disorders may result from the ingestion (intoxication) or reduction in use (withdrawal) of various pharmacological agents.

Acute intoxication with barbiturates produces general depression of the central nervous system, with dizziness, ataxia, confusing slurred speech, stupor and coma. Chronic intoxication may produce syndromes similar to dementia, affective changes and organic personality changes.

Minor tranquillizers such as Valium and Librium are capable of

121

producing acute delirium when given in high doses. Toxic states may produce hyperactivity and rage and occasionally acute maniacal behaviour, with feelings of depersonalization, hallucinations and delusions. When taken with alcohol, smaller doses of minor tranquillizers can lead to death.

Synthetic hypnotics include methyprylorchloral, hydrate flurazepam and methaqualone; these drugs are more potent than the minor tranquillizers and can therefore produce delirium, convulsions and death.

Intoxication from bromides can produce mental disorders and symptoms may be transitory schizophreniform psychosis with paranoia and bromide hallucinations. Simple bromide intoxication is characterized by progressive dulling of awareness, forgetfulness, irritability, tremors, ataxia and slurred speech.

Amphetamines may produce mild withdrawal, severe fatigue and mental depression and sometimes suicidal ideation.

Chemical or environmental-related organic mental disorders can be caused by poisons, or a variety of gases, noxious vapours, solvents, heavy metals and insecticides. Symptoms may last for days and months and include depression, anxiety, irritability, phobias and the presence of paranoid delusions (Kaplan and Sadock, 1985).

Psychoactive substance-induced organic mental disorders (DSM-III-R) and drug dependence (ICD–9)

Psychotic substance-induced organic mental disorders can be caused by 11 classes of substances that are most commonly all taken non-medicinally to alter mood or behaviour; they include alcohol, amphetamines, caffeine, cannabis, cocaine, hallucinogens, inhalant, nicotine, opioids, phencycline (PCP) and sedatives, hypnotics or anxiolytics (DSM-III-R, 1987).

Drug abuse is the taking of drugs at dosages and in circumstances and settings that increase their potential for harm so that they can produce psychological dependence, which is a craving for the drug, or drugs, and which when taken into the body can alter consciousness or state of mind (Kaplan and Sadock, 1985). These drugs, taken for their pleasurable effects, can in some cases produce psychosis and these types of psychoses are said to be on the increase. The increase of incidence of drug dependency is possibly due to the increasing availability of illicit drugs (Evans, 1982). Cremona (1988) lists psychoses with marked paranoid ideas resulting in some cases from the affects of drug abuse.

Alcoholism is classified under the general term of a psychoactive substance use disorder and the specific syndromes that relate to alcoholism (for example, dependency and abuse, and alcohol-induced organic mental disorders). The term 'alcoholism' is in common use and can be defined as a disease marked by chronic, excessive use of alcohol that produces psychological, interpersonal and medical problems (Kaplan and Sadock, 1985). Alcoholic hallucinosis is an organic hallucinosis, either visual or auditory, usually beginning within 48 hours after cessation of drinking and persisting after a person has recovered from the symptoms of alcohol withdrawal. (The hallucinations are not part of alcohol withdrawal delirium.) The hallucinations are unpleasant and might take the form of voices or unformed sounds such as buzzing; they may last for several weeks or months or may be permanent. This condition is considered to be rare (Kaplan and Sadock, 1985). Treatment for alcohol hallucinosis might include the use of benzodiazepines, adequate nutrition, and fluids if necessary, and in some chronic cases antipsychotic drugs may be used.

Cannabis is the general term for the various forms of psychoactive products of marijuana and it is referred to as a hallucinogen. Experiences reported by users are that of distorted perception of various part of the body, spatial and temporal distortions, and depersonalization. There can be an increased sensitivity to sound, heightened suggestability and a sense of thinking more clearly and having a deeper awareness of the meanings of things. Anxiety and paranoid reactions are sometimes seen. There is some dispute over whether marijuana, when used moderately, can produce physical or mental deterioration (Kaplan and Sadock, 1985). Some assent that it may led to psychosis, others suggest that taking the drug might precipitate a schizophrenic breakdown and therefore those susceptible to mental dysfunctioning are at risk but not necessarily suffering from a cannabis psychosis. Cannabis-induced toxic psychosis can result if the cannabis is ingested in a large dose (Kaplan and Sadock, 1985).

Amphetamines are synthetic drugs and their use produces energy, an enhanced capacity for work and a feeling of exhilaration. The physical symptoms are numerous, ranging from flushing and pallor, to cardiac problems, increased blood pressure, tremor, ataxia, loss of sensory abilities, convulsions, coma and death. The psychological effects produce restlessness, dysphoria, logorrhea, insomnia, confusion, tension and anxiety. Amphetamine psychosis, once rare, is another effect and distinguishing amphetamine psychosis from paranoia schizophrenia depends upon the duration of the symptoms.

Treatment usually only requires supportive measures as the psychosis is self-limiting. Antipsychotics may be prescribed in the short term and, as the ampthetamine psychotic patient may be assaultative, it may be necessary to treat the patient in hospital. The withdrawal depression may be treated with tricyclic antidepressants.

Cocaine is taken most commonly by injecting or sniffing and the effects are similar to those of amphetamines; the effects last only for about an hour, while those of amphetamines last for several hours. After the initial feeling of euphoria, feelings of irritability and lassitude lead to the need for more of the drug. Symptoms of high blood pressure, racing heart, anxiety and paranoia exist. The more severe effects are tactile and other hallucinations and delusions (which are considered uncommon), and rarely cases of psychosis are reported; these will be habitual intravenous abusers and the cocaine psychosis is similar to that of amphetamine psychosis.

Treatment is difficult, particularly in chronic cases as cocaine abuse does not usually appear as a medical problem, but for those who do attend a clinic their anxiety, underlying depression and feelings of inadequacy might respond to psychotherapy combined with anxiolytics or antidepressants.

Phencyclidine (PCP) is a marketed drug sold under the name of Sernyl and is a cross between a psychodelic drug and a tranquilliser or sedative. It can be taken orally, intravenously and by sniffing and is often sprinkled onto joints of marijuana. The 'high' lasts for about 4–6 hours and gives rise to mild depression, paranoia and occasionally irrational assaultative behaviour. Treatment once again depends upon diagnosis as it may include sedative or narcotic overdose, psychosis as a consequence of the use of other psychodelic drugs, and acute schizophrenic disorder.

Psychodelics or hallucinogenic drugs are either natural or synthetic. Mescaline, derived from the peyote cactus, and psilocybin, derived from several of the mushroom species, are natural drugs while lysergic acid diethylamide (LSD) is synthetic. LSD produces the widest range of effects and the reaction varies with personality, expectations and setting. It produces profound alteration in perception, mood and thinking. True hallucinations are rare but visual distortions and pseudo-hallucinations are common. Another common effect of hallucinogenic drugs is the flashback, which is a spontaneous transitory recurrence of drug-induced experience in a drug-free state. Prolonged adverse reactions to LSD can produce anxiety disorders, depressive disorders and psychoses. Treatment resembles that given for other drug abuse and long-term abuse is considered uncommon (Kaplan and Sadock, 1985).

Alcoholic disorders, which include alcohol amnestic syndrome (Wernicke-Korsakoff's syndrome), usually occur in people who have been drinking heavily for many years and so rarely occurs before the age of 35. The irreversible memory deficit, Korsakoff's psychosis or alcohol amnestic syndrome, often follows an acute episode of Wernicke's encephalopathy, and ophthalmoplegia, nystagmus and confusion. Once this syndrome is established, the course is chronic and impairment is always severe. Life-long custodial care is often required and prevalence is rare but the syndrome is irreversible (Kaplan and Sadock, 1985).

AFFECTIVE (MOOD) DISORDERS

Affective or mood disorders are a large group of conditions in which a disturbance of affect – either depression or elation – is prominent. Illnesses in which the prevailing effect is depression are commoner than those based on an elevation of mood, and people who suffer from manic illnesses almost invariably suffer from depression as well at some stage (Kendell, 1988). For the purpose of this chapter, consideration will only be given to those disorders serious enough to include psychotic symptomatology and therefore depression will be considered separately in Chapter 6.

Kendell (1988) draws attention to the fact that both mania and melancholia are two of the six types of madness recognized by Hippocrates in the fourth century BC and were recognized for the next two thousand years, although the meanings of these terms have varied through the ages. But the modern concept of the affective disorders was originated in 1896 by Emil Kraeplin, who separated manic depressive insanity from dementia praecox (schizophrenia). The terms 'unipolar' and 'bipolar' were introduced in the 1960s and this has been followed by more recent concepts as expressed in the classification of diseases ICD–9 in 1979 and the *Diagnostic and Statistical Manual* third revision 1980 (DSM-III).

DSM-III-R classifies mood disorders into bipolar disorders and depressive disorders. The essential feature of bipolar disorders is the presence of one or more manic or hypomanic episodes; these are mood disturbances that are sufficiently severe to cause marked impairment in social functioning or to require hospitalization and these are usually accompanied by one or more major depressive episodes. The essential feature of depressive disorders is one or more periods of depression without a history of either manic or hypomanic episodes. Major depression and bipolar disorders are subclassified as either mild, moderate or severe, without psychotic features or with psychotic features.

The ICD–9 classifies affective psychoses into mental disorder, usually recurrent, in which there is a severe disturbance of mood (mostly compounded of depression and anxiety but also manifested as elation or excitement) which is accompanied by one or more of the following: delusions, perplexity, disturbed attitude to self, disorder of perception and behaviour; these are all in keeping with the patient's prevailing mood (and are hallucinative when they occur). There is a strong tendency to suicide.

In 20–35% of cases, there is a chronic course to the illness, with residual symptomatic and social impairment.

Severe depressive disorder

This disorder has previously been referred to as endogenous, endomorphic, psychotic, retarded, vital and naive depressive depression but none of these terms are considered satisfactory and hence the revival of the term melancholia in DSM-III (1980).

Severe depression is a lowering of mood accompanied by greatly reduced energy and activity. There is a general loss of enjoyment and interest in life. The depression is often episodic, the patient returning to a normal state in between episodes of ill health. Abnormalities of mood include sadness, tearfulness, anxiety, worthlessness, hopelessness, self-blame and loss of feeling. These symptoms show limited reactivity to external events. Biological symptoms include sleep disturbance, diurnal variation of mood, loss of appetite and weight, loss of libido and, in women, amenorrhoea. Appendix 5.1 outlines the diagnostic criteria for severe depressive disorder in more detail.

Abnormalities of speech and thought are demonstrated by slow, monotonous speech, brief utterances and a limited range of expression, increased pauses before answering and an increased poverty of speech, marked poverty of thought content and little spontaneous speech. This characteristic is called retardation and is accompanied by slowed body movements and reduced facial expression and restricted gestures with speech. The voice becomes quieter, dull and monotonous. The changes can be slight or so marked that the patient is mute and motionless for hours on end, which understandably results in impaired attention and concentration. Thoughts match the low mood and are pessimistic and distressive in content. Patients view themselves negatively, develop low self-esteem and view the past as worthless and the future as hopeless. Suicidal ideas are common. Patients also complain of difficulty thinking and express problems when attempting to concentrate and their beliefs are often of delusional intensity, hence the past association with psychotic depression. Delusions of guilt, poverty and persecution occur, and the patient will accept blame unnecessarily. Perceptual abnormalities are often present and can be severe enough to present as hallucinations. The overall picture is one of avoidance of social interaction, impaired work performance, self-neglect, not meeting responsibilities and possibly suicide attempts.

Mania

Mania is the elevation of mood, with the possibility of a wide range of accompanying abnormalities. Episodes of mania appear between bouts of normal behaviour and sometimes manic bouts are interrupted by brief episodes of depression. Abnormality of mood presents in feelings of well-being and expansiveness, and is possibly not in keeping with the circumstances. This mood can last for some time and in some patients there might be a tendency towards irritability and anger and even at times aggressive responses towards others. Appendix 5.2 outlines the diagnostic criteria for manic episodes in more detail.

Abnormalities of speech and thought present as garrulousness or pressure of speech, flights of ideas, distractability, and grandiose and persecutory delusions. Speech is likely to be too rapid, too much (pressure of speech), unnecessarily loud and not taking into account the present social setting; it is, in addition, difficult to interpret and full of jokes, puns, plays on words and amusing irrelevancies. It may become theatrical and full of dramatic mannerisms and singing. Sounds rather than meaningful conceptual relationships may govern word choice (clanging). If the person's mood is more irritable than expansive, his or her speech may be marked by complaints, hostile comments and angry tirades (DSM-III-R, 1987).

Frequently there is a flight of ideas, which is a nearly continuous flow of accelerated speech, with abrupt changes from topic to topic, usually based on understandable associations, distracting stimuli, or play on words. When the flight of ideas is severe, speech may be disorganized and incoherent. However, loosening of association and incoherence may occur even when there is no flight of ideas, particularly if the person is on medication. Ideas are expansive, extravagant, reckless and often accompanied by grandiose and other delusions. Delusions usually disappear within days. Insight is usually also impaired, the patient seldom thinks he is ill and so sees no need to receive treatment.

Biological symptoms lead to disturbed sleep; after a brief period of sleep the patient wakes full of energy and ideas and does not display exhaustion. Appetite is increased and in the case of hyperactive patients, in spite of the increased food intake, there might even be a weight loss. Sexual activity increases and with grandiose ideas may lead to sexually disinhibited behaviour that can lead to unlawful acts.

Perceptual abnormalities include illusions, misinterpretations and hallucinations – the hallucinations may be auditory or visual and related to the patient's euphoric mood.

Abnormal behaviour is presented as hyperactivity with sudden unrealistic plans and activities, aggressive acts with minimal provocation, sexual disinhibition, over-familiarity and unlawful acts. In the most severe cases there is a frenzied over-activity, thinking is incoherent, delusions become increasingly bizarre and hallucinations are experienced, Gelder *et al.* (1986) emphasizes that this description is merely a guide and that there is no invariable sequence.

In the foreword of David Wigoder's book *Images of Destruction*, Anthony Storr quoted the author's summary of his own life: 'By the time I was forty I had destroyed two successful careers, served a prison sentence, been made legally bankrupt, lost a treasured professional qualification, attempted to kill two people, and isolated myself from most of my family and friends'. Anthony Storr went on to write that 'any psychiatrist reading these words would guess that the man who wrote them was suffering from a major form of psychiatric disorder which afflicts at least one in a hundred individuals in our society – that is, mania'.

Incident and aetiology

Results of studies of the adult population currently suffering from depressive disorders report rates ranging for females from 9% to 26%, and for males from 5% to 12%, in studies in the USA and Europe (DSM-III-R, 1987).

The cause of depressive disorder is suggested through family studies which have shown that major depression is 1.5–3 times more common among first-degree biological relations with this disorder than among the general population.

Incidence of bipolar disorders suggest that from 0.4% to 1.2% of the adult population have bipolar disorder and recent studies in the USA indicate that the disorder is equally common in males and females (DSM-III-R, 1987).

In the study of the aetiology of bipolar disorders there is some evidence for genetic differences between bipolar disorders and unipolar affective disorders. Patients with bipolar illness are likely to have relations with the same form of disorder, while those with unipolar disorders have relations both with unipolar and bipolar conditions (Catlan, 1988). Other biological factors in addition to genetic factors might be electrolyte disturbances, neurophysiological alterations, dysfunction and faulty regulation of autonomic nervous system activity, neuroendocrine abnormalities and neurochemical alterations in the neurotransmitters.

Psychosocial factors include life events and environmental stress – research has proved that there is a relationship between life events and depression. It is thought that some personality traits predispose towards affective disorders. Personality and psychodynamic factors suggest that people prone to depression suffer low self-esteem and there are those features in the personality which predispose towards depression. Psychodynamic theory believes that mania is a defence against depression, but Gelder *et al.* (1986) do not find this explanation convincing.

Psychoanalytic factors include pre-morbid factors such as introversion, dependency, narcissism and insecurity which are thought to lead to feelings of guilt. Manic patients tend to have more normal pre-morbid personalities than depressed patients. Finally learned helplessness is mentioned as a possible factor in the cause of bipolar disorders (Kaplan and Sadock, 1988). (For further information see Chapter 6.)

There appears to be a slightly higher incidence among upper socio-economic classes than among other classes and it has been found that bipolar disorders may be more common amongst divorced persons than others. The age of onset is from late adolescence and usually before the age of 30. There is no conclusive evidence to prove that there is any difference between black and white races with affective disorders.

Manic-depressive disorders can occur in childhood and adolescence and are generally associated with a family history of functional psychosis, and if they occur before puberty are likely to recur later in life. The clinical manifestations and treatment are similar to those for adult patients.

SCHIZOPHRENIA

Schizophrenia is a term which can be defined broadly or narrowly and means different things to different people – some even doubting the existence of the condition. The concepts of schizophrenia are still criticized by some and are stated as being medical fiction. Others stress the negative aspects of receiving a diagnosis of schizophrenia, as once a person is diagnosed as schizophrenic this can considerably alter his relationships with others. Nevertheless, it is thought that due to the failure to discover the aetiology of schizophrenia there will continue to be confusion as to its meaning. There are also psychiatrists who are not satisfied with the current classification of the functional psychoses (those psychoses which do not have an organic aetiology), feeling that there is no alternative to the term schizophrenia, and it may cover several different conditions (Murray, 1986). However, Tidmarsh (1990) agrees that schizophrenia is a disease and that the medical model is appropriate and useful. He states that in 1973 the World Health Organization initiated a pilot study of schizophrenia and it demonstrated conclusively that psychiatrists in different countries do agree about what they observe, even though they do not all make the same deductions from their observations. When a standard method was used to arrive at a diagnosis, then both the incidence of schizophrenia and its symptoms were remarkably similar in all of the nine countries taking part in the study.

Freeman (1988) states that schizophrenia is a condition which seems to be associated with a fundamental biological fault – a fault in the processing by the brain of stimuli from the outside world, and it means that the affected person is less able to cope with stress or with intense and complex relationships. Kendell (1988) states that schizophrenia is the heartland of psychiatry and the core of its clinical practice. It is a relatively common condition which often cripples people in adolescence or early adult life, and probably causes more suffering and distress that most other illnesses. Until recently about 10% of all hospital beds were occupied by schizophrenics (Kendell, 1988) and so this condition places an enormous burden on the health services. Blakemore (1988) talked of 1% of the world's population as suffering from schizophrenia, and stated that it is a disease of the brain and mind, it causes global impairment and disrupts personality. Blakemore added that one-third of the people who suffer one or two episodes recover, another third respond to therapy and the last third do not and become chronically sick.

Definition

The DSM-III-R definition of schizophrenia states that the essential features of this disorder are the presence of characteristic psychotic symptoms during the active phase of the illness and functioning below the highest level previously achieved (that is, in both children and adults, failure to achieve the expected level of social development), and a duration of at least six months that may include characteristic prodromal or residual symptoms. Prior to the manifest onset of the psychosis, as well as during many stages of its course, many patients present a disturbance of attention. In quite a large number of patients there is inability to keep attention fixed for any length of time and they may hear what is said to them, but they do not register the meaning of the words (Arieti, 1974).

At some phase of the illness schizophrenia always involves delusions, hallucinations, or certain characteristic disturbances in affect and the form of thought. The diagnosis is made only when it cannot be established that an organic factor initiated and maintained the disturbance. Delusions and hallucinations involving the five senses are apparent, the patient's affect is disturbed and his global behaviour is affected. He withdraws from social contact and loses interest in other people, his actions may appear bizarre or inexplicable and he may display behavioural abnormalities of catatonia, muteness or become stuporose. In the chronic stage the delusions and hallucinations may disappear; this may be temporary or a complete recovery, but the more episodes the patient has the more likely there is to be residual damage and this is considered a serious state. The patient may become apathetic, lose determination and interest in others and will therefore talk less so that his inability to form long-lasting relationships is reduced.

It is the apathy and emotional blunting which makes schizophrenia the terrible illness it is, according to Kendell (1988), and he goes on to say that it is the permanent changes in the personality which handicap the subject in every sphere – from the ability to get and keep a job, to be an effective husband, wife or parent, or to achieve or fully enjoy anything. The symptoms can be described as solitariness, impaired empathy and emotional detachment, increased sensitivity, suspiciousness and unusual or odd styles of communicating (Wolff and Cull, 1986). Most of these patients will have recurrent psychotic episodes, suffer depression and some 10% of schizophrenics die by suicide, usually in the early years of their illness (Miles, 1977).

Content of thought

Content of thought is a major disturbance and involves delusions that are often multiple, fragmented or bizarre. More detail of delusions has already been given under the heading 'Disorders of thinking' at the beginning of this chapter.

Form of thought

If there is disturbance in the form of thought it is called 'formal thought disorder'. This is different from a disorder in the content of thoughts. An example is loosening of associations, in which ideas shift from one subject to another, completely unrelated or only obliquely related to the subject. Statements that lack a meaningful relationship may be

131

juxtaposed, or the person may shift idiosyncratically from one frame of reference to another. When loosening of association is severe, a person may become incoherent; that is, his or her speech may become incomprehensible and there may also be poverty in content of speech, in which although adequate in account it conveys little information because it is vague, abstract, concrete, repetitive or stereotyped. Less common disturbances include neologisms, perseveration, clanging and blocking.

Other symptoms listed by DMS-III-R are disturbances of perception, such as auditory, tactile, somatic, visual, gustatory and olfactory hallucinations. Other perceptible abnormalities include sensations of bodily change, hypersensitivity to sound, sight and smell, and illusions. Disturbances of affect often involve flat or inappropriate mood; the disturbed sense of self or loss of ego boundaries, and a perplexity of one's own identity; characteristic disturbance of volition, and an impaired interpersonal functioning and relationship to the external world; and finally disturbed psychomotor behaviour (for example, rigid posture, excited motor movements, bizarre postures, odd mannerisms and grimacing) are other symptoms.

The ICD–9 defines schizophrenia as a group of psychoses (see Table 5.4) in which there is a fundamental disturbance of personality, characteristic distortion of thinking, often a sense of being controlled by alien forces, delusions which may be bizarre, disturbed perception, abnormal affect out of keeping with the real situation, and autism. Nevertheless, clear consciousness and intellectual capacity are usually maintained. The disturbance of personality involves its most basic functions which give the normal person his feeling of individuality, uniqueness and self-direction. The most intimate thoughts, feelings and acts are often felt to be shared by others and explanatory delusions may develop. Perception is frequently disturbed, as is thinking which becomes vague, elliptical and obscure, and its expression in speech sometimes incomprehensible. Breaks and interpolations in the flow of consecutive thought are frequent and the patient may think that his thoughts are being withdrawn by some outside agency. Mood may be shallow, capricious and incongruous and catatonia may be present. Diagnosis of 'schizophrenia' should not be made unless there is, or has been evident during the same illness, characteristic disturbance of thought, perception, mood, conduct or personality.

Table 5.4 DSM–III–R Classification 1987

Schizophrenia

Catatonic
Disorganized
Paranoid
Undifferentiated
Residual

ICD–9 Classification 1975

Other psychoses

Affective psychoses
Paranoid states
Other non-organic psychoses
Psychoses with origin specific to childhood

Schizophrenic psychoses

Simple type
Hebephrenic type
Catatonic type
Paranoid type
Acute schizophrenic episode
Latent schizophrenia
Residual schizophrenia
Schizoaffective type
Other

Incidence

Studies have found that statistics showed higher expectations of schizo-phrenia among four peoples – the Tamils of southern India and Sri Lanka, the people of northwest Croatia, Roman Catholics in Canada, and the southern Irish – but reasons for these findings are uncertain. Studies also suggest that people who migrate are more susceptible to schizophrenia (Murphy, 1968). There are differences in the symptoma-tology across cultures, although apparently not enough to make schizo-phrenic illness unrecognizable. Paranoid illnesses are seen more fre-quently in urban populations; religious delusions in Christian populations, and less frequently in Buddhists or Hindi populations; catatonic symptoms less frequently in Euro-American; and delusions of grandeur are most frequent in rural populations and in the Japanese. This information is based on anecdotal and impressionistic studies from the work of 40 psychiatrists in 27 countries (Murphy *et al.*, 1963).

The onset of schizophrenia can occur in people from 7 to 70 years old, but the most usual onset time is early adolescence or early adult

133

life and it can develop gradually over months or years or the onset can be acute. Before the age of 35 years, males are affected more than females; after this age the reverse is true and, due to the late onset of the condition, women are more likely to be married at their initial hospitalization (Murray, 1986).

DSM-III-R (1987) states that in Europe and Asia, using a relatively narrow concept of schizophrenia, there is a reported prevalence rate of from 0.2% to almost 1%. Studies in the USA using broader criteria surveyed urban populations and have reported higher incidence rates.

Aetiology

Genetic inheritance is considered a convincing predisposing factor associated with the risk of developing schizophrenia. Genetic studies have found that the lifetime expectancy of developing schizophrenia in relatives of schizophrenics is 8–16% in first-degree relatives, over 40% in identical twins and children of two schizophrenic parents, and 2–4% in second-degree relatives (grandfather, nephews, first cousins, etc.) (Rose, 1988).

Stressful life events are thought possibly to precipitate schizophrenia in those already predisposed to the condition, and social and family circumstances may maintain an illness by maintaining stress or depriving a patient of opportunities for help. Over-critical families, isolated living conditions, unemployment and financial problems might also be responsible maintaining factors (Rose, 1988). Studies have established the fact that many schizophrenics come from disturbed families, and a patient who lives with a family with high levels of tension is more likely to relapse than a patient whose family is more tolerant. Systematic studies have demonstrated that the under-privileged social status of schizophrenics is due to the gravitation down the social scale. This may follow the onset of symptoms or it may be a result of the personality disorder already present in many of those who will develop a schizophrenic illness (Roth and Kroll, 1986).

Biochemical approaches to schizophrenia have been given consideration, one theory being that schizophrenia results from an imbalance of central neurotransmitters in the brain, which may be caused by a variety of influences. This theory is supported by the observation that dopamine receptors are blocked by drugs which control schizophrenic symptoms, but as yet there is no evidence that this is the underlying malfunction in schizophrenia (Rose, 1988). It is known that there are no consistent neurological abnormalities in this condition although some schizophrenics have enlarged cerebral ventricles, some have abnormal EEGs and others have abnormal sensory neurological signs.

The prognosis of schizophrenia varies according to the style of onset. The more acute the onset, the better the prognosis for recovery. If a life event has triggered true breakdown the chances are more favourable towards recovery. The younger the patient is at the onset the worse his prognosis; patients who breakdown in childhood or early puberty seldom recover completely. Married schizophrenics have better prognosis than single, divorced or widowed patients. Those patients who relate well to people in their environments and who are capable of emotional warmth and natural reactions have a good chance for reintegration (Kaplan and Sadock, 1985).

DELUSIONAL (PARANOID) DISORDER

Delusional (paranoid) disorders are otherwise referred to as paranoid states; the term paranoid refers to a morbid distortion of beliefs or attitudes concerning relationships between one's self and others. They may occur with a primary organic, affective or schizophrenic disorder but can also occur in a wide range of abnormal conditions as a secondary disorder. Paranoid symptoms can be classified as arising in one of three circumstances: as paranoid symptoms secondary to another disorder (schizophrenia, affective disorders or organic mental disorder); paranoid symptoms as part of a primary paranoid state, and not secondary to another disorder (acute paranoid reactions, morbid jealousy and erotomania); and paranoid symptoms as part of a paranoid personality disorder (Rose, 1988).

Paranoia has a longer psychiatric history than schizophrenia and the changing meaning attached to it over two centuries is due to its fluctuating position in diagnostic schemas (Cutting, 1986). The DSM-III-R classifies delusional (paranoid) disorders of six types; the ICD–9 classification of paranoid states also has six types (see Table 5.5). There is generally a dissatisfaction with the terms used and the DSM-III-R definition of delusional (paranoid) disorder is that there should be a persistent non-bizarre delusion that is not due to any other mental disorder and that no organic factor initiated or maintained the disturbance. The ICD–9 definition of paranoid states excludes acute paranoia reaction, alcoholic jealousy and paranoid schizophrenia and does not offer a broad description. Many people with paranoid illness show very little, if any, intellectual or social deterioration over the years of their illness and can function as well as everyone else. Yet, there is an area

Table 5.5 DSM–III–R Classification, Delusional (Paranoid) Disorder 1978

Delusional (paranoid) disorder
Types: Erotomania Grandiose Jealous Persecutory Somatic Unspecified
ICD–9 Classification, Paranoid States 1975
Paranoid states
Paranoid state, simple Paranoia Paraphrenia Induced psychosis Other Unspecified

of their functioning and thinking which is clearly dominated by intensely held delusional beliefs which appear to colour their entire being.

There is another small group of other non-organic psychoses (ICD–9) that is restricted to psychotic conditions that are largely attributable to recent life experience and include depressive types, excitative type, reactive confusion, acute paranoid reaction and psychogenic paranoid psychosis. The course can be variable; for example, it may be chronic in the persecutory type or there may be periods of remission followed by relapses, and in other cases the disorder may remit without relapse. Impairment in daily functioning is rare, as it is in intellectual and occupational functioning; the major area of difficulty is within relationships.

Assessment towards diagnosis may be difficult; in some cases the delusions are obvious while in others the symptoms may be difficult to elicit. If the patient is suspicious or angry he may offer little speech, or if more at ease he might talk fluently and convincingly about other things or may even deny delusional beliefs and ideas (Gelder *et al.*, 1986).

The major issue in treatment is whether the patient is likely to behave dangerously as a result of his delusions, which necessitates careful study of the patient's personality, delusions and associated hallucinations.

Incidence

Delusional disorder or paranoid states are considered to be relatively uncommon. It is estimated for a population prevalence of the disorder to be around 0.03% which, due to the late onset of this disorder, suggests a lifetime morbidity risk of between 0.05% and 0.1% (DMS-III-R, 1987). However, the epidemiology of paranoid disorders is difficult to estimate due to people's denial of their condition and the lack of valid statistics on the syndrome of paranoid disorders, which is due to poor definition, imprecise instruments and haphazard investigations (Kaplan and Sadock, 1985).

Aetiology

Apparently there is no conclusive evidence to indicate that either hereditary factors or neurophathological abnormalities cause paranoid disorders, but it is thought that psychological factors are important in the development of this disorder. Predisposing factors towards paranoid disorders are immigration and emigration, deafness, other severe stresses and low socio-economic status. People with paranoid, schizoid or avoidant personality disorder may also be more likely to develop delusional disorders (DSM-III-R, 1987).

THE 'PSYCHOSES' IN CHILDHOOD

Psychoses in childhood, which were introduced in Chapter 2, include the disintegrative psychosis and a group of poorly understood conditions which are also known as childhood psychoses. Schizophrenia and manic-depressive disorders are occasionally seen in older children. The prevalence of childhood psychosis in the general population is 4% per 10 000 children.

The most common form of 'childhood psychosis' is infantile autism, and even so this is a rare disorder. Wing and Gould (1979) state that approximately three boys to every one girl suffer this disorder and between 70% and 80% also have general mental retardation.

Prognosis is poor: only one in six children have a reasonably satisfactory work and social adjustment in adolescence and over 50% may, in adult life, need long-term residential care. The DSM-III-R (1987) states that the prevalence of developmental disorder (autistic disorder and pervasive developmental disorder not otherwise specified) has been estimated at 10–15 children in every 10 000.

The ICD–9 definition of psychoses with origin specific to childhood states that this category should only be used for psychoses which begin before puberty and that adult-type psychoses such as schizophrenia and manic-depressive psychoses when occurring in childhood should be coded elsewhere under the appropriate heading.

There are thought to be a wide range of pre-, peri- and post-natal conditions causing brain dysfunction and pervasive developmental disorders.

Childhood disintegrative disorder is a disorder related to conditions where there has been two years of normal early development followed by a marked regression with loss of language, social and other skills with the qualitatively abnormal functioning resembling autism.

Adult-type schizophrenia, like manic-depressive psychosis, can start around puberty and occurs very rarely in younger children. The overall picture, cause and outcome are similar to that of adult psychosis.

Schizoid disorder of childhood is a disorder likely to be classified as a pervasive disorder in ICD–10 as it resembles those features of autism. Schizoid children usually come to medical attention during their school years due to educational failure and poor social relationships with others. They are withdrawn, aloof, solitary and unable to make normal emotional contact with others, and their lack of interest, motivation and competitiveness leads to school failure in often highly intelligent children. Some of these children are quiet, secretive and silent at school. Others are superficially communicative but express themselves oddly and metaphorically (Wolff, 1988).

Definition of childhood psychoses

Autism

Recent work and literature suggests that early infantile autism is in a sense a man-made syndrome, that it is a useful shorthand communication of a clinical picture between mental health professionals or educationalists but not a syndrome having a unitary cause or even a unitary symptomatology (Tanguay, 1984). Autism is a descriptive rather than an aetiological diagnosis (Rutter and Lord, 1987) marked by social withdrawal, a desire for sameness and communicative impairment. This latter is evident in both verbal and non-verbal development. Although in the past these children have been described as uncommunicative there is an increasing body of literature supporting the theory that they use what appear to be abnormal or bizarre behaviours in a communicative way (e.g. Wetherby, 1986; Prizant and Rydell, 1984). In the DSM-III-R 'pervasive developmental difficulties', symptoms range from classically autistic to less and less 'autistic' until arriving at mentally handicapped with no autistic features or those children who have serious disorders of communication and little disturbance relating to others. The DSM-III-R definition of pervasive development disorders is 'the impairment in the development of reciprocal social interaction, in the development of verbal and nonverbal communication skills and in imaginative activity. Often there is a restricted repertoire of activities and interests, which are frequently stereotyped and repetitive'. It is the language/communication behaviours seen in autistic children that most often first lead to referral. Intellectual skills, comprehension of meaning of language and the production of speech, posture and movements, patterns of eating, drinking or sleeping and responses to sensory input are likely to be affected. Impairment in communication includes verbal and non-verbal skills, language may be absent, immature, delayed or echolalic or idiosyncratic. The melody of speech may be abnormal, monotonous or with inappropriate inflexions particularly at the ends of phrases.

Childhood schizophrenia

Tanguay (1984) states that 'childhood schizophrenia' does exist, not only in the 'late-onset childhood psychosis' but in the three symptoms described by Cantor (1984): the 'disorganized type'; the 'undifferentiated type' which is the most common type; and finally the 'paranoid type', in which there are delusions of either persecutory or grandiose types or both. In this last type, by the time the child reaches the seventh or eighth year, although the child has previously been verbal and asked questions, he will no longer value others enough to ask questions and will invent his own answers based on faulty information and this, according to Cantor, is the beginning of true paranoia.

Cantor (1984) is of the opinion that all schizophrenic disorders are thought disorders and the normal 3–4-year-old child is aware of 'what goes with what', whereas the schizophrenic child appears to be completely unable to note context; in other words, all incoming information is learned and stored but is devoid of context. The children will learn but the pace at which they learn is modified by their tendency to perseverate, fragment, ignore context and be oppositional. Of course thought disorder will be reflected in disordered language, and Cantor goes on to suggest that there are two extremes in communication styles: children whose speech is sparse and impoverished, and children with marked pressure of speech. Children with impoverished speech may talk a lot and make little sense and those with pressure of speech may find themselves experiencing expressive difficulty. Their speech styles include neologisms and word approximations; that is, making up new words and articulating near approximations to the real word. Word salad, echolalia and unintelligible speech, including whilst talking to him or herself, are common. Finally, the schizophrenic child often speaks so softly that he is difficult to hear but is still able on occasions to produce a good and powerful voice.

ASSESSMENTS OF PSYCHOSES

Assessments are hindered as patients do not usually believe that they are ill and so are reluctant to seek help; some cases therefore present in a serious condition and the psychiatrist will need to make decisions quickly. The knowledge that perhaps up to half of the patients suffering from these conditions will have some degree of long-term handicap, either as residual symptoms or a tendency to relapse, needs to be taken into account in order to minimize chronic disability (Rose, 1988). Psychological tests can be used to indicate, confirm or rule out a diagnosis of schizophrenia. A diagnosis is supported if tests reflect unusual or bizarre perceptual and conceptual processes. Tests that might be used, for example, are the Rorschach (1942), Thematic Apperception Tests (TAT) (Murray, 1943) and the Wechsler Adult Intelligence Scale (WAIS) (Wechsler, 1981). Self-report inventories such as the Minnesota Multiphasic Personality Inventory (MMPI) (Hathaway and McKinley, 1970) can also be helpful. (These tests are discussed in Chapters 7 and 10.) Some psychiatrists are of the opinion that such tests seldom add anything towards diagnosis. The Rorschach and the TAT are used to examine thought processes, and The Grid Test of Schizophrenic Thought Disorder (GTSTD) is a diagnostic instrument designed to test whether a patient is thought disordered or not (Bannister and Fransella, 1966, 1967) and also add some useful information. Psychometric assessments may add little to the diagnosis but quantitative assessments of specific abnormalities of behaviour are useful for planning and evaluating social relationships (Gelder *et al.*, 1986).

COMMUNICATION AND SPEECH IN PSYCHOTIC DISORDERS

It is not an exaggeration to state that all aspects of communication and speech can be affected by those suffering from psychotic disorders. Changes in speech behaviour can have a profound influence on some or all aspects of communication, in both verbal and non-verbal, where mutism is one extreme, and the over-productive, excitable speech of the manic patient is the other. Incongruency between verbal and non-verbal channels has been noted in clinical descriptions of schizophrenia.

140

The quantity and quality of personal interaction and the resulting effect on communication is possibly partly governed by the perceptual changes caused by the illness, reducing and distorting visual and listening skills.

Communication and speech disturbances can be divided into three possible areas for consideration: firstly, the communication and speech pathology evident prior to the onset of the illness and possibly maintained and exacerbated by the psychosis; secondly, communication and language disruption/disorder caused predominantly by the psychosis; and finally additional problems resulting from drug and physical treatments and organic conditions.

Communication and speech problems that developed prior to the onset of the psychotic illness can be present for any number of reasons: for instance, as a result of residual developmental speech problems when they may be represented by expressive language problems; vocal disorders or vocal misuse (including faulty phonation); language and articulation disorders caused by organic conditions which are not associated with psychosis; sensory impairment such as deafness; dysfluency/stuttering; and psychogenic communication and speech difficulties. If the onset of the psychosis was in adolescence, the development of the symptoms might well influence communication breakdown by gradual social withdrawal and isolation, caused by the developing psychosis, even before the realization and eventual diagnosis of the psychosis. These factors play an important part in inhibiting the continuing development of adult language. Restricted life experiences will restrict language use; if, for instance, a person is damaged enough to be unable to live a full adult life it is possible that adult language is unlikely to continue to develop normally.

Those patients whose primary problem is that of communication and speech difficulties may well have contact with a speech therapist at a number of levels: on an individual basis to work predominantly on the speech and language pathology, and in group work to concentrate on communication difficulties. The need or motivation to communicate is of primary importance and so often individual speech therapy may wait until patient and therapist have established a good working/communicative relationship through group work or individual sessions when little emphasis will be put on clarity of speech. As happens in many therapeutic settings, the very fact that a speech therapist is present tends to produce spontaneously heightened effort to be understood.

Arieti (1974) states that language and its relations with thought processes are so characteristic in schizophrenia as to lead in typical cases to a prompt diagnosis, and in the most pronounced cases schizophrenic language appears obscure or utterly incomprehensible. In mild cases of schizophrenia, patients may show very little, if any, change in the form of their speech, whereas the very sick may show every variety of speech and language abnormality.

Voice may demonstrate changes in pitch, volume and quality, and vocalization can be influenced by bizarre behaviour, such as vocalizing on inspiration rather than expiration, affecting nasalized speech, and subvocal speech (producing voice and superimposing appropriate inflections on the voice without articulation or normal vocal resonance). This latter condition is fairly rare and there are a number of theories as to its provenance. One such theory is that the patient is subvocalizing his auditory hallucinations and/or his replies. Breathiness and tension, irregular volume and uncontrolled pitch may also be features. Abnormal language content and style are very much a part of psychoses and may present as rigid, stilted or unusual. Articulation may be affected by subvocalization and by tardive dyskinesia. The rhythm, delivery and fluency of speech, its speed, smoothness and musical quality may also be abnormal.

Thought disorder

It is probably appropriate here to consider thought disorder in more detail as this is the term that is used to describe abnormality of the form rather than the content of speech and is particularly relevant in schizophrenia. Thought disorder has never been satisfactorily defined nor any fundamental psychological or linguistic deficit identified to account for the various observable abnormalities of schizophrenic speech (Kendell, 1988). It has been suggested that the cause of the listener's difficulty in comprehension is brought about by the patient's failure to provide normal cohesive links between one sentence and the next. The problem is often compounded by the patient's preoccupation with abstruse themes and his failure to appreciate his listener's difficulties. It was popularly believed that thought disorder involved the semantic content rather than the syntactic structure of speech and that the latter remained intact until a very late state of the illness. Morice and Ingram (1982) proved that this is not so as it has been demonstrated by detailed linguistic analysis that the syntactic structure of schizophrenic speech is quite different from that of both manics and of normal controls.

Schizophrenic speech

Schizophrenic speech may be more difficult to understand in the acutely ill patient as the patient is often excited and preoccupied with odd themes and delusional ideas. Speech is considered more normal in the chronic stage but overall the total quantity of speech is reduced. Andreasen (1979) attempted to define thought disorder by suggesting that it should be retitled 'disorders of thought, language and communication'. Kendell (1988) speculates whether, in the future, modern linguistic analysis will illuminate the fundamental nature of thought disorder, particularly if it is now thought to be based on linguistic concepts like cohesion, lexical density and dysfluency rather than on ancient clinical metaphors like derailment. Harrow and Quinlan (1985) draw attention to the fact that their observations lead them to believe that bizarre idiosyncratic verbalizations and thinking are not exclusive to schizophrenia and that it is also common in acute manic patients and occasionally in other acute psychotic patients too.

Some of the features of schizophrenic language are that it is restricted in range of words, and that the patient may repeat what has recently been said, which applies to syllables as well as words. There are times when a patient ceases to speak in the middle of a sentence; this pause may last seconds or minutes and the patient may then have difficulty picking up the thread of his conversation again. Some schizophrenics create new expressions or neologisms when there is a need to express a concept for which no satisfactory word of phrase exists. Occasionally echolalia is part of the speech pattern, which is an echoing of words or phrases just heard, or part of an answer to a question. Speech mannerisms may be apparent, shown in grimacing or tic-like movements, particularly in the perioral area. Mutism, which is the inhibition of all speech, may last for hours or days and in a few rare cases for years in the chronic schizophrenics of the catatonic type (Kaplan and Sadock, 1985). Speech tempo might be uneven, with periods of acceleration and deceleration, and the patient may 'jump' steps in the dialogue, or give 'tangential' responses which are misleading to the listener.

The interest in communication and speech problems in psychoses is already generating a vast literature, and many publications and research projects endorse this knowledge. Hirsch (1988) states that during the last decade there has been a radical change in the direction of psychiatric research into schizophrenia, with increasing emphasis on neurobiology, and he states that each specialty has something to contribute and so there should be an exchange of information and ideas between disciplines. Frith and Allen (1988) state that neuropsychology has a long tradition in the study of schizophrenia in establishing whether it is a functional or organic disorder. They hypothesize that all schizophrenic language disorders are a manifestation of restricted cognitive processes.

Rutter's research into language in schizophrenia (1985) was guided by two main assumptions – the first that language disturbance is widespread among schizophrenic patients and easy to detect and measure, and secondly that schizophrenia is fundamentally a cognitive disorder in which language disturbance is part of an inability or failure to regulate one's thoughts. Rutter found that in conversations, just as in mono-logues, the problem for schizophrenic patients was much less the cognitive processes of regulating and organizing their thoughts than the social processes of expressing and communicating those thoughts in a way which the listener could understand and follow. Where their difficulty really lay was in taking the role of the other and it is that which seems to be the key.

In a comparative study of manic versus schizophrenic speech disorganization, Hoffman *et al.* (1986) state that manics as well as schizophrenics demonstrate major difficulties in generating a coherently organized stream of speech, that schizophrenics tend to produce less speech content than manics, and that utterance length is greater for manics compared to schizophrenics. But, the more a speaker talks, the more chaotic his speech is likely to become.

Undoubtedly communication, speech and language in the psychoses offer many interesting and important opportunities for treatment and research. As already discussed, Kendell's speculations as to whether modern linguistic analysis could well help in understanding thought disorders and perhaps in so doing aid the discovery of the origins of illnesses such as schizophrenia is definitely worth further consideration.

MANAGEMENT AND TREATMENT OF PSYCHOSES

Autism

The speech therapist may see pre-school autistic children, but diagnosis is often delayed or referral for specialist language therapy not made. Frequently it is the therapists working within special units or schools who see these children. Differential diagnosis is difficult and should be a team decision; suggestions have been made that empirical measures of communicative behaviour may be of value in the diagnostic process (Wetherby, 1986). Rutter and Lord (1987) suggest that 'precise categorization is less important than careful assessment of a child's strengths and weakness and the identification of factors most likely to enhance learning and development'.

Treatment may be medical, educational and/or family based, to help parents understand and develop realistic expectations. Speech therapy provision should be considered for each child. In the past most inter-

144

vention has been largely based on operant conditioning theory, providing structure via the use of reinforcement, with varying degrees of success (Baltaxe and Simmons, 1981), and Rutter (1985) offers an excellent introduction to the use of behavioural and educational approaches. Recently there has been a move towards alternative approaches, partly due to an increased interest in psycholinguistics, which has resulted in attempts to use signing and symbols (e.g. Kiernan, 1983), computer programs and non-verbal linguistic systems (e.g. Lovaas, 1968).

Research into the pragmatic aspects of communicative failure in autism has led to suggestions of language intervention programmes that base on communicative intentions and that deviate from normal developmental models on the basis of evidence that there is a pattern of autistic development. Such programmes stress the need to consider the social context and to use pragmatic rewards if operant methods are followed (Wetherby, 1986).

In summary it is true to say that there are no strict answers to the problem of developing appropriate management strategies for use with autistic children. Individual considerations must direct all therapy measures.

Other psychoses

Generally aetiological factors need to be taken into consideration when planning treatment and thinking in terms of future prevention of the illness. Treatment methods might also differ according to whether the illness is acute or chronic – if acute, the aims are to treat the illness as rapidly as possible and to provide support and counselling to the patient and his relations. Hospital admission is usually indicated, particularly if behaviour is severely disturbed. If behaviour is less disturbed, the patient may be managed at home, provided conditions there are satisfactory for support and rehabilitation. In the past, rehabilitation resources were located in large institutions where patients used the on-site facilities such as occupational therapy programmes and industrial workshops; however, times are changing and acute care tends now to be provided in small district-based acute units, whilst rehabilitation and long-term care is provided on a more local basis away from the hospital (Rose, 1988). An aspect of treatment is to develop a supportive relationship with the patient in order to help him through the frightening psychotic experiences. It is during an acute phase that the patient may become assaultative or cause self-harm and it is then that there might be need for compulsory admission under the Mental Health Act 1983 (Rose, 1988).

Management of both post-acute and chronic patients needs to be considered. The possibility of the recurrence of the illness needs to be taken into account as well as considering the best way to rehabilitate the patient to the best level of functioning. The aims of rehabilitation will vary according to individual needs and will usually need to be on a long-term basis. Rehabilitation will aim to cover both social and psychological aspects of the patient's disabilities but will also include maintenance treatment for medication if necessary. There is still some controversy as to whether all schizophrenics should receive maintenance therapy. Studies find that patients with a poor prognosis should receive maintenance therapy as they tend to relapse despite receiving drugs, whilst those with a good prognosis tend not to relapse even without drugs.

Treatment with drugs

The neuroleptic drugs, otherwise known as antipsychotic agents or the major tranquillizers, are used both in schizophrenia and mania. All neuroleptics block dopamine receptors in the brain; this is responsible for their tendency to produce extrapyramidal movement disorders as side-effects. There are three groups of antipsychotic drugs: phenothiazines, thioxanthenes and butyrophenones. Chlorpromazine, one of the phenothiazines, is a popular drug which may be prescribed initially during the acute phase of the illness. It acts as a sedative within hours, although its effect on the psychotic symptoms usually takes about three weeks and has a full effect in about six to twelve weeks. These drugs produce sedation, and reduce anxiety; suppress spontaneous movement and complex behaviour; but preserve intellectual functioning so that incoherent thinking and thought disorder tend to clear, leading to more intelligible language production, but less spontaneity and more circumscription in speech. Mutism tends to disappear (see Appendix 5.3).

Side-effects from the neuroleptics are of three types of extrapyramidal symptoms – Parkinsonism, dystonia and akathisia – and these symptoms can all usually be relieved by anti-Parkinsonian agents. The effects of Parkinsonism on speech is that it produces jerky, dysrhythmic phonation, poor articulation, monotonous intonation, and a soft voice. Other side-effects may also be distressing, including blurring of vision, producing difficulty in reading, and decreased salivation which leads to a dry mouth and difficulty in articulation, but it is important to note that not all patients on neuroleptic drugs develop side-effects.

Tardive dyskinesia is produced by a prolonged high-dosage neuroleptic medication and is characterized by slow, irregular movements in the region of the mouth, such as grimacing, smacking of lips and protrusion of the tongue. It also results in poor articulation of speech, but produces loud phonation and hyperkinetic dysarthria. Dysarthria has been reported as being similar to a stutter but is really of basal ganglion origin and scanning speech has been noted in some patients recovering from toxic doses of drugs. Stopping the medication does not necessarily lead to the disappearance of the dyskinesia and may sometimes make it worse.

Drug treatment for the major affective (mood) disorders include antidepressant drugs and lithium therapy and it is considered that these drugs play an important role in treatment. It is thought that the tricyclic antidepressants are particularly effective in unipolar depression but it is thought that they may in some cases precipitate manic episodes.

Psychological treatments

Psychological treatments for depressed patients can be divided into supportive methods, dynamic psychotherapy, interpersonal methods and cognitive therapy. It is thought that supportive treatment is essential in the management of all depressed patients as it is intended to sustain them until they are well enough to accept other forms of therapy. Dynamic psychotherapy is often restricted to the less severe cases but during intervals between acute episodes such therapy may be valuable. Cognitive therapy is directed towards the patient's way of thinking about life problems, and is considered in more detail in Chapters 7 and 10.

There is nevertheless a divergence of psychiatric opinion as to whether psychotherapy in any or all of its many forms actually offers effective treatment to this group of patients. It is even considered by some psychiatrists as being harmful, the pressure of treatment creating enough stress to cause remission. Others think that with careful monitoring and sensitive handling benefits result and progress can be achieved, even if at a slow and limited pace. In other cases considerable progress can be made and patients themselves appreciate the opportunity to join in and be accepted in the therapeutic milieu.

Psychotherapy is thought by many to be essential even if only to supplement drug treatments, and if a patient suffers a basically physiological form of the illness then psychotherapy is essential to treatment

147

(Kaplan and Sadock, 1985), and it may take the form of analytical (dynamic) or supportive care. Milieu therapy, although regarded as inconclusively researched as to its effectiveness, with the use of modern psychotropic drugs can often deepen insight, or provide new social patterns, particularly for the patient in hospital care. Milieu therapy (the therapeutic effects from the environment in which the patient is living) may be added to by group meetings aiming to increase self-reliance, to share responsibility for treatment, and to help other patients. This can include a wide range of rehabilitation programmes to help domestic and social skills towards living a more independent life.

Psychoanalytic (dynamic) therapy

Psychoanalytic (dynamic) therapy is aimed at effecting a change in personality structure or character and so does more than just reduce symptoms. Psychotherapy is thought, by an increasing number of psychiatrists, to be of benefit, although it has no place in active psychoses. The therapeutic relationship needs to be flexible, direct, sincere, and respecting of privacy. The aim is to convey a need to understand the patient, however disturbed, hostile or bizarre in behaviour. The author has observed that group therapy combined with drug treatment produces better results than drug treatment alone, and positive results are more likely when treatment focuses on real-life plans, problems and relationships, on social and work roles and interaction, or cooperation with drug therapy and discussion of its side-effects and on recreational or work activities (Kaplan and Sadock, 1985). This type of group encompasses rehabilitation, communication, support, problem solving and sharing and is an ideal setting for a speech therapist to share skills with nursing staff and/or with other professional staff such as psychologists, social workers and psychiatrists.

Behaviour therapy

Behaviour therapy is also successful as a method of reducing frequency of bizarre, disturbing and deviant behaviour by increasing adaptive and normal behaviour; direct work on reinforcing appropriate behaviour and training in social skills can offer remedial support. It is known that schizophrenics are deficient in a number of components of social skills. Their social behaviours exhibit greater levels of anxiety and less skill than non-sufferers and they are less efficient in decoding non-verbal cues and in their judgement of appropriateness of social behaviour, but they appear to be aware of their deficient social behaviour (Monti and

148

Fingeret, 1987). Trower *et al.* (1978) bases the need for treatment on the patient's social inadequacy and this will tend to show a particular style of behaviour; the patient will probably appear rather cold, unassertive and unrewarding to others, will show little expressive variation in face, voice and posture, will look rather infrequently at the other person, will make little effort to produce a spontaneous and interesting flow of speech, and will take little part in the management of conversations. Once again a speech therapist has skills and expertise to offer here, particularly if in cooperation with a psychologist, as it appears that the problem is as much of communication as overall social deficiencies.

Family therapy

Family therapy can play an important role as the patient's illness is usually accompanied by serious family problems. This treatment can be extended from hospital (see Chapter 10).

Personal construct psychotherapy

The personal construct approach to treatment, as already explained, can be particularly useful for assessing schizophrenic patients as well as offering an increasingly useful means of treatment. Van den Bergh, De Boeck and Claeyes (1986) give details of work and research in this area and are also optimistic that personal construct psychotherapy with schizophrenic patients will continue to develop and become more widely used. Bannister and Fransella (1966) found that schizophrenics differed from normal people in that they had low correlations between different constructs, and Bannister (1962) theorized that as a result of being repeatedly invalidated in their attempts to develop a meaningful personal construct system, schizophrenics may end up with a very loose construct system. If true, this theory would provide a mechanism whereby abnormal family interaction such as 'double-bind' communication might, by weakening a child's construct system, eventually lead to thought disorder (Murray, 1986). It is known that schizophrenics respond to personal construct psychotherapy (Button, 1986).

Communication and language disruption or disorders that are predominantly caused by the psychoses have been discussed throughout this chapter, and experience proves that with an understanding and sensitive approach improvements can be made. The speech therapist's appreciation and reinforcement of cooperation, effort and motivation help to maintain progress and can, in some cases, be enough alone to produce improvement. Certainly the therapist's expectation of clear, intelligible speech will be necessary and might even be part of the contract for treatment. Further details on treatment techniques are discussed more fully in Chapter 10.

REFERENCES

Andreason, N. C. (1979) Thought, language and communication disorders. *Archives of General Psychiatry*, **36**, 1315–25.

Arieti, S. (1974) *Interpretation of Schizophrenia*, 2nd edn, Crosby Lockwood Staple, London.

Baltaxe, C. A. M. and Simmons, J. Q. (1981) Disorders of language in childhood psychoses: current concepts and approaches, in *Speech Evaluation in Psychiatry* (ed. J. K. Darby), Grune and Stratton, New York, pp. 285–328.

Bannister, D. (1962) The nature and management of thought disorder. *British Journal of Social Clinical Psychology*, **5**, 95–102.

Bannister, D. and Fransella, F. (1966) A grid test of schizophrenic thought disorder. *British Journal of Social Clinical Psychology*, **5**, 95–102.

Bannister, D. and Fransella, F. (1967) *A Grid Test of Schizophrenic Thought Disorder. A Standard Clinical Test*, Psychological Test Publications, Barnstaple, Devon.

Blakemore, C. (1988) *Madness (Programme 6)*, The Mind Machine, BBC2, UK, 18 October.

Button, E. (1986) *Personal Construct Theory and Mental Health*, Croom Helm, London.

Cantor, S. (1984) *The Schizophrenic Child*, Open University Press, Milton Keynes.

Catlan, J. (1988) Affective disorders, in *Essential Psychiatry* (ed. N. Rose), Blackwell Scientific Publications, Oxford, pp. 62–72.

Cremona, A. (1988) Substance abuse, in *Essential Psychiatry* (ed. N. Rose), Blackwell Scientific Publications, Oxford, pp. 94–104.

Cutting, J. (1986) Atypical psychosis, in *Essentials in Postgraduate Psychiatry*, 2nd edn (eds P. Hill, R. Murray and A. Thorley), Grune and Stratton, New York, pp. 425–43.

DHSS Mental Health Statistics for England (1986) *Mental Illness Hospitals and Units in England: Diagnostic Data. Booklet 12* A Publication of the Government's Statistical Service.

DSM-III (1980) *Diagnostic and Statistical Manual of Mental Disorders*, 3rd edn, American Psychiatric Association, Washington, DC.

DSM-III-R (1987) *Diagnostic and Statistical Manual of Mental Disorders* 3rd edn – revised, American Psychiatric Association, Washington DC.

Evans, J. (1982) *Adolescent and Pre-Adolescent Psychiatry*, Academic Press, London

Freeman, H. (1988) The long term treatment of schizophrenia with neuroleptic drugs, in *Perspectives in Psychiatry* (eds P. Hall and P. Stonier), Wiley, Chichester, pp. 167–76.

Freud, A. (1936) *The Ego and the Mechanisms of Defence*, Hogarth Press, London (1958); Adolescence 1: adolescence in the psychoanalytic theory, in *The Psychoanalytic Study of the Child*, (ed. A. Freud), International University Press, New York.

Frith, C. D. and Allen, H. A. (1988) Language disorders in schizophrenia and their implications for neuropsychology, in *Schizophrenia: The Major Issues*

150

(eds P. Bebbington and P. McGuffin), Heinemann Professional Publishing, London, pp. 172–86.

Fulford, K. W. M. (1988) Diagnosis classification and phenomenology of mental illness, in *Essential Psychiatry* (ed. N. Rose), Blackwell Scientific Publications, Oxford, pp. 4–16.

Gelder, M., Gath, D. and Mayou, R. (1986) *Oxford Textbook of Psychiatry*, Oxford University Press, Oxford.

Harrow, M. and Quinlan, D. M. (1985) *Disordered Thinking and Schizophrenic Psychopathology*, Gardener Press, USA.

Hathaway, S. and McKinley, J. (1970) *Minnesota Multiphasic Personality Inventory*. NFER Nelson, Windsor.

Hill, P. (1986) Child psychiatry, in *Essentials of Postgraduate Psychiatry*, 2nd edn (eds P. Hill, R. Murray and A. Thorley), Grune and Stratton, New York, pp. 81–184.

Hirsch, S. R. (1988) Essential aspects of the research problem in schizophrenia. *Journal of the Royal Society of Medicine*, **81**, 691–7.

Hoffman, R. E., Stopek, S. and Andreasen, N. C. (1986) A comparative study of manic versus schizophrenic speech disorganisation. *Archives of General Psychiatry*, **43**, 831–8.

International Classification of Diseases (1975) *Manual of the International Statistical Classification of Diseases, Injuries and Causes of Death*, Vol. 1, World Health Organization, Geneva, 1977.

Kaplan, H. and Sadock, B. (1985) *Modern Synopsis and Comprehensive Textbook of Psychiatry IV*, 4th edn, Williams and Wilkins, Baltimore.

Kaplan, H. and Sadock, B. (1988) *Clinical Psychiatry from Synopsis of Psychiatry*, Williams and Wilkins, Baltimore.

Kendell, R. E. (1988) Schizophrenia, in *Companion Guide to Psychiatric Studies*, 4th edn (eds R. E. Kendell and A. K. Zealley), Churchill Livingstone, Edinburgh, pp. 310–44.

Kiernan, C. (1983) The use of non-vocal communication techniques with autistic individuals. *Journal of Child Psychology and Psychiatry*, **24**, 339–75.

Kraeplin, E. (1896) *Psychiatric, ein Lehrbach fur Studierende und Arzte*, 5th edn, Barth, Leipzig.

Lovaas, I. (1968) A programme for the establishment of speech in psychotic children, in *Operant Procedures in Remedial Speech and Language Training* (eds H. N. Sloan and B. D. MacAulay), Houghton Mifflin, Boston.

Mental Health Act (1959) HMSO, London.

Mental Health Statistics for England (1986) *Booklet 12: Mental Illness Hospitals and Units in England, Diagnostic Data, DHSS*, a publication of the Government's Statistical Service.

Miles, C. P. (1977) Conditions predisposing suicide. *Review Journal of Nervous and Mental Disease*, 164–231.

Monti, P. M. and Fingeret, A. L. (1987) Social perceptions and communication skills among schizophrenics and non-schizophrenics. *Journal of Clinical Psychology*, **43** (2), 197–204.

Morice, R. D. and Ingram, J. C. L. (1982) Language analysis in schizophrenia: diagnostic implications. *Australian and New Zealand Journal of Psychiatry*, **16**, 11.

Murphy, H. B. M. (1968) Cultural factors in the genesis of schizophrenia, in

The Transmission of Schizophrenia, (eds D. Rosenthal and S. Kety), Pergamon Press, Oxford.

Murphy, H. B. M., Wittower, E. D., Fried, J. and Ellenberger, H. (1963) A cross-cultural survey of schizophrenic symptomatology. *International Journal of Social Psychiatry*, **9**, 237–47.

Murray, H. A. (1943) *Thematic Apperception Test TAT*, Harvard University Press, Cambridge, Massachusetts.

Murray, R. (1986) Schizophrenia, in *Essentials of Postgraduate Psychiatry*, 2nd edn (eds P. Hill, R. Murray and A. Thorley), Grune and Stratton, New York, pp. 339–79.

Ostwald, P. F. (1981) Speech and schizophrenia, in *Speech Evaluation in Psychiatry*, (ed. J. K. Darby), Grune and Stratton, New York, pp. 329–48.

Prizant, B. M. and Rydell, P. J. (1984) Analysis of functions of delayed echolalia in autistic children. *Journal of Speech and Hearing Research*, **27**, 183–92.

Rorschach, H. (1942) *Rorschach Inkblot Test Psychodiagnostics*, Hans Huber, Berne.

Rose, N. (1988) Schizophrenia, in *Essential Psychiatry*, (ed. N. Rose), Blackwell Scientific Publications, Oxford, pp. 48–60.

Roth, M. and Kroll, J. (1986) *The Reality of Mental Illness*, Cambridge University Press, Cambridge.

Rutter, D. (1985) Language in schizophrenia: the structure of monologues and conversations. *British Journal of Psychiatry*, **146**, 399–404.

Rutter, M. and Lord, C. (1987) Language disorders associated with psychiatric disturbance, in *Lanauge Development and Disorders*, (eds W. Yule and M. Rutter) MacKeith Press, London, pp. 206–33.

Schneider, K. (1959) *Clinical Psychopathology*, Grune and Stratton, New York.

Storr, A. (1987) Foreword, in *Images of Destruction* (ed. D. Wigoder), Routledge and Kegan Paul, London.

Tanguay, P. (1984) Preface, in *The Schizophrenic Child* (ed. S. Cantor), Open University Press, Milton Keynes.

Tidmarsh, D. (1990) Schizophrenia and crime, in *Principles and Practice of Forensic Psychiatry*, (eds R. Bluglass and P. Bowden), Churchill Livingstone, Edinburgh.

Trower, D., Bryant, B. and Argyle, M. (1978) *Social Skills and Mental Health*, Methuen, London.

Van den Bergh, O., De Boeck, P. and Claeys, W. (1986) Schizophrenia: what is loose in schizophrenic construing, in *Personal Construct Theory and Mental Health* (ed. E. Button), Croom Helm, London, pp. 59–81.

Wechsler, D. (1981) *The Wechsler Adult Intelligence Scale*, Psychological Corporation, Sidcup, Kent.

Wetherby, A. M. (1986) Ontogeny of communicative functions in autism. *Journal of Autism and Developmental Disorders*, **16** (3), 136–295.

Wigoder, D. (1987) *Images of Destruction*, Routledge & Kegan Paul, London.

Wing, L. and Gould, J. (1979) Severe impairments of social interaction and associated abnormalities in children: epidemiology and classification, *Journal of Autism and Developmental Disorders*, **9**, 11–29.

Wolff, S. (1988) Psychiatric disorders of childhood, in *Companion Guide to Psychiatric Studies*, 4th edn (eds R. E. Kendell and A. K. Zealley), Churchill Livingstone, Edinburgh, pp. 505–34.

Wolff, S. and Cull, A. (1986) Schizoid personality and anti-social conduct: a retrospective case note study. *Psychological Medicine*, **16**, 677–87.

APPENDIX 5.1: OUTLINE OF DIAGNOSTIC CRITERIA FOR MAJOR DEPRESSED EPISODE RELATED TO PSYCHOTIC DISORDER

A. At least five of the following symptoms have been present during the same two-week period and represent a change from previous functioning; at least one of the symptoms is either (1) depressed mood or (2) loss of interest or pleasure.

1. Depressed mood
2. Markedly diminished interest or pleasure in all or almost all activities most of the day, nearly every day
3. Significant weight loss or gain when not dieting
4. Insomnia or hypersomnia nearly every day
5. Psychomotor agitation or retardation nearly every day
6. Fatigue or loss of energy nearly every day
7. Feelings of worthlessness and excessive or inappropriate guilt (which may be delusional) nearly every day
8. Diminished ability to think or concentrate, indecisiveness nearly every day
9. Recurrent thoughts of death, recurrent suicidal ideation without a specific plan for committing suicide

B. (1) It cannot be established that an organic factor initiated and maintained the disturbance.
    (2) The disturbance is not a normal reaction to the death of a loved one.

Major depressive episode with psychotic features. Delusions or hallucinations.

Mood-congruent psychotic features. Delusions or hallucinations whose content is entirely consistent with the typical depressive themes of personal inadequacy, guilt, disease, death, nihilism, or delusioned punishment.

Mood-incongruent psychotic features. Delusions or hallucinations whose content does *not* involve typical depressive themes of personal inadequacy, guilt, disease, death, nihilism, or delusioned punishment. Included here are such symptoms as persecutory delusions, thought insertion, through broadcasting and delusions of control.

Based on DSM-III-R (1987).

APPENDIX 5.2: OUTLINE OF DIAGNOSTIC CRITERIA FOR MANIC EPISODES RELATED TO PSYCHOTIC DISORDER

A. A distinct period of abnormally and persistently elevated expansive or irritable mood.

B. During the period of mood disturbance at least three of the following symptoms have persisted (if the mood is only irritable) and have been present to a significant degree.

    1. Inflated self-esteem
    2. Decreased need for sleep
    3. More talkative than usual or pressure to keep talking
    4. Flight of ideas
    5. Distractibility
    6. Increase in goal-directed activity
    7. Excessive involvement in pleasurable activities which have a high potential for painful consequences

C. Mood disturbance sufficiently severe to cause marked impairment in

Based on DSM-III-R (1987).

APPENDIX 5.3: DRUGS USED IN TREATING PSYCHOSES

Group	Non-proprietary name	Proprietary names	Mode of action	Adverse effects
(a) Phenothiazines	Chlorpromazine Thioridazine Trifluoperazine Fluphenazine	Largactil Melleril Stelazine Moditen Modecate (depot)	Sedation, anti-anxiety, suppression of complex behaviour. Lack of initiative and interest in environment. Intellectual function preserved. Incoherent thought clears. Mutism tends to disappear	(a) *Parkinsonism* (effects on speech) jerky dysrhythmic phonation; articulation poor; monotonous intonation; soft voice (b) *Tardive dyskinesia* (effects on speech) poor articulation; loud phonation and hyperkinetic dysarthria
(b) Thioxanthenes	Flupenthixol Zuclopenthixol	Depixol (also depot) Clopixol		
(c) Diphenylbutylpiperidines and butyrophenones	Pimozide Haloperidol	Orap Serenace Haldol Decanoate (depot)		

6

Depression

Jenny France

Overall approximately 3% of the world's population, that is about 100 million people, suffer from depressive states at a given time, according to the World Health Organization (Kelly, 1987a). It has been established that there will be 3–4% men and 7–8% women in the community suffering from a depressive illness at any one time. It is thought that one of the reasons for the discrepancy between the figures for men and women suffering from depression is due to the fact that more women will admit to depressive symptoms than men and that some men will abuse alcohol, thus confusing the diagnosis of depression. In one study depression accounted for 12% of the problems presented to the family practitioner for the first time (Pennell and Creed, 1987). As depressive disorders are so common and are responsible for a high proportion of a total psychiatric morbidity, it is important to include mention of the affective disorders and depression in particular, in this volume.

Depression comes under the heading of the affective disorders, which are so called because the main feature is an abnormality of mood. It therefore includes a wide range from mild to severe states (severe depression or psychotic depression includes features such as delusions and hallucinations and is accompanied by feelings of worthlessness and guilt), a few of which may even be life threatening; these severe depressions were covered in some detail in Chapter 5. Some of the mildest forms may be self-limiting but the more severe forms, which are less common, need recognition due to the possible risk of suicide and in order to receive the present effective treatments as soon as possible. Pennell and Creed (1987) state that approximately 25% of people with depressive illness who attend the family practitioner make a rapid recovery, 50% show a fluctuating course over one year, and 25% show chronic illness.

Depression is the common cold of psychopathology and has touched the lives of everyone; to be depressed is to endure terrible isolation (Seligman, 1975). It is characterized by depressed mood, pessimistic thinking, lack of enjoyment, reduced energy and slowness. The moods may be infrequent and of short duration in some cases and for others the mood is recurrent, pervasive and can be of lethal intensity. Seligman states that one out of every 200 persons affected by depressive illness will die a suicidal death. This estimate is thought to be probably on the low side.

Kelly (1987a) states that depressive disorders are on the increase due to recent progress on the diagnosis of depression and the fact that more people are now seeking help for this condition. The true size of the disorder is difficult to define due to the differing diagnostic definitions. It is known that depressive symptoms are common and are more frequent among women than in men and particularly in those women of the lower socio-economic groups. Symptoms vary with age, the highest rate being between 35 and 45 years, whereas the rate of depression in men increases with age. Surveys suggest that many cases of depression go unrecognized and untreated although depressives are the most treatable of all psychiatric patients.

Kelly (1987b), who states that depression is on the increase, also draws attention to masked depression – a condition which doctors often fail to diagnose as the patient does not necessarily complain of feeling depressed. In the course of various clinical encounters, these people may present with a condition unrelated to depression, but nevertheless deserving vigilant diagnostic skills with the possibility of further referral to ensure appropriate clinical intervention.

Anthony Storr (1983) states emphatically that depression is not an illness, but a psychobiological reaction which can be provoked in anyone. Storr thinks that use of language such as depressive illness or affective disorder and their underlying assumptions have prevented the understanding of depression.

DEFINITION OF DEPRESSION

Psychiatrists find it difficult to agree on the classification of affective disorders. A wide variety of terms are used, resulting in considerable confusion, particularly to those who have no medical training. Kendell (1988) reports that in an attempt to satisfy the widely differing assumptions and traditions of psychiatrists from fifty different countries, a number of alternative classifications have been put together in the ICD–9 (1975). One of the categories within the ICD–9 was provided to accommodate the simple diagnosis of 'depression' or 'depressive illness'.

In the DSM-III-R (1987) all affective disorders have been brought together in a single grouping of mood disorders and terms such as manic-depressive, psychotic and neurotic, endogenous and reactive have been discarded.

In the tenth revision of the ICD it is likely that all mood disorders will be in one section, with the terms manic episode and depressive episode predominating. A distinction will also be drawn between severe and mild depressive disorders. At present the ICD categorizes affective (mood) disorders under two major headings, that of affective psychoses under one heading, and neurotic disorders with personality disorders and other non-psychotic mental disorders, adjustment reaction and depressive disorder not elsewhere classified, disturbance of emotions specific to childhood and adolescence under another heading. Chapter 5 includes more detail of the bipolar disorders and major depression.

AETIOLOGY

The causes and mechanisms of depression are not fully understood but it is thought that depressive illness is not based on a simple pathology but has multifactoral aetiology (Pennell and Creed, 1987).

The causes of depression can be divided into three categories: predisposing factors, precipitating factors and maintaining factors.

Predisposing factors

Genetic factors

Genetic studies report a morbidity rate of 10–15% for a first-degree relative of a patient with depression. This risk is increased in female relations and in the relations of patients who have become depressed before the age of 40. Twin studies and adoption studies provide convincing evidence that there is a genetic aetiology of depression (Checkley, 1986).

Personality factors

Personality factors are not thought to be relevant in cases of unipolar depressive disorders, but features of obsessional traits and anxiety may be as they influence the way people respond to stressful life events.

Early environment

Psychoanalysts have suggested that deprivation of maternal affection through separation or loss predisposes to depressive disorder in adult life (Gelder *et al.*, 1986). Current literature on the relationship between depression and parental loss is large, conflicting and inconclusive and suggests that it is unlikely that death or loss of a parent in childhood does predispose to depression in later life, whereas Brown and Harris (1978) in their studies stated the opposite. It has been found that when attempting to assess a depressed patient's poor family relationships the patient's memories may well be distorted (due to the present depression) and so memories of negative events and relationships are more likely to be quoted than positive ones and so give an unbalanced bias to the past relationships with parents and siblings.

Social factors

Social factors predispose towards depression as it is thought more likely to occur where there is a chronic long-standing stress or illness in the family, unresolved conflicts in family relationships and excessive alcohol consumption. Brown and Harris (1978) show that mothers are at special risk from depression if they lost their own mother before adolescence, have three or more children under the age of 14, have marital difficulties, and do not have a job outside the home. These 'at risk' women cannot easily cope with adverse life events or continuing difficulties. Adverse events with a long-term threat, such as a spouse threatening to leave or who becomes unemployed, if there is family bereavement, and caring for a physically or mentally handicapped child or adult may provoke a depressive episode in an 'at risk' mother. Depression may also be provoked by financial, housing or other difficulties and it is known that poor housing conditions prevent a woman recovering from depression, and women from low-income families are at much greater risk from depression because they have more 'at risk' factors, and more persistent difficulties (France, 1988).

Precipitating factors

Precipitating factors include adverse life events such as threat and loss, and death or separation are thought to be of particular relevance. The maintaining factors of depression may include many of the factors that predispose towards and precipitate depression (Catlan, 1988).

Organic factors

Organic factors such as cerebral diseases including senile dementia, arteriosclerosis, brain tumour, epilepsy and post-traumatic disorders are thought to cause depression (Kielholz, 1987).

Physical factors

Physical factors, for example, after a viral infection such as influenza or glandular fever, following intoxication, an operation, or of sleep deprivation, anaemia, and endocrine disorders such as diabetes can also cause depression (Kielholz, 1987).

Drug and alcohol abuse

Drug and alcohol abuse are known to induce depression. Selected drugs, particularly the steroids, amphetamines, barbiturates and central nervous system depressants, are known to produce depression after periods of heavy use. A chronic depression secondary to heroin use or long-term methadone use has also been described. Kaplan and Sadock (1985) suggest that drugs of various kinds have often been blamed for causing depression. The contraceptive pill and neuroleptic drugs, particularly intramuscular Depo preparations, are mentioned as causing depression (Kendell, 1988). Kaplan and Sadock (1985) draw attention to the high percentage of chronic alcoholics who develop secondary depression, the rates ranging from 25% to 50%.

Social factors

Social factors can cause depression in childhood. A child whose mother is depressed may well become apathetic and depressed due to lack of maternal comforting and warmth, maternal anger and inconsistent discipline. Conflict within the parental relationship commonly causes depression. Parental standards set above the child's abilities, producing failure and low self-esteem in some children, and those suffering from epilepsy, brain damage or diabetes are more likely to develop depressive disorders (Thursfield, 1987).

Psychological theories

These theories are concerned with the psychological mechanisms by which recent and past life experiences can lead to depression (Gelder et al., 1986).

Psychoanalysis

The psychoanalytic theory was developed by Freud in 1917 and published in an essay called *Mourning and Melancholia*. Freud suggested that mourning results from loss by death, so melancholia results from loss of other kinds. The role in depression of the super-ego (a structure in the unconscious built up by early experiences), of ambivalence and of narcissistic identification (extreme self-love), were ideas developed by Melanie Klein and others and described the depressive position to which patients are thought to regress (Klein, 1934).

Klein suggests that the infant must acquire confidence that when his mother leaves him she will return, even when she has been angry, and this stage is called the 'depressive position'. If this stage is not passed through successfully, the child will be more likely to develop depression in later life.

Behavioural therapy

Many of the behavioural formulations are based on Skinner's ideas (1953). He proposed that depression could be understood as an extinction of normal behaviour due to lack of positive reinforcement from the social environment. Depression is also seen to be due to a low rate of positive rewards and a high rate of negative rewards based on arousive interactions with the environment producing distress, for example negative sexual and marital experiences and experience of incompetence in any field.

Cognitive theory

Beck (1967) states that mood is determined by a central cognitive process (scheme) which filters all incoming stimuli from the environment and determines the way in which they are interpreted. He has proposed that three particular thinking patterns are common. Firstly, depressed people have a negative concept of self; secondly, they interpret their experiences in a negative way; and thirdly, they take a negative view of the future. Depression is therefore primarily a disorder of thinking and secondarily of mood.

DESCRIPTION OF DEPRESSION

Psychological and behavioural symptoms of depression include loss of ability to enjoy life, feelings of sadness, grief and regret accompanied by crying and possible suicidal ideas when the mood is at its lowest. There is a loss of mental energy, indecision, slowness of thinking and memory disturbance. Feelings of guilt and pessimism, a reduced desire and interest in life, self-isolation and avoidance of people, and carelessness in appearance all add to the picture. Some of the associated symptoms present as anxiety, tension and headaches, phobias, panic attacks or obsessional symptoms.

Worrying may give rise to somatic symptoms such as insomnia, weight loss or gain associated with appetite loss or gain, loss of libido, menstrual disorders and other psychosomatic disturbances. Alcoholism may also be an added problem. Depression in children may present as a normal mood change of sadness in response to difficulties or it may occur as an illness with an identifiable aetiology and outcome, with one of the symptoms being depressive thinking. As the patient's moods vary the mental state at interview may appear normal; it is therefore difficult to diagnose and at times may well be mistaken for an anxiety state. The mood changes may last a few days or long enough for the practitioner to experience difficulty distinguishing between depression and personality disorder. Occasionally antisocial and/or aggressive behaviour which is out of character may signal the onset of depression. Depressions are variable in symptomatology, severity and duration and are extremely common, as previously stated.

ASSESSMENTS

Emphasis is placed upon the patient's case history and behaviour prior to the onset of depression, examining both physical and mental states. Investigators need to establish that there is no organic disease present and that the patient has not previously received drugs in other treatments that would be likely to induce depression. The diagnosis is further confounded by the fact that many psychiatric patients with schizophrenia, borderline personality disorders, organic brain syndromes, paranoid disorders and other various physical illnesses may also suffer varying degrees of depression. Storr (1983) comments that learned helplessness is also a feature of the apathetic variety of chronic depression which accompanies institutionalization and which, if prolonged, makes the individual incapable of living an ordinary life. Psychoanalytic thinking has emphasized the role of self-esteem in depression. Self-esteem may be lost if someone important withdraws their attention or concern; similarly, self-esteem may also suffer if a person loses status or position. Many depressed people do, of course, view themselves as ordinary people who are suffering from a severe impairment in their capacity to sleep, eat, concentrate and function normally.

Detecting depression is obviously important as it may not be directly presented to the doctor and so non-verbal cues such as poor eye contact and moist eyes, excessive anxiety and choking or pausing during sentences may be indicators of existing depression (Pennell and Creed, 1987).

Kupfer *et al.* (1987) suggest that there are four methods of assessing depression. The first is through the patient's body movement, which may provide cues that would help improve reliability and validity towards assessing diagnosis in affective disorders. Dittman (1987) calls for a series of research studies to refine and enhance our knowledge base in this area. The second is facial expression: indeed, it seems logical to measure the face in studies of affective disorder because the face is one of the main emotion signal systems, and Ekman and Fridlund (1987) state that it is surprising that there have been so few studies on this topic. Thirdly, vocal assessments of affective disorders are seen as being increasingly important. Scherer (1987) points out that clinicians are trained to be sensitive to the sound and annunciation of speech and are aware that the tempo of speech and the non-linguistic elements of communication and other aspects of vocalization can play an important part in the diagnosis of affective disorders. Finally, the tempo or pacing of speech in depressed individuals is important as observations of tempo could serve as objective markers for major affective disorders and it is suggested that depression is possibly associated with high pause times and slow speech rates (Siegman, 1987).

The Beck Depression Inventory (BDI)

The Beck Depression Inventory (Beck *et al.*, 1979) can be used for measuring depression and might usefully be part of the initial assessment prior to treatment as well as being used on occasions during the course of treatment. The inventory is an extremely useful monitor of the patient's present condition as it is designed to measure the behavioural manifestations of depression. It is a quantitative inventory which assesses the intensity of depression and can reflect changes of depression after an interval of time, but it is important to point out that this inventory does not set out to distinguish among standard diagnostic categories. The inventory can be used frequently at varying intervals; it takes a modest amount of time to complete and assess results. Furthermore it provides information that can usefully form part of the treatment plan or perhaps direct the course of treatment.

Grids

The personal repertory grid (described more fully in Chapters 5 and 10) is a further useful means of assessing the patient's present state, monitoring progress and in particular identifying objectives and determining where change is needed (Fransella and Bannister, 1977).

163

COMMUNICATION AND SPEECH PROBLEMS ASSOCIATED WITH DEPRESSION

As psychiatrists have noted that depressed patients have difficulty communicating within their social environment, it is therefore important for speech therapists to take into account the overall communication problems of the patient as well as those of speech and language. The patient's reluctance to talk of their distress, problems, hopes and fears, and their denial of difficulties is often seen to be the easiest and simplest 'way out'. To admit to problems is thought, by the patient, to be a sign of weakness and it may also promote unwanted change and produce further difficulties, thereby adding to the patient's feelings of hopelessness. Patients may talk about other symptoms as these are perceived to be respectable, such as physical symptoms of feeling tired or ill, but they are unlikely to discuss the major problem. Feelings of low self-esteem and the risk of being rebuffed prevent disclosure.

Depression of mood can be manifested by sadness, tearfulness, hopelessness and gloominess, together with feelings of despair, conflict and alienation thus creating social changes and difficulties. The depressed person is more likely to avoid social intercourse, is therefore less likely to seek help and through reduced non-verbal communication will signal 'keep your distance' and so limit social approaches and resulting interactions.

Non-verbal communication

The patient's non-verbal communication will emphasize how he or she feels. Changes in posture, gesture and facial expression may give the appearance of dejection by displaying slow and restricted body movements: a stooped or hunched posture with the head held low minimizes eye contact. Facial expression may be 'mask like' and immobile and therefore displaying little expression or with obvious expressions of sorrow. There might be accompanying tensions demonstrated by rigidity of posture and movement and set facial expression. In other patients agitation may be common, accompanied by restlessness and pacing up and down and nervous fidgeting movements of the hands.

Speech and language

The speech style of agitated patients is often demonstrated by their asking the same question repeatedly, which hints at poor concentration, and talking in short staccato-like phrases. The less active depressed person uses a slow speech tempo with frequent pauses and hesitations and so the overall effect is a 'dead', 'listless' voice with reduced volume, stress and rhythm. Pitch changes of the voice will be narrower due to less emotional expressions and resonance will sometimes be abnormally nasal or pharyngeal. Language tends to be limited to convey the minimum of information and the response is short or non-verbal and little speech is initiated. Those suffering from 'chronic states of gloom,' are said to show a different speech pattern from those with other depressions. Rather like the masked depression, articulation can be clear and normal and vocal pitch described as relatively lively, tempo normal and pauses infrequent. These people often look normal, smile and even seem happy but it is known that this is deceptive behaviour as demonstrated through their reduced use of language and avoidance of communication situations. Depressed or low mood restricts language and renders it colourless and limited. During the course of treatment it will be observed that there is a reduction in the negative content of the patient's speech. Language will become more descriptive and expressive, vocal volume will increase and become more normal, with increased flexibility of pitch, stress and rhythm and more obvious appropriate accompanying non-verbal gestures.

Breznitz and Sherman (1987) found that speech of depressed patients is often punctuated by long pauses due possibly to the interjection of depressed thoughts that interfere with the patient's speaking rather than being reflective of overall motor retardation. It has been hypothesized by Breznitz and Shermon that such slowing down would be apparent in the interaction of depressed women and their children in that the depressed women would respond more slowly than normal mothers to the cessation of speech of their children. They go on to state that children adapt to their unwelcoming mothers and the negative effects on the child's continued social, emotional and cognitive development may be profound. Research is needed to discover the effects on the speech behaviour of the young child as a result of living with a depressed mother.

Speech changes in depression have been described in a number of studies and one of the approaches to measuring psychomotor function in depression is to assess the voice functions of depressed people, as the intricate neuromuscular system of the larynx is likely to be affected by changes in neural motor function, due to depression. Acoustic properties of the voice can be analysed instrumentally to show voice changes associated with depression.

Nilsonne (1988) draws attention to areas of research of the effects of medication on speech, variable voice changes, and word finding difficulties, and further elucidation of the complex relationship between

165

speech and depression which would be of theoretical and clinical value. It is also thought that the acoustic study of voice may contribute to the differentiating of emotions and moods as well as various other psychopathological states.

MANAGEMENT AND TREATMENT

The patient's lifestyle is usually severely impaired; therefore as well as medical care a special programme of rehabilitation is required in most cases if full function, health and happiness are to be restored. The aims of the programme will be to change faulty habits, restore self-esteem, reduce social isolation by joining self-help groups, restore family relationships and achieve a return to work, by structuring the day thereby changing the negative to positive and achieving goals very gradually. Therapists need to show empathy, genuineness and warmth for results. The emphasis is on restoring self-esteem and avoiding isolation as this is disruptive (Kelly, 1987c).

The biological treatments of depression with antidepressant drugs can restore a normal sleep pattern, reduce tearfulness, lighten the patient's pathological mood and improve coping behaviour. Depressive illness is associated with biochemical changes in the brain and other parts of the body. These changes involve the brain amines (neurotransmitters), the electrolytes sodium and potassium, and certain hormones, particularly thyroid and adrenocorticosteroid hormones (Silverstone and Turner, 1988). Antidepressant drugs not only have therapeutic effects on depressive illness but also have mood-stimulating effects. The two main groups of drugs that have antidepressant properties are the tricyclic antidepressants and the monoamine oxidase inhibitors (MAOIs) although the effects of MAOIs are questioned. Of considerable interest are the recently introduced selective 5-hydroxytryptamine reuptake inhibitors, although their exact place in therapy is yet to be determined.

Tricyclic antidepressant drugs remain the cornerstone for treatment of depressive illness. Amitriptyline has marked side-effects as well as working as an antidepressant and so is helpful if the depressive illness is accompanied by anxiety or agitation, as it has a sedating quality and is thought to be one of the best drugs for most patients. These drugs are rapidly absorbed and have a long action and need to be given only once a day. Dosage will be adjusted to individual clinical response and to the side-effects of the drug. The side-effects may include a dry mouth and disturbance of visual accommodation and affect communicative ability if severe. Tiredness and drowsiness may affect concentration and motivation; memory impairment has also been noted in some cases. Speech blockage (difficulty in word retrieval) has been reported. Dysarthria has also been reported of a kind that is similar to a stutter but really of basal ganglion origin. Speech scanning has been noted in patients recovering from toxic doses (Maguire, 1986). Once a therapeutic effect has been achieved the drug is continued for at least six weeks; it is then reduced for a further six months, all being well.

MAOIs are drugs thought to have anxiolytic properties and possibly a weak antidepressant action too, and are likely to be prescribed for the less severe depressive disorders. The therapeutic effects in depression are therefore considered to be modest. The side-effects include a dry mouth and this again can be a handicap to speech (see Appendix 6.1).

Psychological therapies for depression might include supportive psychotherapy, as supportive treatment is an important part of the management of every depressed patient and is intended to sustain the patient until other treatments have their effect, or natural recovery occurs (Gelder et al., 1986). Interpersonal psychotherapy, which is a treatment approach to relationships and life problems, is also found to be helpful in certain cases. Other therapies might include behavioural, cognitive, personal construct and psychodynamic therapy, of which there will be more detail in Chapter 10.

Speech therapists are unlikely to be referred a clinical case with depression as the major problem; it is much more likely that depression is discovered as one of the presenting clinical problem associated with speech pathology that might have resulted from either cerebral trauma, organic illness (which might result in major surgery such as a laryngectomy), physical or mental handicap, degenerative illness or a long-standing speech disability such as a severe stutter.

In a formal psychiatric setting where communication problems rather than speech pathology are associated with depression, the speech therapist could be involved in either individual or group work as part of the treatment plan. Group work is generally favoured as the support offered by the group is possibly the most important aspect of the treatment in the early stages. Few demands need to be made of the patient except to attend and survive the session with the knowledge that he is safe, wanted and valued as a group member and when ready to participate in group activities he will be encouraged and rewarded. The group is a place where treatment can focus on current rather than past problems and the patient is helped to cope with everyday living. When adjusted to the group, past problems can be explored and feelings shared openly. The group is somewhere to cry, laugh and grieve, talk about anger, frustration, loving, hating, failure and success, past and present relationships and eventually hopes and plans for the future.

Recognition of depression during the course of treatment of speech pathology is important as conventional speech therapy methods can be developed to encompass both problems. Without doubt the depression is the most important of the two problems and, if unrecognized or ignored, little progress is likely to result in other areas. During the course of therapy it might be possible to help the patient to assess beliefs objectively and reject those thinking patterns that make him depressed, working towards changing negative patterns of thinking to positive ones.

REFERENCES

Beck, A. T. (1967) *Depression: Clinical, Experimental and Theoretical Aspects*, Harper and Row, New York.

Beck, A. T., Rush, A. J., Shaw, B. F. and Emery, G. (1979) *Cognitive Therapy of Depression*, Wiley, Chichester.

Breznitz, Z. and Sherman, T. (1987) Speech pattern of normal discourse of well and depressed mothers and their young children *Child Development*, **58**, 395–400.

Brown, G. and Harris, T. (1978) *The Social Origins of Depression*, Tavistock Publications, London.

Catlan, J. (1988) Affective disorders, in *Essential Psychiatry* (ed. N. Rose), Blackwell Scientific Publications, Oxford, pp. 62–72

Checkley, S. (1986) Affective disorder: depression, in *Essentials of Postgraduate Psychiatry*, 2nd edn (eds P. Hill, R. Murray and A. Thorley), Grune and Stratton, London, pp. 381–403.

DSM-III-R (1987) *Diagnostic and Statistical Manual of Mental Disorders* 3rd edn – revised, American Psychiatric Association, Washington, DC.

Dittman, A. T. (1987) Body movements as diagnostic cues in affective disorders, in *Depression and Expressive Behaviour* (ed. J. D. Maser), Lawrence Erlbaum Associates, London, pp. 18–36.

Ekman, P. and Fridlund, A. J. (1987) Assessment of facial behaviour in affective disorders, in *Depression and Expressive Behaviour* (ed. J. D. Maser). Lawrence Erlbaum Associates, London, pp. 37–56.

France, R. (1988) *Symposium on Depression for Speech Therapists*, Speech Therapy Special Interest Group in Psychiatry, Broadmoor Hospital.

Fransella, F. and Bannister, D. (1977) *A Manual for Repertory Grid Technique*, Academic Press, London.

Freud, S. (1917) *Mourning and Melancholia: Standard Edition*, Vol. 14, Hogarth Press, London, pp. 243–58.

Gelder, M., Gath, D. and Mayou, R. (1986) *Oxford Textbook of Psychiatry*, Oxford University Press, Oxford.

International Classification of Diseases (1975) *Manual of the International Statistical Classification of Diseases, Injuries and Causes of Death*, Vol.1, World Health Organization, Geneva, 1977.

Kaplan, H. I, and Sadock, B. J. (1985) *Modern Synopsis of Comprehensive Textbook of Psychiatry*, 4th edn, Williams and Wilkins, Baltimore.

Kelly. D. (1987a) Introduction in *A Practical Handbook for the Treatment of Depression* (eds D. Kelly and R. France), Parthenon Publishing Group, Lancs, pp. 15–16

Kelly, D. (1987b) Diagnosis of masked depression, in *A Practical Handbook for the Treatment of Depression* (eds D. Kelly and R. France), Parthenon Publishing Group, Lancs, pp. 25–7.

Kelly, D. (1987c) Overcoming depression, in *A Practical Handbook for the Treatment of Depression* (eds D. Kelly and R. France), Parthenon Publishing Group, Lancs, pp. 57–64.

Kendell, R. E. (1988) Affective (mood) disorders, in *Companion to Psychiatric Studies*, 4th edn (eds R. E. Kendell and A. K. Zealley), Churchill Livingstone, Edinburgh, pp. 335–61.

Kielholz, P. (1987) The classification of depression, in *A Practical Handbook for the Treatment of Depression* (eds D. Kelly and R. France), Parthenon Publishing Group, Lancs, pp. 41–3.

Klein, M. (1934) A contribution to the psychogenesis of manic-depressive states, reprinted in *Psychiatry*, 130–282. Contributions to psycho-analyses 1921–45, *Developments in Child and Adolescent*, Hogarth Press, London.

Kupfer, J., Maser, J. D., Blehar, M. C. and Miller, R. (1987) Behaviour assessments in depression, in *Depression and Expressive Behaviour* (ed. J. D. Maser), Lawrence Erlbaum Associates, London, pp. 1–15.

Maguire, T. (1986) *Pharmacological Effects in Speech and Language*, paper presented at Speech Therapy Special Interest Group Seminar, Broadmoor Hospital.

Nilsonne, A. (1988) Speech characteristics as indicators of depressive illness. *Acta Psychologica Scandinavica* **77**, 253–63.

Pennell, I. and Creed, F. (1987) Depressive illness, *Medicine International*, August 1987.

Scherer, K. R. (1987) Vocal assessments of affective disorders, in *Depression and Expressive Behaviour* (ed. J. D. Maser), Lawrence Erlbaum Associates, London, pp. 59–82.

Seligman, M. E. P. (1975) *Helplessness: On Depression, Development and Death*, Freeman, San Francisco.

Siegman, A. W. (1987) The pacing of speech in depression, in *Depression and Expressive Behaviour* (ed, J. D. Maser), Lawrence Erlbaum Associates, London, pp. 83–102.

Silverstone, T. and Turner, P. (1988) *Drug Treatment in Psychiatry*, 4th edn, Routledge, London.

Skinner, B. F. (1953) *Science and Human Behaviour*, Free Press, New York.

Storr. A. (1983) A psychotherapist looks at depression. *British Journal of Psychiatry* **143**, 431–5.

Thursfield, D. (1987) Childhood depression, in *A Practical Handbook for the Treatment of Depression* (eds D. Kelly and R. France), Parthenon Publishing Group, Lancs, pp. 122–6.

169

APPENDIX 6.1: DRUGS USED IN TREATING DEPRESSION

Group	Non-proprietary name	Proprietary names	Mode of action	Adverse effects
(a) Tricyclic Antidepressant i sedative	Amitriptyline Dothiepin Doxepin Trimipramine	Tryptizol Prothiaden Sinequan Surmontil	Block the receptake of noradrenoline and serotonin	Dry mouth, blurred vision. Convulsions in overdose
ii non-sedative	Imipramine Lofepramine Nortriptyline	Tofranil Gamanil Aventyl		
(b) Trazodone	Trazodone	Molipaxin	? Antiserotonin and receptor antagonist	Less anticholinergic side-effects than tricylics. Less convulsive and cardiotoxic
(c) MAOIs	Phenelzine Isocarboxid	Nardil Marplan	Prevent breakdown of monoamine neurotransmitters	Drowsiness, weakness, fatigue. Serious reactions with other drugs and some foods.

Group	Non-proprietary name	Proprietary names	Mode of action	Adverse effects
(d) 5-HT Reuptake inhibitors	Fluvoxamine Fluvoxetine	Faverin Prozac	Block receptake of 5-hydroxytryptamine	Virtually free of noradrenegic and cholinergic side-effects, may cause somnolence, agitation and convulsions
(e) Lithium salts	Lithium carbonate	Priadel Phasal	?Decreases noradrenergic release and enhances uptake	Tremor, diarrhoea and weakness. Skin and kidney effects REGULAR BLOOD TESTS NEEDED

7

Personality disorder

Jenny France

Personality disorder is considered a controversial problem in psychiatry. There are those who do not in fact consider personality disorder as a mental illness due to the fact that social maladjustment, or deviance, does not equate with disease or illness unless it is a consequence of only partial function of that person (Hibbert, 1988). Nevertheless, Hibbert goes on to state that psychiatrists often attempt to treat people with personality disorders even though there is no evidence of only partial function; this may be due to the demand for medical intervention by patients, relatives and society. Although many psychiatrists are uneasy about treating these disorders, it is possibly as a result of their offer to help these problems that personality disorders are treated as psychiatric illnesses. Tyrer (1988) states that not much is known about personality disorders, and much that is written about them is speculative and anecdotal. In the opinion of Tyrer the separation of personality disorder from other forms of mental illness in current classifications is important as it prevents clinicians thinking of the terms as mutually exclusive.

Gelder *et al.* (1986) report that in abnormal personality unusual behaviour occurs even in the absence of stressful events and at times these anomalies of behaviour may be so great that it is difficult to decide whether they are due to personality or neurotic illness. Extreme cases of abnormal behaviour are obvious as, for example, in cases of violence and repeated behaviour of harming others and showing no remorse. Abnormality of personality causes problems to both the patient and others due, in the severest cases, to the unacceptable, anti-social behaviour exhibited by the patient which may lead to dislike of that person and the possibility of rejection. These people may profoundly affect other people, often in subtle and unconscious ways, and may also affect a merging of personal boundaries. There have always been people who have suffered with personality disorder and those who work with these people need to consider the positive qualities as opposed to the negative ones when considering management and treatment. It needs to be stressed that a diagnosis of personality disorder in some cases will occur with affective disorders, organic states or schizophrenia and it is frequently found in association with neurotic disorders.

The antisocial or sociopathic personality disorder was until recently the most familiar and commonly studied section of personality disorder and therefore those patients with whom the psychiatrists and psychologists were likely to have most contact. Many of the less serious personality disorders might never seek help and therefore the cause of their conditions and alleviation of their problems are seldom faced either by psychiatrists or other authorities, unless problems escalate to such a degree where help is sought. Those with antisocial/sociopathic personality disorder are on occasions most likely to cause social disruption and in some cases come into contact with the law; they may even receive considerable publicity and at times their behaviour will result in tragic consequences. There is confusion of the terms psychopath or psychopathic personality and antisocial or sociopathic personality disorder, as often the term psychopath is used when describing all personality disorders rather than referring to the severest of the personality disorders. This confusion is possibly associated with the evolution of the terminology and redefining of the classification of personality disorder with particular emphasis on psychopathy. There is also confusion about whether psychopathy refers to all those with personality disorder or only those who are classified as suffering from antisocial/sociopathic personality disorder. The term sociopathic disorder is referred to in the Mental Health Act 1983, which also still uses the term psychopathic disorder.

The Mental Health Act 1983 defines psychopathic disorder of mind as 'a persistent disorder (whether or not including significant impairment of intelligence) which results in abnormality or seriously irresponsible conduct on the part of the person concerned'. This is a legal definition and not a diagnosis although the term 'psychopath' is still used widely today to represent the more severe personality disorders. It dates back to the earlier difficulties of finding an appropriate term for those people with marked abnormalities of behaviour in mental illness. Sir David Henderson (1939), who published *Psychopathic States*, defined psychopaths as 'people who, although not mentally abnormal, throughout their lives or from a comparatively early age, have exhibited disorders of conduct of an antisocial or social nature, usually of a recurrent or episodic type which in many instances have proved difficult to influence by methods of a social, penal and medical care or for whom

173

we have no adequate provision of a preventative or curative nature'. He defined three groups of psychopaths, as predominantly aggressive, predominantly passive or inadequate and the creative psychopath.

PERSONALITY

The type of personality disorder is likely to be described not in the diagnosis but in descriptive account of the patient's problems as based on the classifications from ICD–9 (1975) and DSM-III-R (1987), and so in order to understand personality disorders a description of normal personality will be attempted. Normal personality will include personal features that have been apparent since adolescence, have been stable despite mood changes, observable in different environments and recognizable to others known to the person. Personality is that which makes one person different from another and this will include characteristic patterns of behaviour and thinking that include intellectual functioning, attitudes, beliefs, moral values, emotional reactivity and motives acquired in the process of growing up (Freeman, 1988). Trethowan and Sims (1983) consider personality subjectively – in other words what the patient believes and describes about himself as an individual – and objectively, in terms of what an observer notices about his more consistent patterns of behaviour. Personality is a unique quality and is the characteristic behaviour that allows others to predict how a person will act in a particular circumstance. It is emphasized that personality, which includes prevailing attitudes and opinions, is manifested in social relationships and must be assessed by observing what people actually do in a social context. It was thought that behaviour which is determined by personality rather than illness is consistent over time and from situation to situation, but research has failed to show as much consistency as was believed (Freeman, 1988). It has been found that people behave in a certain way because of the situation they find themselves in, but many qualities do remain constant, for example physical appearance, gestures and way of speaking (Freeman, 1988).

Abnormal personality

Those with abnormal personality and/or personality disorder are said to display no apparent guilt, tend to be impulsive, manipulate others, are often aggressive and accused of being unloving. Nevertheless it is important to recognize that even those with abnormal personalities will have positive traits as well as negative ones and these positive traits (as has been said) need recording and taking into account when planning treatment. Therefore as part of collecting a full history a complete description of an individual's personality might include factors such as intellectual ability, attitudes, beliefs, moral values, emotional reactivity and motives acquired in the process of growing up – hence the importance of gaining a full medical and social history and the desirability of interviews with others who know or have known the patient previously.

Doren (1987) reports that psychiatrists in Canada filled in a questionnaire that ranked the most significant characteristics of personality disorder as being: does not learn from experience; lacks a sense of responsibility; unable to form meaningful relationships; lacks control over impulses; lacks a moral sense; chronologically or recurrently antisocial, punishment does not alter behaviour; emotionally immature; unable to experience guilt; and being self-centred. Other observations listed by workers include having superficial charm and good intelligence; poor judgement; unthruthfulness and insincerity; making suicide threats; failure to follow any plan; unable to show empathy or genuine concern for others; lack of feeling or affection; and lack of shame accompanied by aggressiveness.

The importance of the DSM-III-R classification (see Appendix 7.1) is that it excludes severe mental retardation, schizophrenic and manic episodes; it has also been important in research into personality disorder and it highlights further areas of research. WHO (1975) defines abnormal personality in ICD-9 as 'deeply ingrained maladaptive patterns of behaviour generally recognizable by the time of adolescence or earlier and continuing throughout most of adult life, although often becoming less obvious in middle or old age. The personality is abnormal either in the balance of its components, their quality and expression or in its total aspect. Because of this deviation or psychopathy the patient suffers or others have to suffer and there is an adverse effect upon the individual or society' (Appendix 7.2 lists the ICD–9 personality disorders). In ICD–10 (when published) many of the personality disorders will be equivalent to DSM-III-R and the term sociopathic will be replaced by dyssocial personality disorder.

Antisocial personality

It is apparent by now that by far the most detailed information results from the particular interest paid to the antisocial (psychopathic) personality disorder. More articles and books are written about this personality disorder than any other and the reason for this is the profound effect these people make on society, due possibly to their criminal propensities. McCord (1982) quotes results of studies which estimated that approximately 20% of incarcerated criminals could be labelled 'psychopathic' and English psychiatrists thought that their prisons contained 18% of 'psychopaths' (Hyland, 1942). In the 1980 survey McCord found that institutions for juvenile delinquents held approximately 30% of psychopaths and it has been suggested therefore that about 10% of all criminals are, on a cross-cultural basis, psychopathic (McCord, 1982). It is likely that most of these individuals treated, particularly in secure units or secure hospital settings, are psychopaths, or suffering from the severest forms of personality disorders and this may in some cases be associated with other forms of mental illness. McCord (1982) agrees that there has been an attempt to change the term 'psychopath' to 'sociopath', and then to antisocial personality; he argues that the 'psychopath' is not 'antisocial' but 'asocial' and to use the term antisocial is likely to 'lump' all criminals, drunkards and many other deviants together. The term antisocial personality disorder will be used in this chapter as it occurs in both DSM-III-R and ICD–9 classifications.

The DSM-III-R states that to record a diagnosis of antisocial personality disorder a person must have demonstrated an antisocial history before the age of 15 years. This may include truancy, expulsion or suspension from school, legal infractions and theft, vandalism, delinquency, antisocial history, interpersonal transgressions, persistent lying, repeated sexual intercourse in casual relationships, initiation of fights, under-achievement in school, drunkenness and substance abuse. After the age of 18 years and for five previous years there needs to be a demonstration of significant antisocial activity.

The DSM-III-R goes on to define adult forms of antisocial personality disorder as including any set of four of the following: inability to sustain consistent work behaviour, poor responsibility as a parent, illegal behaviour, poor ability to endure interpersonal relationships, irritability and aggressiveness, failure to honour obligations, impulsivity or failure to plan ahead, lying, 'conning' or the use of aliases, and recklessness. After the age of 30, the more flagrantly antisocial behaviours may diminish.

ICD–9 states that predominantly sociopathic or asocial manifestations are characterized by disregard for social obligations, lack of feeling for others and impetuous violence or callous unconcern. Behaviour is not readily modified by experience, including punishment. These people are often affectively cold and may be abnormally aggressive or irresponsible. Their tolerance level is low, and they blame others or offer plausible rationalizations for the behaviour which brings them into conflict with society.

McCord (1982) defines a 'psychopath' as an asocial, emotionally and psychologically insensitive person, who feels no guilt and is unable to

176

form emotionally affectionate relationships with people. McCord goes on to state that the core 'psychopath' exhibits all of these characteristics, but he or she is a rare type, resting at one end of a continuum which stretches from 'normal', displaying all of these traits, to an extreme degree and in such a manner that they constantly direct or inform his or her life.

Personality disorders in children and adolescents include disorders of childhood or adolescence such as conduct disorder, avoidant disorder of childhood or adolescence, identity disorder and personality disorders, antisocial personality disorder, avoidant personality disorder and borderline personality disorder. The diagnosis of conduct disorder, rather than antisocial personality disorder, should be made if the person is under 18 years of age.

Gelder *et al.* (1986) see the necessity to classify abnormal personalities for the purpose of collecting statistics. They are of the opinion that it is better to give a description of the main features of personality such as being sensitive, lacking in self-confidence, being abnormally aggressive, showing little evidence of feelings for other people or feeling remorse. It is also stated that clinicians should be careful not to be misled into thinking that they understand any more about the patient just because they have assigned a personality to one of the classification categories.

In view of these previous statements further description of the individual personality disorders will not be included here, but attention is drawn to the DSM-III-R and ICD–9 references, where full descriptions of similarities and differences will be found.

INCIDENCE OF PERSONALITY DISORDER

Generally speaking, study of the epidemiology of personality disorders has included statistics across the range of personality disorders rather than isolating each disorder accordingly. Problems of obtaining true statistics are due to the difficulties of diagnosis of personality disorders as well as their distribution; that is, for example, whether the population studied is from the mental hospitals or the community. Worldwide epidemiological studies of personality disorder may vary due to inconsistency of the statistics, as in some studies a wider diagnostic range of disorders has been used and some figures include admissions and readmissions to hospital, thus accounting for the large discrepancy of prevalence of personality disorder. The problem of studying personality disorder in populations is compounded by alcohol and substance abuse as these occur frequently in antisocials and it is difficult to separate these from those leading to antisocial personality (Cadoret, 1986). Cadoret goes on to give details of recent population studies in several major American cities, including some rural areas in one survey; these studies showed that there was a male predominance of the diagnosis of personality disorder with male to female ratios varying from 4:1 to 7 or 8:1. There is little reliable difference between races (that is, between blacks and non-blacks), with a lower prevalence of antisocials among college graduates, as many antisocials drop out of formal schooling early. The highest prevalence of personality disorders is said to be in central city populations, rather less in inner suburbs and less still in smaller towns, but the reasons for this distribution are not clear.

AETIOLOGY

It is widely thought that if personality disorders were better understood perhaps the concomitant behaviours could be brought under control, but since little is known about the factors accounting for normal variations in personality it is not surprising that difficulties are encountered when studying abnormal personality. Gelder *et al.* (1986) stresses that both constitutional and environmental influences affect personality development. Most theories of the causes of personality disorders have both strengths and weaknesses.

Genetic causes

Slater (1948) studied nine pairs of identical twins who had been raised in separate environments since birth; seven people had turned out to be 'psychopathic', and others to be neurotic. He found that only two pairs of twins possessed similar life histories and so concluded that a genetic basis for the disorder might exist but that environmental forms played the dominant role, but generally there is not conclusive evidence to suggest that there is a genetic contribution to personality disorders.

Biological/neurological influences

Close relationships have been observed between behaviours of those suffering from antisocial personality disorder and those suffering brain injuries (Gelder *et al.*, 1986). It has been quoted that 'almost all of the clinical features of the psychopath can be produced by physical disorders of the brain' (Elliott, 1978). There is a possibility that personality disorder might result from delay in the development of the brain, and electroencephalographic abnormalities consistent with maturational delays have been reported in people with antisocial personalities. A previous study by Hare (1970) confirmed that antisocial personalities have atypical wave patterns and EEG research shows that there is widespread slow wave activity. This led earlier workers to suggest that psychopathy was caused by cortical immaturity, and that these people supposedly have the brain of a child and therefore exhibit the behaviour of a child. Nevertheless 15% of the population apparently have similar brain waves to the antisocial personality and they are normal.

It is thought by some that 'psychopaths' suffer from a dysfunction in the underlying temporal and limbic mechanisms (Hare, 1970). The limbic system has inhibitory effects on behaviour, particularly that related to fear, hence lesions in the limbic mechanisms could well interfere with learning to inhibit a punished response and so a person suffering from a dysfunction in the limbic system would tend to respond with the same behaviour, even if it had previously been inhibited because of punishment (McCord, 1982).

Psychological theories

Psychological theories stress the importance of the first five years of life. According to Gelder *et al.* (1986) if during development the child passes successfully through the oral, anal and genital stages, normal personality development will proceed. Other theorists consider personality development as a life-long process and so changes occurring later in life might also have an influence on personality development. There have been many modifications and reappraisals of the psychoanalytic approaches to personality, and it has been stressed that the unconscious and the id (which is the primitive pre-formed psychic force in the unconscious – the source of the instinctive energy necessary for self-preservation and propagation) were less powerful than Freud had thought. They felt that personality was shaped more by the individual's life experiences than by instincts (Freeman, 1988). Rogers' (1951) 'self-theory' is based on the individual's view of himself – his self-concept – and this determines his view of the world and his behaviour. The self consists of all the cognitions and perceptions related to the 'I' or 'me' and the individual evaluates every experience in relation to this self-concept.

Social and environmental influences on personality development

There is no evidence to prove that disturbances in parent-child relationships, and in particular maternal deprivation, have any influence on personality disorders other than in the antisocial personality. The antisocial personality disorder is considered to begin during childhood as findings demonstrate that it is more frequent in childhood than adult life and becomes less so during adolescence. Only a minority of conduct disorders in childhood go on to become antisocial personality disorders in adult life but antisocial personality disorder in adult life is almost always preceded by antisocial behaviour in childhood. Conduct disorders which are the most prevalent of child psychiatric disorders are behaviours that excite social disapproval (Hill, 1986). One of the major problems is how to tell which conduct disorders in childhood will go on to become antisocial personality disorder in adult life (Rutter and Garmezy, 1983: Rutter and Giller, 1983).

During the course of working with personality-disordered patients it has been found that many of these patients might previously have attended a child guidance clinic, exhibited difficult behaviour, might have had a father with a criminal record or was alcoholic, or have been taken into care and/or repeatedly moved during childhood. Research into psychopathology has been limited predominantly to the study of aggressive criminal or delinquent 'psychopaths', due possibly to psychopathy in its more violent forms presenting a threat to human life. The non-criminal 'psychopath' is difficult to distinguish from the rest of society.

There is also some evidence to support the hypothesis that there is a relationship between psychopathy and hyperactivity in children (Freeman, 1988). It is also thought that these people have a low degree of cortical arousal rather than suffer from brain damage. Added to this, helplessness increases the condition as the person is both rewarded and punished for the same behaviour. There is poor attention to environmental cues as they see people as objects and objects to be overcome; they are thought to have a limited behaviour repertoire and a preoccupation with control and challenge.

ASSESSMENTS

Initial assessments rely upon careful interviewing of the patient and members of their families, as it is not possible to judge the personality of these patients in the same way as judging other forms of mental illness. Those with personality disorder seldom complain of any difficulties and so the diagnosis can rarely be made just by listening to the patient. Personality therefore can only be judged by reliable accounts of the person's behaviour. As usual, accurate historical information is essential, so all available records should be checked, and if the patient is unable to give a good account of his behaviour, assessment may rely on information obtained from other informants, such as relatives, partners or employers, and from social workers and public officers (Hibbert, 1988). It is commonly thought that reliable information of personal history and past behaviour can be obtained from other inform- ants and it is necessary to obtain a detailed account of the patient's behaviour in the past and under a wide range of circumstances. Hibbert states that observations of behaviour in a hospital setting may not be an accurate guide to a patient's normal behaviour.

The patient's self-given history cannot always be relied upon due to their propensity for lying or denying, but the diagnosis might well be aided by the therapist's feeling of frustration and helplessness brought about by the verbal battle and 'push' on the emotions during inter- actions (Doren, 1987). This is a typical experience with personality- disordered patients, and this emotional reaction is considered an invalu- able tool towards diagnosis – if 'battling' then there is a possibility that the person has an antisocial personality disorder.

It has been reported that many patients will fall into a passive, dependent or antisocial group and perhaps little more diagnosis is needed, but what is important is understanding the individual's prob- lems in order to understand the chaos in the patient's life (Thorley, 1986). During this process several consultations may be necessary. Strengths and weaknesses need to be ascertained and investigation and detailed observation of undesirable behaviour, over a period of several weeks, might be necessary. Problems that are not apparent, but perhaps reported by others, or suspected, should also be noted, and this infor- mation is an aid to treatment.

Medical and case histories

A full medical history is necessary together with investigation of poss- ible physical illnesses and organic brain disease (with access to CAT scan and EEG, if thought necessary), and an intellectual assessment. Psychosis, neurotic disorders and knowledge of alcohol and substance abuse also need investigation.

A social history is also important as knowledge of the family, the accommodation and living conditions, educational and occupational history may also be a useful guide to management. A legal history will immediately suggest the seriousness of the problem so the current forensic status, recent offences, prison and institutional experience and delinquent behaviour and trouble with the police need to be known.

Personality

Identification of circumstances that provoke undesirable behaviour may indicate practical ways of reducing the frequency of behaviour (Hibbert, 1988). Therefore a number of questions need to be asked, such as: is there evidence of empathy and ability to form a rapport; is the patient able to tell the truth and degrees of truth; does the patient lose his temper, fight or become violent; or is the patient excessively shy; and what are the general relationship problems?

Personality testing

A need for a battery of psychological tests arises, not because of the possible invalidity of any single test, but because a relationship between the tests reflects the person's multilevel system of functioning (Kaplan and Sadock, 1985). Personality and intellectual functioning assessments may well give a lead towards detecting abnormal traits in personality. Traits are considered to be universal to differing degrees in people as they influence behaviour in the same ways in different situations and at different times, so that trait measures can be used predictively. The trait approach is popular in psychology as a number of apparently valid objective personality tests have been derived from it (Freeman, 1988), such as the 16 Personality Factor (16PF) questionnaire. In the 16PF 12 factors were obtained from factor analysis of ratings of one person by another and four from self ratings. These were combined to form the 16PF, which is a hundred question yes/no test, and by plotting the scores a personality profile results (Cattell and Butcher, 1968). (Further information on the 16PF is found in Chapter 10).

The Eysenck personality system is made up of four dimensions: extraversion-introversion; neuroticism-stability; psychoticism-stability; and intelligence (Eysenck and Eysenck, 1963). These measures apply not just to normal and abnormal personality but to mental illness, criminals and those suffering from antisocial personality disorder (Freeman, 1988). From this personality system a succession of personality inventories have been produced to measure such traits: the Eysenck Personality Inventory (EPI) and, more recently, the Eysenck Personality Questionnaire (EPQ) (Eysenck and Eysenck, 1975), which also contains items for measuring psychoticism and has a lie scale.

The Minnesota Multiphasic Personality Inventory (MMPI) (Hathaway and McKinley, 1970) measures traits such as depression, hypochondriasis, hysteria, psychopathic deviation, masculinity, femininity, paranoia, psychasthenia, schizophrenia, hypomania and finally social introversion. The inventory has 550 statements about attitudes, emotional reactions, physical and psychological symptoms and past experiences to which the subject answers 'true', 'false', or 'cannot say'. Items on the scale differentiate between eight clinical groups, and other scales test for the reliability and consistency of the responses which are subject to deliberate false reporting. The final score is plotted on a profile and any score that is two standard deviations above the mean is considered potentially pathological. The test was designed to identify people with serious personality disorders but it is also widely used in studying normal populations (Hathaway and McKinley, 1970). Further mention of these assessments will be made in Chapter 10.

The Rorschach (1942) is a test in which a standard set of ten inkblots serve as a stimulus for associations. The series of inkblots is administered in order and they are reproduced on cards which are numbered one to ten. A verbatim record is kept of the patient's responses with reaction times and total time spent on each card. Each response reflects what there was about the blot that made it look the way the patient thought it looked, and the content areas (human, animal, anatomy, sex, food, nature and so on) reflect the breadth and range of interests (Kaplan and Sadock, 1985). This test is a particularly useful diagnostic tool as the thinking and associational patterns of the patient are highlighted or brought more clearly into focus, largely because the ambiguity of the stimulus provides relatively few areas for what may be conventional or standard responses.

Tyrer and Alexander (1979) developed a structured interview, the Personality Assessment Schedule (PAS) for rating of personality disorder, and this is conducted with a relative or close friend. These assessments are aimed to help highlight strengths as well as weaknesses as treatment is based on attempting to build favourite features as well as modify unfavourable ones (Gelder *et al.*, 1986).

Once a diagnosis is arrived at the usual battery of pre-treatment assessments might also be completed, which will be carried out by those who will be involved in the treatment and will vary according to the overall treatment plan. They might include behavioural and cognitive assessments, investigation into the suitability for dynamic psychotherapy – either in groups or for individual treatment – educational assessment and general assessment of overall communicative ability, with particular emphasis on language and its use.

COMMUNICATION PROBLEMS ASSOCIATED WITH PERSONALITY DISORDERS

History

There is no specific communication problem associated with personality disorders, but a general difficulty which is likely to be identified during the course of assessment and treatment. Details of the patient's history, acquired from his family, may include their observations such as a lack of maternal/infant bonding, or rearing a placid, quiet, unresponsive or rejecting baby; the child who develops temper tantrums and frustrations that later lead to the inability to discuss, negotiate or share feelings and information are found to be a regular part of the background to personality disorder. This all adds further useful information in discovering the origins of some of the problems and also helps towards deciding upon areas of treatment. Parents often tell of difficulty communicating with their child stemming from early childhood and the problems associated with this, particularly when other children in the family do not present in the same ways. Patients themselves report similar difficulties when talking about the past – 'I couldn't talk with my family'; 'I felt like an outsider'; 'I was a loner for as long as I could remember' – are the sort of comments regularly heard. During the course of talking about these details in treatment the patient discovers that the family isolation was often engineered by the patient himself. It is interesting to note how in many cases there is a 'close' relationship built between the patient and a member of the extended family (such as an aunt, grandmother or close family friend), which has produced friction within the family and has provided a certain 'power' for the patient. Reference to these people features regularly during the course of therapy.

Few personality-disordered people excel academically, although intellectually they are often capable of achieving successful educational standards. Educational interest and competence decline during adolescence when truanting (a regular addition to the history), delinquency, alcohol and substance abuse take the place of formal education. The result is poor literacy and numeracy skills, linked with equally poor language skills. Many patients have reported experiencing difficulty concentrating at school, their minds always being on other things, suggesting an active fantasy life. Maturing verbal skills are also handicapped as formal peer group and teacher-organized groups will be shunned. This seldom leads to social and educational accomplishments and so the communication problems increase. If perhaps there should be a period of enforced detention resulting from criminal behaviour, the patient will have lived in close contact with others whose histories are similar to his own. He will have been exposed to the tough, 'macho' communication style of prison life where the use of prison jargon, swearing and obscene language is normal and social refinements are scorned and ridiculed.

Patients may give the impression of being verbally capable, for example saying 'I've always been good with words. I had a better vocabulary than most, it was how I used those words that was wrong; all the words were negative and I used them to intimidate'. Another young man stated that he could not talk about his feelings as all he ever felt was anger; this was demonstrated by his inability to use or find words related to his anger. Yet another young man said that he 'hadn't got anything to say', and some time later was to remember that statement with incredulity. Some patients unable to express anger verbally may state their difficulties with silence, a mute refusal, and in some extreme moments of tension self-expulsion from the therapeutic situation. The patient usually returns for the next session and explains his dilemma, which might be a chain of negative thoughts or panic and eventual helplessness compounded by a paucity of adequate accompanying expressive language.

A limited vocabulary might be accompanied by non-verbal communication abnormalities with a seeking of greater body distance than is usual, a reluctance to be touched, with gestures which are minimal or when accompanied by anger are exaggerated or intimidating. Facial expressions tend to be more limited than normal, and in cases of antisocial personality disorder thunderous looks accompanied by tension and aggressive postures with harsh, loud and perhaps abusive speech are used to keep others at bay.

Cleckley (1976) speculates that antisocial personalities suffer from a deep-rooted semantic disorder in which the normal connections between semantic and affective components of language are missing or dysfunctional. There is also an assertion that the left hemisphere of 'psychopaths' (and schizophrenics) are damaged or dysfunctional and that there is something 'odd' about the way in which psychopaths use language. Their behaviour is often strikingly inconsistent with their verbalized thoughts, feelings and tensions, and there may be something pathological about the structure and dynamics of this person's language processes. Recent research suggests that there may be subtle deficits or anomalies in the interhemispheric organization of the 'psychopath's' language processes (Hare, 1986).

Particular problem areas

Speech problems may be more to do with lack of experience through restricted exposure to the usual variety of speech situations. In some cases these difficulties are accompanied by speech pathology, such as a severe stutter, voice disorders and continuing articulatory disorders inherited from childhood, all of which help to complicate the general impoverished language pattern. From case histories it is found that many patients have received formal speech therapy either before or during the early years at school, or during attendance at a special school or unit, and in some cases these patients may still demonstrate an inadequate use of both expressive and receptive language. It would appear that even with early treatment and support, full resolution of the speech and communication problems was not achieved, as during the course of development difficulties maintaining and developing adequate adolescent and adult use of language continued. The patient's preoccupation with his own position and problems might well reduce his listening skills which may, as a result, become overselective and handicapping. Poor concentration and language development and maturation are unlikely to improve, unless these problems are addressed early in treatment.

In some cases working in groups with these patients can be difficult as there are those patients who attempt and succeed, through inappropriate laughing, grunting, and voicing unpleasant and derogatory comments, in making others feel uncomfortable. This behaviour can prove both destructive towards other group members and exhausting for the therapists. In individual sessions silence might also be used to control, confront and demonstrate hostility or to bring about some response such as anger in the therapist. In these cases the session will be concluded with a statement of recognition of the silence and an invitation to meet as usual for the next session.

MANAGEMENT AND TREATMENT

There is a difference of opinion about the usefulness of treating personality-disordered patients – many say that this work is unrewarding but it is known that a substantial number of patients improve with time and the intervention of treatment.

Management

It has been suggested that the management of personality disorder should concentrate on helping individuals find a role and a situation in which they can live with less dissonance and conflict, rather than attempting to change long-standing and deeply ingrained personality patterns – concentrating on situations and situation-specific behaviours rather than attempting to alter the traits themselves (Freeman, 1988). In many cases it is thought that medical help is often denied these patients due to the ingrained nature of their personality features and their apparent non-compliance to medical treatment and direction.

On the whole the management these patients are offered will depend on where and when they are seen. These patients are found in certain settings and are unlikely to be found in others; for instance, they rarely refer themselves for treatment and so are unlikely to be treated in the community, and if referred by others will resist help as in some cases they perceive that the problems are not theirs. A patient can spend a great deal of time attempting to change the environment rather than himself and is reluctant to discuss his problems with a stranger and yet equally resists prolonging a relationship in order to develop a satisfactory environment for discussion. A substantial number of these people will be seen in a locked or controlled environment, either prison or special (forensic) hospitals, regional secure units or other specialized units. Once in such an environment the patient's options for affecting his environment are substantially decreased.

Resistance to treatment

Boredom is a major problem and, added to the initial reluctance to accept a treatment regime, the resistance to conform might well be channelled into seeking stimulation he enjoys and so creating frustration and difficulties for others. Eventually, once it is found that the system cannot be 'beaten' and that the patient can be partly responsible for himself, the carers are given opportunity to offer and provide help. This realization will vary in time from patient to patient and in some cases resistance to treatment will be maintained indefinitely, whereupon treatment will eventually be terminated. Even so, offers to help the patient will be tested by the patient, and so the therapist also needs to test by setting tasks and assignments to complete between treatment sessions. The excuse for not completing these tasks are legion but without doubt their completion is a rewarding sign of positive motivation and acceptance of treatment.

It is known, to this author, that these patients when seen in speech therapy out-patient clinics pose extra problems; they see their rights to receive treatment yet are often poor attenders, some manipulate numerous appointments within the local services, not always presenting with the same speech symptoms, and they allow little chance for the therapists to establish a diagnosis, let alone collect all the relevant medical and psychiatric notes. In the case of one young man it was not until he was admitted to a special hospital that the size of the problem and the energy he expended seeking his idea of the ideal treatment came to light. Five different speech therapy appointments for assessment in five different centres were manipulated, whilst intermittently attending a psychiatric out-patient clinic and occasional short-stay in-patient treatment. The result presented confusion for the professional carers as well as the patient and could well have continued, but for admission, at which point care was organized by a clinical team. There was no opportunity to manipulate treatment or the therapists, and no choice of therapy, and so with compliance the therapeutic results were eventually rewarding, including satisfactory remediation of the speech pathology.

Treatment

Few therapists will agree that they enjoy working with personality-disordered patients. This is probably due to the results of treatment being less observable than with other patients and the additional frustration of observing the patient persistently performing self-destructive and self-defeating behaviour (Doren, 1987). The patient–therapist relationship is also less rewarding as responsiveness is negative, but this can also be a guide to progress when emotional responsiveness improves and becomes more normal. Lion (1981) states that treatment and rehabilitation of personality disorder, when carried out with realistic optimism, empathy and enthusiasm, leads to slow but significant change and improvement. Drugs have little part to play in personality disorder; the aim is to build up a trusting relationship so that the patient can talk openly. Treatment is not aimed at altering personality but altering the behaviour or unacceptable symptoms resulting from the personality and associated with the abnormality. The treatment is not hopeless – just difficult. Many therapists persist in this work as they find it so interesting and this interest leads to reward and satisfaction.

Treatment might involve various types of psychotherapy as angry and antisocial people often value a contract that allows access to staff or a place where they can discharge their anger safely or verbally ventilate their feelings (Thorley, 1986). Individual and group psychotherapy might be appropriate; cognitive and behavioural approaches are particularly helpful in cases where patients experience social anxiety and fear and for those with low self-esteem. The passive dependent personalities are often helped by assertiveness training and almost all patients may benefit from some degree of social skills training (Argyle *et al.*, 1974). It is thought that in some cases patients will benefit from a total therapeutic environment such as in a special unit or hospital where treatment can be organized towards gradual changes and where the aims should be modest. It should also be recognized that there are some patients, as already mentioned, who due to their resistance will not benefit from treatment, however sensitive and skilful the therapist, and therefore sessions should not continue. The prerequisites to treatment are that the patient 'needs' to be there proving that he is motivated and that he sees the advantage of developing this particular interpersonal relationship. The therapist should be able to exploit the patient's positive qualities, to help put them to use, and must not fear the treatment and so should be able to confront the patient in order not to be manipulated.

The multidisciplinary team possibly offers the greatest scope for treatment and has the advantage of supporting individual team members constantly throughout their endeavours. This support is vital for the continuation of therapeutic energy and inspiration, as well as monitoring 'across the board' progress and may possibly be the only way, in some cases, to receive rewards in this work. The therapeutic team has a great deal to offer. No one person will make a decision and this helps to reinforce and support any therapeutic decision made on behalf of the patient. This also endorses an eclectic approach to treatment and so gives the patient every opportunity to make progress. A highly coordinated team effort is needed for treatment.

The younger the patients the more likely they are to respond to treatment. This is thought to be due to the more recent onset of symptoms than, for instance, in the cases of hardened antisocial criminal adults where a 'cure' is unlikely but treatment towards a more adaptive functioning for daily living might be achieved. There is a need to stress that most of the treatment programmes assume, at the least, a modest linguistic skill as without this ability the more sophisticated psychodynamic treatments present problems for the patient. The behavioural treatments, and in particular cognitive therapy and speech therapy, may help to address these linguistic difficulties as they may introduce and develop a vocabulary that can be extended for daily use as well as in various group therapy settings. An area of great difficulty for many patients concerns feelings where the paucity of vocabulary limits the patient's ability to participate fully in treatment. A variety of treatments can be organized to take place side by side if necessary.

Psychotherapy

Verbal skills in group psychodynamic therapy need to be adequate to allow for personal development and progress for both the patient and the group, and linguistic imbalance in a group is not only a handicap to the patient but to the group as a whole. Although many people progress and develop language skills in this kind of group it is a slow process and supplementary treatment to assist the development of language competence is desirable in some cases. Individual psychotherapy offers the chance to continue development of language use and incorporate the more conventional psychodynamic approach. The personality-disordered patient demonstrates a pronounced reluctance to commit thoughts to paper, but if prepared to do so a diary is a means of setting and maintaining a regular task demonstrating an investment in treatment. Both patient and therapist share the contents and this helps to develop an important level of trust. It is another way of monitoring the developing use of language, gives permission for therapeutic direction and ultimately is a clear way of demonstrating to the patient a number of fundamental points of importance and interest. The diary may become spontaneously more elaborate and emphasis develop from self to others. Attitudes change with mellowing of opinions; expansion, flexibility and creativity of language is ongoing; and feelings rather than actions prevail. There might be an occasional bonus of sharing a dream, joke, sad or happy event and occasionally there might be a written reward or compliment for the therapist's persistence.

Supportive psychotherapy

Supportive psychotherapy might be the gentle way towards initiation into more formal psychotherapy and offers the chance to experiment with talking in a group and getting the 'feel' of group dynamics, learning that a group *can* be supportive, like a family, and that it can also produce a few pressures aiding personal growth.

Personal construct psychotherapy

Personal construct psychotherapy (which is covered in more detail in Chapter 10) offers the choice of where to begin in therapy as a result of viewing where the patient is on his personal construct grid. It is a way of monitoring change and development, reducing suspicion and developing trust and is often seen by the personality-disordered patient as being a safe method of treatment. It is a particularly useful means of working on language development and the development is demonstrated on subsequent grids.

Cognitive therapy

Cognitive therapy focuses on cognitive processes as mediators of behaviour and emotion and suggests that disordered behaviour and emotion are largely consequences of various cognitive deficiencies. It relies chiefly on speech as the vehicle for identifying and remediating these deficiencies (Barley, 1986). During their recent cognitive work with personality-disordered patients, Beck and Podesky (1989) focus on the person's main beliefs and strategies such as the avoidant personality's belief that it is terrible to be rejected, that people don't really know them and that they cannot tolerate unpleasant feelings, for example. Or the antisocial personality patient who believes he is entitled to break the rules, sees that other people are weak and are capable of being exploited and so his main strategy is to attack, rob, deceive and manipulate.

Behaviour therapy

Behaviour therapy may be introduced in a group setting and might include social and communication skills, assertiveness training, anger control and work on interpersonal skills (which will also include a cognitive approach.

Formal educational programmes and specialized programmes such as sex education, family therapy, groups for alcohol and substance abuse problems, community skills programmes and domestic and social rehabilitation might be some of the appropriate therapies offered. Not all of the patients will need all of these treatments; some might well be involved in a number of complementary groups or individual sessions. The speech therapist's skills can be used in many of these treatment areas as well as to help augment programmes by providing formal treatment for any speech pathology, either as a separate treatment or within a structured group. This will be discussed again in more detail in Chapter 10.

REFERENCES

Argyle, M., Trower, P. and Bryant, B. (1974) Explorations in the treatment of personality disorder and neurosis by social skills training. *British Journal of Medical Psychology*, **47**, 63–72.
Barley, W. D. (1986) Behavioural and cognitive treatment of criminal and delinquent behaviour, in *Unmasking the Psychopath* (eds W. H. Reid, D. Dorr, J. I. Walker and J. Bonner), Norton, New York, pp.159–90.
Beck, A. and Podesky, C. (1989) *Cognitive Therapy of Personality Disorders*, World Congress of Cognitive Therapy, Oxford, June 1989.
Cadoret, R. (1986) Epidemiology of antisocial personality, in *Unmasking the*

Psychopath, (eds W. H. Reid, D. Dorr, J. I. Walker and J. Bonner), Norton, New York, pp. 28–44.

Cattell, R. B. and Butcher, H. J. (1968) *The Prediction of Achievement and Creativity*, Bobbs-Merrill, London.

Cleckley, H. (1976) *The Mask of Sanity*, 5th edn, Mosby, St Louis.

DSM-III-R (1987) *Diagnostic and Statistical Manual of Mental Disorders*, 3rd edn – revised, American Psychiatric Association, Washington, DC.

Doren, D. M. (1987) *Understanding and Treating the Psychopath*, Wiley, Chichester.

Elliott, F. A. (1978) Neurological aspects of antisocial behaviour, in *The Psychopath* (ed. W. H. Reid), Brunner/Mazel, New York, p. 146.

Eysenck, H. J. and Eysenck, S. B. G. (1963) *Eysenck Personality Inventory* NFER Nelson, Windsor.

Eysenck, H. J. and Eysenck, S. B. G. (1975) *Manual of the Eysenck Personality Questionnaire (Junior & Adult)*, Hodder and Stoughton, Sevenoaks.

Freeman, C. P. (1988) Personality disorder, in *Companion to Psychiatric Studies*, 4th edn (eds R. E. Kendall and A. K. Zealley), Churchill Livingstone, Edinburgh, pp. 407–32.

Gelder, M., Gath, D. and Mayou, R. (1986) *Oxford Textbook of Psychiatry*, Oxford University Press, Oxford.

Hare, R. D. (1970) *Psychopathy: Theory and Research*, Wiley, Chichester.

Hare, R. D. (1986) Twenty years of experience with the Cleckley psychopath, in *Unmasking the Psychopath* (eds W. H. Reid, D. Dorr, J. I. Walker and J. Bonner), Norton, New York, pp. 3–27.

Hathaway, S. and McKinley, J. (1970) *The Minnesota Multiphasic Personality Inventory*, University of Minnesota NFER Nelson, Windsor.

Henderson, D. (1939) *Psychopathic States*, Norton, New York.

Hibbert, G. A. (1988) The personality disorders, in *Essential Psychiatry* (ed. N. Rose), Blackwell Scientific Publication, Oxford, pp. 86–91.

Hill, P. (1986) Child psychiatry, in *Essentials of Postgraduate Psychiatry*, 2nd edn (eds P. Hill, R. Murray and A. Thorley), Grune and Stratton, London, pp. 195–259.

Hyland, H. H. (1942) Psychoneuroses in the Canadian Army Overseas. *Canadian Association Journal*, **47**, pp. 432–40.

(WHO) International Classification of Diseases (1975) *Manual of the International Statistical Classification of Diseases, Injuries and Causes of Death*, Vol. 1, World Health Organization, Geneva 1977.

Kaplan, H. I. and Sadock, B. J. (1985) *The Modern Synopsis of Comprehensive Textbook of Psychiatry*, 4th edn, Williams and Wilkins, Baltimore.

Lion, J. R. (1981) A comparison between DSM-III and DSM-II personality disorders, in *Personality Disorders: Diagnosis and Management*, 2nd edn (ed. J. R. Tonin), Williams and Wilkins, Baltimore.

McCord, M. W. (1982) *The Psychopath and Milieu Therapy: A Longitudinal Study*, Academic Press, New York.

Rogers, C. (1951) *Client Centred Therapy*, Houghton Mifflin, Boston.

Rorschach, H. (1942) *Rorschach Inkblot Test Psychodiagnostics*, Hans Huber, Berne.

Rutter, M. and Garmezy, A. (1983) Developmental psychopathology, in *Socialisation, Personality and Social Development*, Vol. 4, 4th edn (ed. E. M. Heatherington), Wiley, New York, pp. 775–911.

Rutter, M. and Giller, H. (1983) *Juvenile Delinquency: Trends and Perspectives*, Penguin, Harmondsworth, Middlesex.

Slater, E. (1948) Psychopathic personality as a genetical concept. *Journal of Mental Science*, **94**, p. 277.

Thorley, A. (1986) Neurosis and psychopathic disorder, in *Essentials of Postgraduate Psychiatry* (eds P. Hill, R. Murray and A. Thorley), Grune and Stratton, London, pp. 195–260.

Trethowan, W. and Sims, A. C. P. (1983) *Psychiatry*, 5th edn, Baillière Tindall, London.

Tyrer, P. (1988) *Personality Disorders: Diagnosis, Management and Course*, Butterworth, London.

Tyrer, P. and Alexander, J. (1979) Classification of Personality Disorder, *British Journal of Psychiatry*, **135**, pp. 163–7.

APPENDIX 7.1: DSM-III-R CLASSIFICATION OF PERSONALITY DISORDERS (1987)

Cluster A   Paranoid
                  Schizoid
                  Schizotypical

Cluster B   Antisocial
                  Borderline
                  Histrionic
                  Narcissistic

Cluster C   Avoidant
                  Dependent
                  Obsessive–compulsive
                  Passive–aggressive
                  Personality disorder
                  Not otherwise specified

APPENDIX 7.2: ICD–9 CLASSIFICATION OF PERSONALITY DISORDER (1975)

Paranoid
Affective
Schizoid
Explosive
Anankastic
Hysterical
Asthenic
Personality disorder with predominantly sociopathic or antisocial manifestation
Other personality disorders
Unspecified

8

The psychiatry of old age

Helen L. Griffiths

Recent years have seen the emergence of a new branch of psychiatry, that is, the discipline of psychiatry of old age. The considerable expansion of psychiatric services for elderly people in the UK has been documented by Wattis (1988), who identified that in the early 1970s there were about a dozen psychiatrists working with elderly people. By the end of 1986 an estimated 250 psychiatrists were working in this area. Associated with the development of such posts has been the improvement of non-medical staffing levels including speech therapy. In 1981, approximately 12% of district psychiatry services for elderly people had access to speech therapy staff (Wattis, Wattis and Airie, 1981), whereas the current level is around 30% with approximately 7% of districts having specialist speech therapy staff (College of Speech Therapists, 1990). Whilst nationally the provision of speech therapy to such services is low, with considerable regional variation, the specialism is in a period of growth.

The author suggests it is essential that the scope of speech therapy intervention in psychiatry of old age is examined as an independent speciality and not subsumed under the rubric of speech therapy in general psychiatry. This chapter will therefore review the mental health problems of elderly people and the development of services to meet the needs of this group before focusing on the contribution which speech therapy can make.

A striking demographic feature of the western world is the changing age structure of the population. In the UK approximately 15% (8 million) are now aged over 65 compared with roughly 5% (2 million) at the beginning of the century. Projections indicate that between the years 2001 and 2021 there will be a further 17% increase in those aged over 65 (Wicks and Henwood, 1988). However, the elderly population is growing not only in numerical terms but also as a proportion of the population as a whole. Furthermore, there will be dramatic changes in the composition of this group. The proportion of very elderly people, that is, those aged 85 and over, is predicted to double from current levels, whilst other age cohorts will see a less marked increase (see Figure 8.1). Approximately 3% of those over 65 years will be individuals who were born outside the UK, mainly in continental Europe, Asia and the West Indies (DHSS, 1981).

Identification of the composition and health and social status of the elderly population is vital because of the implications for policy development. There is general correlation between advancing years and increasing disability, including mental illness. Dementia, for example, occurs in about 5% of people over 65, rising to 20% in those over 80. (Brayne and Ames, 1988). Depressive states of various kinds, however, are more common than cognitive decline, with a significant depression affecting 10–20% of the elderly population (The Nation's Health, 1988).

MENTAL HEALTH PROBLEMS IN OLD AGE

The traditional organization of diagnostic categories has been established with regard to aetiology. A broad division is made between the organic disorders of dementia and delirium and the so-called functional disorders of depression, mania, neuroses and paranoid states. A variety of terms have been used for describing much the same thing and such alternative terminologies reflect the inadequacies of simple classification to cope with the complexities and variabilities of mental illness in old

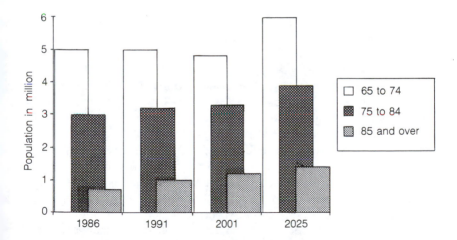

Figure 8.1 UK elderly population growth, 1986–2025. (Based on figures in *Social Trends*, **18**, 1988).

age. Pitt (1982) warns that mental health problems in elderly people rarely present in pure form as often physical and mental health problems co-exist, some arising as a consequence of the other and some quite separate.

Organic disorders

Dementia

Dementia is a descriptive term referring to a constellation of clinical features and is not a disease in its own right. Dementia has been defined by the Royal College of Physicians (1981) as 'the global impairment of higher cortical functions including memory, the capacity to solve the problems of day to day living, the performance of learned perceptuo-motor skills, the correct use of social skills, and control of emotional reactions in the absence of gross clouding of consciousness. The condition is often irreversible and progressive.' Whilst common symptoms can be identified there is great variety in presentation as many disorders may produce the syndrome of dementia.

Alzheimer's disease. By far the commonest of the degenerative dementias is Alzheimer's disease, causing between 50% and 60% of cases (Fraser, 1987). The term Alzheimer's disease has previously been applied only to those who develop this form of dementia before the age of 65. People over 65 with a similar condition have been considered to have senile dementia of the Alzheimer type. This distinction is made less frequently now as present indications favour a unitary disorder. However, the possibility of subgroups within Alzheimer's disease exists. The onset is insidious with a gradual progressive course. The clinical features include memory disturbance, alterations in intellectual processing and personality change. There is progressive involvement of the parietal lobes giving rise to agnosias, language disturbance, apraxias and spatial dysfunction. Social competence tends to be preserved until the disease is advanced. Although Alzheimer's disease causes diffuse cerebral atrophy, focal symptomatology can be found. Indeed, the pattern and temporal course of the cognitive decline is often not uniform (Neary *et al.*, 1986). Characteristic histological changes are described. There is striking cell loss, accompanied by senile plaque and neurofibrillary tangle formation. In addition to these changes, deficiences of cholinergic transmission have been reported (Davies, 1977). The cause of the changes associated with Alzheimer's disease is as yet unknown.

196

Vascular dementia. Vascular dementia, also referred to as multi-infarct or arteriosclerotic dementia, is the second most common type, causing between 15% and 20% of all cases (Fraser, 1987). The course is different from that of Alzheimer's disease in that there may be a more sudden onset, a fluctuating course and less prominent cognitive changes. There is often episodic exacerbation which may be followed by plateau. Dysfunction is typically variable and explicable in terms of the focal deficits. Thus, a variety of clinical pictures may arise in vascular dementia. Personality and insight are often retained until later in the disease and consequently there may be marked affective changes in response to the awareness of the deteriorating cognitive function. It is distinguished clinically from non-vascular dementia by applying the criteria of the Hachinski Ischaemic Index (Hachinski *et al.*, 1975), which refers to features in the history and presentation. The many titles for this type of dementia are indicative of aetiological confusion. The presence of large and small vessel disease has been described by Caplan (1979). Hachinski, Lassen and Marshall (1974) suggest that the evolution of the dementia depends upon the accumulation of deficits from multiple infarcts.

Frontal lobe type dementia. In dementia of the frontal lobe type there is progressive and selective damage to the frontal regions of the brain. The clinical picture is one of change in personality and social behaviour, with disinhibition and lack of concern. The pattern of cognitive change includes variable impairment of memory with relative sparing of parietal lobe functions (Neary *et al.*, 1988). Pick's disease is one such form, in which there is cell loss and the presence of 'balloon cells', that is, distended nerve cell bodies. Onset is typically in the presenium and appears to follow a Mendelian dominant pattern of inheritance.

Alcohol and dementia. Alcohol-related problems are common in older people (Wattis, 1983) and include cognitive deterioration. Lishman's (1987) review of the literature suggests that alcoholic dementia occurs as frequently as vascular dementia. In this syndrome global impairment is described, including memory and personality change. A frontoparietal focus to the dementia has been suggested (Dreyfus, 1974). Wernicke-Korsakoff syndrome, the cerebral response to thiamine deficiency, is more appropriately termed a severe amnesic syndrome rather than a dementia.

Trauma and dementia. Two causes of dementia following trauma are described. The first, due to subdural haematoma, may typically follow

197

a fall, particularly in the elderly. If untreated it may become chronic and affect the mental state. The second described is that of the 'punch drunk' state, typically found in professional boxers. The salient clinical features are ataxia, dysarthria and mental and physical slowing accompanied by memory loss.

Subcortical dementia. The subdivision of the dementia syndrome into two types, cortical and subcortical, is a recent and controversial topic. Although the syndrome of subcortical dementia is a clinical description it is associated with pathological change in the subcortical nuclear structures. The dementias associated with Huntington's chorea, Parkinson's disease and progressive supra-nuclear palsy can be traced to subcortical lesions. Clinically, subcortical dementia manifests itself by emotional and personality changes, slowness in the rate of information processing, reduced ability to manipulate acquired knowledge and memory disorder. There are associated motor system abnormalities. In Parkinson's disease, a dementia syndrome is estimated to occur in 15–20% of individuals (Fraser, 1987). However, neither the precise nature of the intellectual impairment, nor whether Parkinson's disease is responsible for a form of dementia distinct from other types or occurs with an existing Alzheimer's disease, is agreed. Dementia is rarely an early symptom in Parkinson's disease.

Huntington's chorea is associated with a single autosomal dominant gene with onset most commonly between the ages of 35 and 40, although it may present later. Choreiform movements together with dementia are characteristic. Personality changes have been described and the presence of depression is a common psychiatric manifestation.

Reversible dementia. There is a lack of agreement about which conditions underlie a reversible dementia. However, cerebral tumour, normal pressure hydrocephalus, toxins, infections, metabolic and endocrine disturbances have been cited as causes. Indeed, the use of the term dementia to describe the cognitive changes arising from these disorders has been questioned. This in part reflects the lack of agreement on the essential criteria for diagnosis. As the name suggests, such dementias are treatable, and therefore potentially reversible.

Delirium

Delirium or acute confusional state is generally of abrupt onset and arises as a result of an underlying systemic disease which interferes with cerebral activity. Causes include infections, hypoxia, endocrine and metabolic disorders and the toxic effects of drugs. Confusion, comprising memory impairment and disorientation, is present, with clouding of consciousness, limited concentration and impairment of perception. It is important that delirium is distinguished from dementia, as delirium once diagnosed is treatable.

Dementia and an acute confusional state may co-occur, as may different types of dementia. For example, approximately 20% of individuals with dementia show both vascular changes and signs of Alzheimer's disease.

Functional disorders

Depressive illness

The main features of depressive states are described in detail in Chapter 6 of this book. Depressive illnesses experienced by elderly people are much the same as in younger people but studies have suggested that depression in the elderly may be overlooked or misdiagnosed as dementia (Pitt, 1988). The detection and treatment of a depressive illness is essential as the prognosis for depression in old age is good, with the majority responding to treatment (Baldwin and Jolley, 1986).

Pseudo-dementia is the term used to refer to the cognitive impairment which may be seen in association with a number of psychiatric disorders. In elderly people it has been estimated that pseudo-dementia occurs in as many as 10% of those admitted to hospital with depressive illness. There is considerable dispute as to the nature of the disorder and many conceptual difficulties arise with this diagnosis. Mahendra (1984) suggests that the situation is rather more complex than the notion of 'pseudo-dementia induced and sustained by depression and dependent upon its course for its own symptomatology' and urges changes in the nomenclature. However, the presence of a group of individuals with a cognitive disorder which does not arise from any discernible organic cause and is potentially reversible is of great clinical importance. It is important to note that depression may herald and co-exist with dementia, with some 25% of individuals with vascular dementia also suffering from depression (Roth, 1983).

Other functional disorders include neurosis, anxiety states and paranoid conditions. The reader is referred to the relevant chapters in this book for further discussion of these disorders.

DEVELOPMENT OF SERVICES

It is essential that those planning services take account of the social circumstances as well as the health status of elderly people and the increasing demands being placed upon both community services and families providing continuous care to elderly relatives. The 1981 census indicated that 95% of the over–65s lived in private households whilst the other 5% lived in institutions or residential care. The overall number of residents in homes has gradually grown, with an increase of approximately 20% in the number of elderly people in local authority homes or supported by the Department of Social Security in private or voluntary organization homes. The age of admission to such homes has been rising steadily and the average age is now approximately 82 years (DHSS, 1981). Increasingly, residents are suffering from mental and physical disabilities. Two-thirds of residents in local authority accommodation are found to be suffering from dementia (Murphy, 1986). However, the majority of elderly people with mental illness live in private households, with less than one in seven people with moderate to severe dementia in receipt of institutional care. There is therefore a growing need for support for those living in the community, where the responsibility for care frequently falls to female relatives (Age Concern, 1980).

That services have arisen in response to the changing need and expectations of the population is clear. In 1975 a DHSS Command urged the identification of rational and systematic priorities in provisions for the elderly and mentally ill. The development of specialist psychiatric services for elderly people was encouraged. Hence the progression from the asylum model of care that was then being provided on a multi-district basis in mental illness hospitals to the current social policy of care in the community. It is proposed that by 1991 each health district should have a coordinated programme for community care. Strategies which facilitate and prolong independent living in the community, particularly at home, are stressed. Consequently there has been local level development, evidence of which is the rise in the number of specialist units at district level and in the provision of day-care and community-based accommodation for those no longer able to manage at home. It is stated that support should be available, not only for the individual but also for the family and other informal carers. The need for an expansion of personal social services, closer links between social and health care teams and significant improvements in staffing to enable patients to be assessed and reviewed on a multi-professional basis to provide for earlier intervention and preventative work is evident.

It is within this context that speech therapy is beginning to provide a service. As yet little detail about the activity of speech therapists with specific client groups in psychiatry of old age has emerged. However, it is anticipated that the majority of a clinician's case-load will be concerned with people suffering from chronic organic psycho-syndromes (Griffiths and Baldwin, 1989). Thus this chapter is concerned as much with the possibilities of intervention with this group as the range of expertise developed to date.

The 'medical model' remains the dominant philosophy for many speech therapists, but is largely inappropriate to the needs of the elderly mentally ill person, as it is characterized by a disease-oriented approach to care, aimed at bringing about changes in particular physiological systems or anatomical parts by restitution of function. Under this regime, strategies are selected by which the impairment may be most effectively 'cured'. A more appropriate model for this group would be one which values attempts at decreasing the levels of disability and therefore handicap arising from an impairment, taking into account not only the medical but also the social and psychological implications of mental illness in old age. Thus the need to develop an alternative conceptual framework or model to provide 'guidelines within which to explore the appropriateness of particular approaches to care' (Aggleton and Chalmers, 1986) becomes evident. It should embrace the World Health Organization's objectives (WHO, 1988) which holds maintenance and enhancement of quality of life in relation to promoting independence as central values.

The speech therapy model developed for this client group should harmonize with and form part of the philosophy of the unit in which the therapist works. It is quite likely that nursing staff in such a unit will have selected one or more models for care and, in spite of the fact that they have been devised as ways in which nursing intervention may be explained and structured, it nevertheless would seem that some of the basic tenets of these models could apply to speech therapy. Roper, Logan and Tierney (1980) have identified 12 'activities of living', including communication, which are related to fundamental human needs. They argue that individuals differ in the way in which they involve themselves in these activities of living and a central concern within the model is the degree to which the individual can carry out activities independently. Where there is some inability to do so, the need for intervention arises, by which means the individual can be helped to achieve a state of total or relative independence, supported by the nurse, other therapists and the individual's family, friends and other carers. Within Orem's model (1980) six ways have been identified in which the individual can be assisted in achieving 'self care': that is, doing or acting for, guiding or directing, providing physical support, providing psychological support, providing an environment which supports development and teaching another. These principles encompass those which the speech therapist will adopt in working in this area.

It is proposed that a holistic approach which regards communicative competence 'not as something inherent in the patient but as existing between the patient and each of the communicative partners within his or her environment' (French, 1986) is relevant. Thus intervention should focus not only on the individual but also the linguistic environment. The model also needs to value research-based practice and should strive for clinical and professional advancement through this medium. Therefore, there needs to be a commitment to a continuing process of evaluative research.

It can be argued with much justification that speech therapy in old-age psychiatry is at a point where there are a number of competing schools of thought, none of which had universal acceptance. The conflict between competing schools and the inability of the existing paradigm to explain phenomena suggest that a new and unique set of theory is required.

ASSESSMENT

The interview is central to the psychiatric assessment of the individual, as the way in which the person communicates provides information on the integrity of language functioning, the affective state, the coherence of thought processes, motor activity, memory and attention (Roberts, 1984). The contribution of the speech therapists to the assessment process is considered here.

It is only recently that communication processes in elderly persons with psychiatric disorders have been subject to systematic investigation. As currently there is a lack of adequate descriptions, there is a need for prospective studies to provide clearer delineation of patterns of communication breakdown. This being the case the primary aim of assessment is to provide a detailed description of communicative behaviour. This aim differs from that traditionally pursued in the field of acquired communication disorders where the identification of deficits for diagnosis and treatment is paramount.

The descriptive assessment aims to facilitate an understanding of the person's communication needs and encourages the identification of intact skills which may be of value in devising compensatory strategies. Assessment data should be stated in such a way as to be clearly relevant to activities of daily living and to take account of the person's cognitive level. This functional approach is only tenable for the particular environment in which communication takes place. Therefore, communication should be assessed in those contexts and in those acts that are relevant to each individual and because of their interactive role would include various communicative partners, as their skills must be part of the definition of communication handicap. These principles give direction to assessment methods, which involve the therapist in observation of and participation in activities of living. Although during such activities the success of communication is influenced by other variables, these are an integral part of the assessment and the speech therapist can seek to identify factors influencing performance. The views of both informal and formal careers must be sought, including an analysis of those situations and activities in which the carer experiences difficulties in communicating with the patient.

The speech therapist is able to establish whether there is any evidence of an acquired language disorder, which would indicate the presence of organic damage. In doing so, it becomes possible to exclude those changes in mental state which can cause alteration in patterns of communication but are not associated with known organic pathology, such as normal ageing and depressive illnesses, and to identify potentially reversible disorders such as pseudo-dementia. Consequently there is a need for the clinician to be familiar with the communication changes in these areas, for the knowledge base to be expanded and for age-appropriate normative data to be developed. In testing a population of normal elderly people, Walker (1982) demonstrated quantitive changes on the Minnesota Test for Differential Diagnosis of Aphasia with increasing age. Maxim (1982) supported claims for a change in linguistic ability in normal ageing when she demonstrated that elderly people find complex sentences containing an adverbial subordinate clause harder to understand and produce than younger people. The performance of a depressed elderly population was found to be similar to that of the normal elderly on a number of language measures (Maxim *et al.*, 1989). Where there is evidence for an acquired language disorder it is essential to distinguish between symptoms which superficially appear homogeneous but in fact may represent pathologically and clinically distinct groups. Neary *et al.* (1986) suggest that clinical distinctions between patients with different syndromes of dementia are possible and between subgroups within one diagnostic category. It follows that distinctions need to be made between the patterns of language breakdown in a classic aphasic syndrome (in the context of a focal lesion) and that occurring in dementing illnesses or that arising from a localized cerebral atrophy (Mesulam, 1982; Goulding *et al.*, 1989). That these distinctions can be made rests on the assertion that the language breakdown is different in each. Some authors have described the patterns of language breakdown in dementia as being similar to those found in classic aphasic syndromes and describe the language disorder in such terms (Obler and Albert, 1981; Cummings *et al.*, 1985). However, other authors (Bayles and Kaszniak, 1987) have said that 'Alzheimer's and other dementia patients have linguistic communication deficits that are fundamentally different from the classic aphasia syndromes'. Hence the use of the term aphasia to describe the language breakdown in dementia has been questioned. The underlying assumption for many speech therapists is that aphasia is due to focal damage, usually of acute onset, and is disproportionate to the impairment in other cognitive functions. The use of the term aphasia therefore reinforces the idea of the presence of a specific language disorder rather than a feature of general intellectual deterioration. Alternatively, the use of the term does not necessarily infer similarity of underlying primary deficits, only of clinical manifestation. A description of the language disturbance associated with dementia is required to enable comparison with and differentiation from the classic aphasia syndromes. Although the speech therapist's assessment findings are of value in the identification of psychiatric syndromes it is important to remember that factors such as onset, mood, the presence of other cognitive deficits and behaviour will be as relevant in the process of differential diagnosis as is the communication assessment. Thus, it must not stand alone but form part of a multidisciplinary assessment.

The effects of dementia on communication

Language disorder has been commonly reported in dementia (Appel, Kertesz and Fisman, 1982; Cummings *et al.*, 1985; Hier, Hagenlocker and Shindler, 1985), and may occur as the presenting and dominant feature as in the cases described by Wechsler (1977), Kirshner *et al.* (1984) and Pogacar and Williams (1984). As those with dementia do not form a homogeneous group, it is essential to describe the patterns of breakdown associated with particular forms of dementia. Much of the available data refer to individuals with Alzheimer's disease.

It is suggested that language disturbance is present at all stages in Alzheimer's disease, and studies show change across a range of language functions with gradual deterioration as the disease progresses. Therefore it has been proposed that language tests may be useful as an index of the severity of dementia (Skelton Robinson and Jones, 1984). Particular components of the language system are susceptible to Alzheimer's disease. In the early stages few problems are experienced with syntactical and phonological processing but there is impairment in semantic and pragmatic knowledge (Irigaray, 1973; Bayles, 1982). Bayles and Kaszniak (1987) propose that fundamental to the change in communication in Alzheimer's disease is the deterioration of the contents and processes of semantic memory, that is, conceptual and propositional knowledge. Evidence cited for this includes the deterioration in performance on tests of the ability to generate, relate and order ideas, for example, linguistic reasoning, generative and visual confrontation naming, vocabulary tests, pantomime and reading comprehension.

The speech of early Alzheimer's disease is often described as fluent, circuitous, empty and vague with incomplete utterances. Word-finding difficulties and semantic paraphasias become apparent in conversation. Naming ability has been extensively investigated. There is agreement that the ability to name is impaired and that this deteriorates as the disease progresses. However, the nature of the impairment on visual confrontation naming tasks is unclear. Errors are frequently semantically related to the target, suggesting a linguistic impairment (Martin and Fedio, 1983; Huff, Corkin and Growdon, 1986). However, the extent to which non-linguistic factors influence performance is controversial. Rochford (1971), for example, regards visual perceptual impairment to be the basis of the misnaming.

As the disease progresses speech becomes increasingly repetitive and egocentric with less adherence to conversational rules. In the later stages there is increased phonological disturbance and emergence of neologisms. Speech becomes largely unintelligible, with jargon, echolalia and palilalia. Mutism may follow. Disorders of reading and writing in Alzheimer's disease have been documented. The consistent finding is of relative preservation of oral reading in the presence of a disorder of comprehension of written material (Cummings et al., 1986). Further research suggests impairment of written spelling, indicating that the phonological route remains relatively intact whereas the lexical route is impaired (Code and Lodge, 1987; Rapcsak et al., 1989).

The communication changes associated with vascular dementia have been less extensively examined than those in Alzheimer's disease and findings appear to be variable. However, there is agreement that the patterns of language associated with the two conditions do differ (Powell et al., 1988, Kontiola et al 1990).

Powell et al. (1988) report that in a vascular dementia there are likely to be fewer characteristics of fluent aphasia. Output is described as less grammatically complex, perseverative and, when compared with Alzheimer's disease, less anomic and therefore more information is conveyed in the same number of words. Kontiola *et al.* (1990), however, conclude that basic language functions, including word recognition, repetition and naming, are impaired in vascular dementia. They therefore do not support the findings of Powell *et al.*

Again in comparison to Alzheimer's disease the speech associated with frontal lobe syndromes tends to be less fluent and telegraphic (Holland *et al.*, 1985). Spontaneous conversation is reduced, brief and unelaborated with occasional word-finding difficulty and few verbal paraphasias. The patient described by Holland *et al.* (1985) appeared to retain access to the semantic store. There is a reduction in vocabulary as measured by verbal fluency. Language becomes increasingly concrete and is characterized by verbal stereotypes and perseveration, both of ideas and linguistic units. In the later stages echolalia, hypophonia and mutism are described (Neary *et al.*, 1988).

There is little detailed documentation of the progressive language disorder secondary to localized cerebral atrophy. It does appear possible though to distinguish between this and a classical aphasic syndrome (Northen *et al.*, 1990).

As it is likely that critical distinctions will be more apparent early on in the disease process, differential diagnosis requires the early referral of individuals. The value of speech therapy assessment can therefore be enhanced by involvement with those with mild cognitive change, such as persons attending memory clinics (Stevens, 1988). It appears clear that early diagnosis is vital if rational therapies are to be implemented. On the other hand, there are considerable difficulties as 'early dementia is difficult to diagnose with any certainty' (Pitt, 1982). The work of Bergmann (1979), who undertook studies with a group of subjects with suspected early dementia, illustrates this. On follow-up (which occurred on average three years later) results showed that only 32% had developed dementia, 37% turned out to be psychiatrically normal subjects and the remainder continued to be only mildly impaired and of uncertain diagnostic status. In the study, the largest number of subjects developing dementia came from previously normal and functionally ill groups. It has been proposed that language tests can identify individuals with dementia and moreover that they can do so at an early stage in the disease (Bayles and Boone, 1982). This is based on the interpretation of research evidence indicating that language impairment is found in all stages of dementia. This finding does not have universal support as Neary *et al.* (1986) described individuals with histologically proven Alzheimer's disease in whom linguistic disturbance was not evident. These conclusions may in part depend upon the definition of language used, and which tools are selected for assessment.

It is unlikely that the aphasia batteries currently available will provide a suitable framework for the comprehensive and valid description of the communication disorders seen in old age psychiatry. However, the selective use of sub-tests from such assessments provide a point from which data collection can start. The language assessments used will require sensitive and qualititative scoring systems which can differentiate between groups being examined as important differences may be missed in a purely quantitative analysis. A neutral framework unhindered by prescriptive terminology is required.

The changing nature of the disease needs to be reflected in a dynamic and continuing assessment process, which highlights the use of assessments in providing a baseline against which change can be measured. In this way the course of the disease may be monitored, the introduction of therapies evaluated and the monitoring of the beneficial and possible side-effects of medication achieved.

As it has been suggested that communication breakdown is a universal feature of dementia, it might be assumed that all persons with dementia referred to the psychiatric service are seen by the speech therapist. This may be both impractical and unnecessary. A person is seen when a need has been identified either by the patient, their carer or a member of the health care team. The ability of other members of the multidisciplinary team to make appropriate referrals is based partially on the speech therapist's involvement in their activities. By participating in ward rounds, case conferences and other discussions, the speech therapist is able to raise awareness within the team of language and communication (Griffiths and Baldwin, 1989).

MANAGEMENT

Planning

Planning involves three steps: clarification of problems identified during assessment, determination of appropriate goals and the prescription of intervention to achieve these goals. If an integrated and effective management programme is to be devised, the speech therapist must plan intervention in the light of the information generated by the assessments carried out by other disciplines. In this way, it becomes possible to capitalize on the patient's strengths, using these to compensate for areas of difficulty.

Although the approach which is emphasized is that of compensation and attempting to adjust to and cope with the changes occurring, it may be inappropriate to assume that all persons with dementia are unable to benefit from linguistic therapy (Walker, 1988). For example, those who experienced language breakdown as an early symptom in the presence of relatively intact cognitive skills may be able to rehearse skills with the possibility of postponing deterioration or avoiding the functional loss of skills. However, as Golper and Rau (1983) state: 'any therapeutic approach that requires the learning of new behaviour or purports to stimulate or re-establish previously learned abilities will, in large measure, be undermined by diffuse disease. Treatment therefore is better directed towards therapies that require little cognitive flexibility or learning'. Plans must aim to maximize the individual's ability to function effectively by reducing the need for lost functions, compensating, where possible, for these and utilizing remaining skills. Goals need to be related to enhancing the communication skills necessary for daily life. This notion is neatly crystallized by Dobson (1989), who states that 'speech therapy needs to become an overall daily living philosophy rather than an individual skill area.'

It is clearly very important to determine goals which are both achievable and measurable, since they will form the basis of subsequent evaluation. In setting the goal, it is also important to set an evaluation or review date, to specify who will be involved in achieving the goal and the conditions under which the goal will be met. Problems and goals need to be stated in terms which can be understood by all involved in the delivery of the plan of care. It may be helpful to avoid diagnostic labels in favour of more behaviourally oriented statements, as such clarity will be of assistance in preventing behaviour being wrongly labelled and therefore misunderstood.

There is increasing recognition of the demands being placed upon the carers in looking after elderly relatives. Most of the literature has shown that caring is stressful and may lead to psychological distress. The needs of carers thus assume a high profile when management plans are being devised. A number of studies have attempted to find out which aspects of caring family members find most difficult and to assess any ill effects on the care givers. Indications are that the behavioural manifestations of dementia upset relatives as much as incapacity to perform self-care skills or the level of cognitive function. Greene et al. (1982) indicated that personal distress in carers is mainly a response to their relative's passive, withdrawn behaviour. Factors in this included not being able to take part in family conversations, not being able to read newspapers and magazines, or start and maintain a sensible conversation, not responding sensibly when spoken to and not understanding what is said. Gilleard (1984) concludes that many carers are as distressed by the loss of meaningful interaction which distorts the relationship as they are by difficult behaviour. That communication problems are commonly encountered is illustrated by Rabins *et al.* (1982), in whose study 68% of carers reported that communication difficulties occurred and 74% reported these to be a problem. However, when examining problems faced by care givers there is a tendency by professionals to focus on overt behaviours, such as aggression, incontinence and wandering. There is a need therefore to establish what is the relative's perception of the difficulties. Furthermore, studies have shown that the majority of care givers felt that they were uninformed as to the nature and implications of the disorder and so could not predict their relative's behaviour. Chenoweth and Spencer (1976) have stated that 'until families received thorough explanations of the progression of the disease they tend to believe that their relatives had more control over their behaviours than was likely, and expected that reasoning and past means of communication would still work'.

It is often assumed that the person with dementia does not 'suffer' from the distress of the illness, thus the need for emotional support may go unrecognized. Much of the assessment process tends to focus on the cognitive abilities of the individual, which may be to the detriment of the 'experiencing feeling self' (Froggatt, 1988). Lee (1981) observed that people with early dementia are often embarrassed about their memory loss and fearful of being rejected. Newroth and Newroth (1980) identified the experience of intermittent fear and anxiety and underline the need for support for the sufferer throughout these periods. Although aware of some difficulty the person may not be able to understand the nature of the problem and be unable to express feelings clearly. The speech therapist's knowledge of language changes can be used to interpret what is being said and to develop sensitivity to the reality of the emotional experience. Feelings can be identified and, in listening, validity and value can be given to the person.

Perhaps one of the most important long-term goals would be to help and support both carers and patient, avoiding increases in stress, enabling care in a manner acceptable to both.

Implementation

The speech therapist's clients may be seen in a number of settings but the emphasis should be on a domiciliary-based service, where intervention can involve both the patient and carers. The provision of support to care givers is a critical step in community care and there is a need to examine the most effective ways in which support can be provided. Zarit *et al.* (1980) found that relatives with least perceived burden were those who received most visits by other family members. Gilhooly (1984) emphasized that some estimate of quality of support is needed in addition to measures of frequency. There is a need for the service to develop a supportive network which will incorporate regular visits and ease of access to staff and information. It is envisaged that this would embrace the provision of psychological and practical support. It is important that the speech therapist coordinates with other team members in this and does not work in isolation.

There is a need to provide information which helps relatives understand the communication difficulties being experienced but more importantly which can be used to predict problems in day-to-day activities. Such information needs to be provided over several visits, both in oral and written form. Valuable sources include the booklet *Coping With Caring* (Lodge, 1981) and the Alzheimer's Disease Society booklet *Caring for the Person with Dementia* (ADS, 1984), which include sections on communication. However, it is anticipated that the speech therapist will provide additional information geared towards the particular needs of the patient. Discussing specific linguistic strategies to manage communication difficulties helps the carer develop their own adaptive skills. Bayles and Kaszniak (1987) suggest that the most effective way of teaching these would include demonstration, role play and the use of video for feedback. As the carer may well be unsure of the best approach to take, the therapist must help them to determine what is most appropriate. For example, when faced with repetitive questioning it is essential to identify the reason why the person does so. Is it related to a failure to retrieve or register the information or due to anxiety and insecurity or a perseveration of ideas? In addition, highlighting those skills through which someone may still be occupied is of value. Encouraging the person to engage in conversation is likely to be perceived as positive.

Providing psychological support enables the carer to share the emotional burden of caring and to discharge some of their frustration, worry and anger. Thus demands will be made on the therapist's skills as counsellor, requiring empathy and a non-judgemental approach. Such support may be achieved through a combination of individual and group approaches. Groups facilitate social contacts, the sharing of experiences and are valuable in helping members realize that they are not alone in coping. Therefore time must be allocated for family contact, possibly in the absence of the patient in order to allow for free discussion. Family therapy, as discussed in Chapter 10, is an approach which is being increasingly explored as a means of intervention. However, as Gravell (1988) points out, speech therapists are not trained in family therapy techniques and should refer patients to qualified counsellors.

In spite of the community orientation of the service, a proportion of the speech therapist's work will be carried out in an institutional setting. The role will include examining ways in which the environment may influence communication. In modifying the physical environment, Peterson *et al.* (1977) demonstrated that altering the seating arrangement could influence the level of social interaction. Conversation levels doubled when chairs were arranged in small groups compared with the traditional organization of chairs around the perimeter of the room. Of interest to the speech therapist are environmental communication cues, examples of which are written signs denoting toilets and orienting information. The possibility of visual misperception and comprehension disorder arise, therefore simplicity and clarity are important. Information needs to be explicit so signs should be used which do not require the reader to make inferences.

Lubinski *et al.* (1981) refer to a 'communication impaired environment' within institutions, in which little opportunity exists for successful, meaningful communication. The speech therapist can influence the level and quality of interaction by helping to clarify the role of care staff with regard to communication. By encouraging a wider definition of a task, its nature can change radically, as the objective of the staff becomes different. For example, regular daily activities such as mealtimes, in which there is no need to communicate, can be exploited. The speech therapist can act as a role model by demonstrating the way in which the task of serving meals may be manipulated to encourage the exercise of normal social roles and decision making. Training for all staff working with the elderly has been recommended and local government training boards are making resources available for social service staff training. Helping staff to develop an understanding of, and sensitivity to, communication enables them to adopt a problem-solving approach in the manipulation of linguistic and environmental variables.

Within institutions group programmes have particular therapeutic value. Group-based activities provide a context for rehearsal and reinforcement of communication skills and opportunities to assess which linguistic strategies are most effective in facilitating understanding or expression. The therapist can model skills to others involved, hence groups should be run on a multidisciplinary basis. Activities should be selected on the basis of known preferences and skills of the group members and where possible exploit real situations rather than representations of reality. Particular therapeutic approaches have found favour when working with this group.

Reality orientation

Reality orientation is an approach which has become associated with the management of people with dementia (Holden and Woods, 1982). It comprises two elements: firstly informal or 24-hour reality orientation, in which carers are involved in presenting current information in every interaction with the person, prompting appropriate behaviour and correcting confused speech and actions. As an adjunct to this, formal or classroom reality orientation provides group-based activity. The approach stresses two components: the interpersonal-interactive aspect, in which a humanitarian approach to care is emphasized; and the prosthetic-environmental element, in which the environment is reorganized to provide orienting aids and to facilitate interaction. The original aims of reality orientation were to improve cognitive and behavioural functioning. Whilst there is some evidence to suggest change on measures of orientation, there is little for changes in other dimensions of behaviour (Burton, 1982). It may be that broader goals than those usually considered can be adopted. For example, reality orientation could be used as a method of facilitating communication, as clients are actively encouraged to engage in successful verbal interaction (Bailey *et al.*, 1986).

Reminiscence therapy

Reminiscence therapy would also appear to facilitate increased interaction and spontaneous conversation, not only with staff but also with fellow patients (Norris and Eileh, 1982). A particular strength of this approach is that it capitalizes on relatively intact knowledge and unlike some activities reminiscence is age appropriate. The growth of reminiscence as a therapeutic approach has been facilitated by the production of 'Recall' packs (Help the Aged, 1984) and other commercially available material. Whilst these may provide a starting point, there is value in obtaining material and discussing subjects which are particularly meaningful to the individual. Personal memories, local archive material and the individual's own possessions can be used. The process of reminiscence may be a way of enhancing self-esteem, self-worth and reinforcing personal identity. Such functions were identified by Norris (1986) and, perhaps through the process of reminiscence, emotional health could be maintained around the cognitive impairment. However, sensitivity is needed in undertaking reminiscence therapy as for some the process of remembering can be painful.

Validation therapy and resolution therapy

Validation therapy, first described by Feil in 1982, requires the therapist to assume that all behaviour has meaning. It aims to support and understand the feelings of disoriented persons by focusing on the underlying meaning of what is said (Jones, 1985). For example, in response to the person looking for a deceased relative, rather than reasserting the facts, the therapist identifies with the sense of loss and loneliness being expressed, then finds ways of helping the person cope with the feelings. Goudie and Stokes (1989) criticize validation therapy for its attempts to interpret behaviour in psychodynamic terms and that it attributes skills to the person which they may no longer possess, for example, analytical skills. They suggest that resolution therapy in which the emotional experience is acknowledged has potential as a form of counselling with this group. Certainly it provides guidelines for a method of communicating with elderly confused persons.

Other activities which require less linguistic ability, for example, music, can be used to encourage interaction with more severely impaired persons.

Evaluation

It is important that the speech therapy service is subject to ongoing evaluation. Two levels of evaluation can be identified. The first focuses on single cases and involves comparing the goals set for the patient and carers at the planning stage with the actual outcome. The second level is concerned with the service as a whole and it may be necessary to first set quality standards to guide service planning and subsequent evaluation. The model which the speech therapist adopts will influence the methods of evaluation used at both levels. Here evaluation will be considered in terms of structure, process and outcome.

Structure evaluation involves examination of the suitability of the facilities for care, including staffing levels and the adequacy of training and education. In order to determine the level of staffing required to serve the population, it is necessary to gather further information as to the epidemiology of communication problems in this group, possibly via a survey of those working in this area. This could form part of a progressive research strategy which would serve to refine assessment and therapeutic techniques. There is a need for longitudinal studies to examine the patterns of communication breakdown and implications for management over time. Undertaking research of this nature would place speech therapy in old-age psychiatry on a firmer theoretical base which could be utilized both in the preparation of speech therapists for work in this area and in the education of others. The foundation for professional growth is in the assessment and evaluation of one's own discipline and indeed the DHSS (1975) has identified the elderly mentally ill as a research priority. The speech therapist therefore needs to secure research and study time. It is likely that speech therapists will be working in relative isolation from their speech therapy colleagues and will need the support of specific interest groups, through which examples of good practice and research can be shared.

Process evaluation is concerned with the quality and nature of the speech therapist's intervention. There is a danger of applying established techniques and emerging with a spurious respectability based on little or no evidence. Therefore it becomes important to take a wide view of process evaluation – one which considers not only the therapist's impression but also the views of the carers, other health professionals and the patient. This is not to denigrate the importance of self-evaluation but to underline the fact that process evaluation should be thought of as an array of approaches rather than as single discrete activities. At the lowest level of evaluation the therapist may provide basic numerical data such as the number of patient contacts, case-load and discharges. Of course, this reveals little about the quality of care delivery and other evaluative methods should be used, for example, interviews and questionnaires in which the carers' perceptions of the delivery of care is sought.

Outcome evaluation deals with the effect of care given. It is at this point that the therapist seeks to determine the extent to which intervention has been successful in achieving the stated goals, whether these be the goals determined for the individual or the service as a whole. The need to determine and make explicit realistic and specific goals has been emphasized above and if this has happened then the process of outcome evaluation is facilitated. In deciding the extent to which intervention has been successful a number of sources of data can be used. It is necessary to seek the opinions of all involved in the patient's care and one useful approach is to ask relatives to record relevant information. The need for management via a multidisciplinary approach has been stressed and part of the outcome evaluation will involve the development of strategies by which the effectiveness of other team members in accessing and using the communication skills developed by the speech therapist can be examined. Evaluation can be facilitated by multidisciplinary record keeping in which all members contribute to a single case record. Such a record helps to integrate care planning and goal setting and act as a focus for team evaluation.

In outcome approaches to evaluation there are two difficulties. The first of these is in determining the extent to which the interventions influenced the movement towards the goal. This is particularly problematic in a multidisciplinary context where more than one individual may be working on aspects of the same problem. The second difficulty is in relating the process to the outcome, in other words deciding whether or not the intervention actually produced the effect seen. These issues are not unique to speech therapy but confront any health professional who wishes to undertake evaluation of their work. As well as indicating the way in which the plan of care might be altered, evaluation inevitably highlights the need for further research. It is through this research that the solution to these problems will be found.

Whatever combination of means the speech therapist uses to evaluate intervention it is quite clear that evaluation can never be considered as an end-point in therapy but as one part of an ongoing and encyclical process.

REFERENCES

Age Concern (1980) *Beyond Three Score and Ten: A Second Report on a Survey of the Elderly.* Age Concern, Mitcham, Surrey.

Aggleton, P. and Chalmers, H. (1986) *Nursing models and the Nursing Process.* Macmillan Educational, London.

Alzheimer's Disease Society (1984) *Caring for the person with Dementia*, Alzheimer's Disease Society, London.

Appel, J., Kertesz, A. and Fisman, M. (1982) A study of language functioning in Alzheimer patients. *Brain and Language*, **17**, 73–91.

Bailey, E. A., Brown, S., Goble, R. E. and Holden, U. P. (1986) 24 hour reality orientation: changes for staff and patients *Journal of Advanced Nursing*, **11**, 145–51.

Baldwin, R. C. and Jolley, D. J. (1986) The prognosis of depression in old age. *British Journal of Psychiatry*, **149**, 574–83.

Bayles, K. A. (1982) Language function in senile dementia. *Brain and Language*, **16**, 265–80.

Bayles, K. A. and Boone, D. R. (1982) The potential of language tasks of identifying senile dementia. *Journal of Speech and Hearing Disorders*, **47**, 204–10.

Bayles, K. A. and Kaszniak, A. W. (1987) *Communication and Cognition in Normal Aging and Dementia*, Taylor & Francis, London, p. 182.

Bergmann, K. (1979) The problem of early diagnosis, in *Alzheimer's disease: Early Recognition of Potentially Reversible Deficits* (eds A. J. M. Glen and L. J. Whalley), Churchill Livingstone. Edinburgh.

Brayne, C. and Ames, D. (1988) The epidemiology of mental disorders in old age, in *Mental Health Problems in Old Age* (eds B. Gearing, M. Johnson and T. Heller),Wiley, Chichester.

Burton, M. (1982) Reality orientation for the elderly: a critique. *Journal of Advanced Nursing*, **7**, 427–33.

Caplan, L. (1979) Chronic vascular dementia. *Primary Care.* **6**, 843–8.

Chenoweth, B. and Spencer, B. (1986) Dementia: the experience of family care givers. *The Gerontologist*, **26** (3), 267–72.

Code, C. and Lodge, B. (1987) Language in dementia of recent referral. *Age and Ageing*, **16**, 366–72.

College of Speech Therapists (1990) *Dementia Working Party Survey*, unpublished, College of Speech Therapists, London.

Cummings, J., Benson, F., Hill, M., and Read, S. (1985) Aphasia in dementia of the Alzheimer type. *Neurology*, **35**, 394.

Cummings, J. L., Houlihan, J. P. and Hill, M. A., (1986) The pattern of reading deterioration in dementia of the Alzheimer type: observations and implications. *Brain and Language*, **29**, 315–23.

Davies, P. (1977) Cholinergic mechanisms in Alzheimer's disease. *British Journal of Psychiatry*, **131**, 318–19.

DHSS (1975) *Better Services for the Mentally Ill*, Command 6233, HMSO, London.

DHSS (1981) *Growing Older*, Command 8173, HMSO, London.

DHSS (1988) *Social Trends 18*, Central Statistical Office, HMSO, London.

Dobson, S. (1989) New skills are needed in adult mental handicap. *Speech Therapy in Practice*, **4**, 19–20, Good Impressions, London.

Dreyfus, P. M. (1974) Diseases of the nervous system in chronic alcohism, in *The Biology of Alcoholism* (eds B. Kissin and H. Begleites), Plenum Press. New York.

Feil, N. (1982) *Validation: The Feil method*, Edward Feil Productions, Cleveland.

Fraser, M. (1987) *Dementia: Its Nature and Management*, Wiley, Chichester.

French, A. (1986) A response: some thoughts on 'functional communication', *Bulletin 411*, College of Speech Therapists, London.

Froggatt, A. (1988) Self awareness in early dementia, in *Mental Health Problems in Old Age* (eds. B. Gearing, M. Johnson and T. Helles), Wiley, Chichester.

Gilhooly, M. L. M. (1984) The social dimensions of senile dementia, in *Psychological Approach to the Care of the Elderly* (eds I. Hanley and J. Hodge), Croom Helm, London.

Gilleard, C. (1984) *Living With Dementia*, Croom Helm, London.

Golper, L. C. and Rau, M. T. (1983) Treatment of communication disorders associated with generalised intellectual deficits in adults, *Current Therapy of Communication Disorders: Language Handicaps in Adults* (ed. W. H. Perkins), Thieme-Stratton, New York. pp. 119–29.

Goudie, F. and Stokes, G. (1989) Understanding confusion. *Nursing Times*, **85**, 35–7.

Goulding, P., Northen, B., Snowden, J. S., *et al.* (1989), Progressive aphasia with right sided extrapyramidal signs: another manifestation of localised cerebral atrophy. *Journal of Neurology, Neurosurgery and Psychiatry*, **52**, 128–30.

Gravell, R. (1988) *Communicative Problems in Elderly People. Practical Approaches to Management*, Croom Helm, London.

Greene, J. G., Smith, R., Gardiner, M. and Timbury, G. C. (1982) Measuring behavioural disturbances of elderly demented patients in the community and its effects on relatives: a factor analytic study. *Age and Ageing* **11**, 121–6.

Griffiths, H. and Baldwin, B. (1989) Speech therapy for psychogeriatric services: luxury or necessity? *Psychiatric Bulletin*, **13**, 57–9.

Hachinski, V. C., Lassen, N. A. and Marshall, J. (1974) Multi infarct dementia: a cause of mental deterioration in the elderly. *Lancet*, **ii** 207–10.

Hachinski, V. C., Iliff, L. D., Kilkha, E., *et al*. (1975) Cerebral blood flow in dementia. *Archives of Neurology*, **32**, 632–7.

Help the Aged (1984) *Recall*, Help the Aged Education Dept., London.

Hier, D. B., Hagenlocker, K. and Shindler, A. G. (1985) Language disintegration in dementia: effects of aetiology and severity. *Brain and Language*, **25**, 117–33.

Holden, U. P. and Woods, R. (1982) *Reality orientation: psychological approaches to the confused elderly*, Churchill Livingstone, Edinburgh.

Holland, A., McBurney, D., Moosey, J. and Reinmuth, O. M. (1985) The dissolution of language in Pick's disease with neurofibrillary tangles: a case study. *Brain and Language*, **24**, 35–58.

Huff, J., Corkin, S., and Growdon, H. (1986) Semantic impairment and anomia in Alzheimer's disease, *Brain and Language*, **28**, 235–49.

Irigaray, L. (1973) *Le Language des Dements*, Mouton, The Hague.

Jones, G. (1985) Validation therapy: a companion to reality orientation. *The Canadian Nurse*, March, 20–3.

Kirshner, H. S., Webb, W. G., Kelly, N. P. and Wells, C. E. (1984) Language disturbance: an initial symptom of cortical degeneration and dementia. *Archives of Neurology*, **41**, 491–6.

Kontiola, P., Laaksonen, R., Sulkava, R. and Erkinjuntti, T. (1990) Pattern of language impairment is different in Alzheimer's disease and multi-infarct dementia. *Brain language*, **38**, 364–83.

Lee, J. A. (1981) Human relatedness and the mentally impaired older person. *Journal of Gerontological Social Work*, **4**.

Lishman, W. A. (1987) *Organic Psychiatry: The Psychological Consequences of Cerebral Disorder*, 2nd ed., Blackwell Scientific Publications, London.

Lodge, B. (1981) *Coping with Caring: A Guide to Identifying and Supporting an Elderly Person with Dementia*, MIND, London.

Lubinski, R., Morrison, E. B. and Rigrodsky, S. (1981) Perception of spoken communication by elderly chronically ill patients in an institutional setting. *Journal of Speech and Hearing Disorders*, **46**, 405–12.

Mahendra, B. (1984) *Dementia: A Survey of the Syndrome of Dementia*. MTP Press, Lancaster.

Martin, A. and Fedio, P. (1983) Word production and comprehension in Alzheimer's disease: the breakdown of semantic knowledge. *Brain and Language*, **19**, 124–41.

Maxim, J. (1982) Language change with increasing age, in *Communication Changes in Elderly People* (ed. M. Edwards), College of Speech Therapists, London, pp. 40–52.

Maxim, J., Beardsall, L., Huppert, F. *et al*. (1989) *Can Spontaneous Language be used to Diagnose Dementia? A Comparison of Demented, Depressed, Aphasic and Normal Subjects.*, personal communication.

Mesulam, M. M. (1982) Slowly progressive aphasia without generalized dementia. *Annals of Neurology*, **11**, 592–8.

Murphy, E. (1986) *Dementia and Mental Illness in the Old*, Macmillan, London.

Nation's Health, The (1988) A strategy for the 1990's: A report from an indepen-

dent multidisciplinary committee (eds A. Smith and B. Jacobson), King Edward's Hospital Fund for London.

Neary, D., Snowden, J. S., Bowen, D. M. *et al.* (1986) Neuropsychological syndromes in presenile dementia due to cerebral atrophy. *Journal of Neurology, Neurosurgery and Psychiatry*, **49**, 163–74.

Neary, D., Snowden, J. S., Northen, B. and Goulding P. (1988) Dementia of the frontal lobe type. *Journal of Neurology, Neurosurgery and Psychiatry*, **51**, 353–61.

Newroth, A. and Newroth, S. (1980) *Coping with Alzheimer's Disease*, National Institute for Mental Retardartion, Ontario.

Norris, A. (1986) *Reminiscence with Elderly People*, Winslow Press, London.

Norris, A. and Eileh, A. E. (1982) Reminiscence groups. *Nursing Times*, **78**, 1368–9.

Northen, B., Hopcutt, B. and Griffiths, H. (1990) Progressive aphasia without generalized dementia. *Aphasiology*, **4**, 55–65.

Obler, L. K. and Albert, M. L. (1981) Language in the elderly aphasic and in the dementing patient, in *Acquired Aphasia* (ed. N. T. Sarno), Academic Press, New York, pp. 385–98.

Orem, D. (1980) *Nursing Concepts of Practice*, 3rd edn, McGraw Hill, New York.

Peterson, R. F., Knapp, T. J., Rosen, J. C. and Pither, B. F. (1977) The effects of furniture arrangement on the behaviour of geriatric patients. *Behaviour Therapy*, **8**, 464–7.

Pitt, B. (1982) *Psychogeriatrics: An Introduction to the Psychiatry of Old Age*, Churchill Livingstone, Edinburgh.

Pitt, B. (1988) Characteristics of depression in the elderly, in *Mental Health Problems in Old Age* (eds B. Gearing, M. Johnson and T. Heller), Wiley, Chichester.

Pogacar, S. and Williams, R. (1984) Alzheimer's disease presenting as slowly progressive aphasia. *Rhode Island Medical Journal*, **67**, 181–5.

Powell, A. L., Cummings, J. L., Hill, M. A. and Benson, D. F. (1988) Speech and language alterations in multi-infarct dementia. *Neurology*, **38**, 717–19.

Rabins, P. V., Mace, N. L. and Lucas, M. J. (1982) The impact of dementia on the family. *Journal of the American Medical Association*, **248**, 333–5.

Rapcsak, S. Z., Arthur, S., Bliklen, D. A. and Rubens, A. B. (1989) Lexical agraphia in Alzheimer's disease. *Archives of Neurology*, **46**, 65–8.

Roberts, J. K. A. (1984) *Differential Diagnosis in Neuropsychiatry*, Wiley, Chichester.

Rochford, G. (1971) A study of naming errors in dysphasic and in demented patients. *Neuropsychologia*, **9**, 437–43.

Roper, N., Logan, W. and Tierney, A. J. (1980) *The Elements of Nursing*, Churchill Livingstone, Edinburgh.

Roth, M. (1983) Depression and affective disorders in later life, in *The Origins of Depression: Current Concepts and Approaches* (ed. J. Angst), Springer – Verlag, New York.

Royal College of Physicians (1981) Organic impairment in the elderly: implications for research, education and the provision of services: report of the Royal College of Physicians by the College Committee on Geriatrics. *Journal of the Royal College of Physicians*, **15**, 141–67.

Skelton Robinson, M. and Jones, S. (1984) Nominal dysphasia and the severity of senile dementia. *British Journal of Psychiatry*, **145**, 168–71.

Stevens, S. (1988) Assessment of dementia has growing importance. *Speech Therapy in Practice*, **4**, 23–4, Good Impressions, London.

Walker, S. (1982) Communication as a changing function of age, in *Communication Changes in Elderly People*, (ed. M. Edwards), College of Speech Therapists, London, pp. 31–9.

Walker, S. (1988) The challenge of dementia: first we need information. *Speech Therapy in Practice*, **3**, Good Impressions, London.

Wattis, J. P. (1983) Alcohol and old people. *British Journal of Psychiatry*, **143**, 306–7.

Wattis, J. P. (1988) Geographical variations in the provision of psychiatric services for old people. *Age and Ageing*, **17**, 171–80.

Wattis, J. P., Wattis, L. and Arie, T. (1981) Psychogeriatrics: a national survey of a new branch of psychiatry. *British Medical Journal*, **282**, 1529–33.

Wechsler, A. F. (1977) Presenile dementia presenting as aphasia. *Journal of Neurology, Neurosurgery and Psychiatry*, **40**, 303–5.

Wicks, M. and Henwood, M. (1988) The demographic and social circumstances of elderly people, in *Mental Health Problems in Old Age*, (eds B. Gearing, M. Johnson and T. Helles), Wiley, Chichester.

World Health Organization (1988) cited in *The Nation's Health. A Strategy for the 1990's*, King Edward's Hospital Fund for London.

Zarit, S. H., Reever, K. and Bach Peterson, J. (1980) Relatives of the impaired elderly: correlates of feelings of burden. *The Gerontologist*, **20**, 649–55.

9

Gender identity problems

Judith Chaloner

INTRODUCTION

There is a line in the musical *Fiddler on the Roof* that refers to the rituals and customs of Orthodox Jewish life in pre-Revolutionary Russia. Tevya the Milkman explains that by observing these codes of behaviour, and also following the rules that separate the roles played by two sexes, 'We know who we are, and what we are, and what God expects us to be'. Although, of course, most people do not follow such rigid discipline of thought, this line does exemplify the idea that the great majority of human beings do fit into the world and society as their social background dictates, and above all as a member of the sex to which they born. They then go on to make the best life possible for themselves as a man or a woman. For people with a gender identity problem, however, this mental acceptance of their sexual identity is an impossible challenge, and it is this lack of acceptance that is the cause of continual conflict, frustration and unhappiness.

TRANSSEXUALISM

The most obvious 'gender identity problem' is that an individual has the conviction that he or she has been born into the body of the opposite sex. They feel that somehow a tragic biological mistake has been made, and that although their physical body may appear entirely male or female, the mind trapped inside that body has all the instincts, feelings and mental and physical desires of the opposite sex.

As Pauly and Edgerton (1986) state: 'These individuals attempt to deny and reverse their original biological gender and pass into and maintain the opposite gender-role identification'. They go on to say that these individuals are, of course, distinct from those born with 'confusing external genitalia' where mistakes of sexual identity assignment may have been made at birth.

These individuals have been termed transsexual, and although they can be of either sex, for the purpose of this chapter, which is a discussion of clients being referred to speech therapists from a psychiatric department, only the male to female clientele will be dealt with in detail. These individuals are termed by some as primary or true transsexuals as opposed to those with other patterns of gender dysphoria. Dolan (1987) describes this latter group of what might be termed secondary transsexuals as belonging to one of the five following types: 'an effeminate homosexual type; transvestitic type; inadequate-schizoid personality type; a psychosis in remission category; and an exhibitionistic-sociopathic type.'

Most transsexuals feel that their happiness and stability depend on the need to live as women. Most of these people also feel that they want to have a sex-change operation. To qualify for this very serious undertaking they must have a psychiatric referral to a surgeon. Some of the factors which the psychiatrist will take into consideration before making this referral will involve an assessment of how convincing the transsexual is in the female role. A referral to a speech therapist may accordingly be an important part of the process involved in preparing the client for the operation.

Although most of these clients are firmly resolved to have the operation, some, for a variety of personal reasons, may decide against it even though they wish to live completely in the female role. There are also a few of these clients who are considered medical risks because of some condition unrelated to the operation as such, and they will not get a surgical referral. These patients, too, may be referred for speech therapy. The object of this chapter is to suggest to speech therapists a few guidelines to consider when working with this type of client. There will be a discussion of the transsexual condition itself, the general management of the patient, the role of the psychiatrist in dealing with this unique type of referral and some suggestions about communication work.

As mentioned earlier, transsexuals feel that they are trapped in the wrong-gender body. In her study on bisexuality, Charlotte Wolff (1979) explains that these are individuals who have a violent clash between their gender and sexuality identities. It should be mentioned that although she uses the term 'bisexuality', this is, as she explains, in fact the concept that has been used 'as an umbrella for many different sexual variations for over 100 years'. It is not, she feels, the qualities of 'masculinity' or 'femininity' that are the upsetting factors to the transsexual, but rather the sense of belonging to the opposite sex. Harry Benjamin (1966) was the first person to use the term transsexual, although as Pauly and Edgerton (1986) mention, 'the concept of gender dysphoria and its specific forms of expression have been known since antiquity and have been described in the classic literature from Heroditus to Shakespeare'. Benjamin, as a psychiatrist working with these clients in America, did much by his publications to create international interest in this condition.

Aetiology

Anyone approaching this problem of transsexualism is drawn to the question of 'what causes it?' As little is probably known about ultimate causality here as in the different area of homosexuality. In both conditions it is clear that there is no simple anatomical causation, nor is any chromosonal abnormality implicated; the problem is essentially psychological. Little enough is known about the programming of normal psychosexual differentiation, and less still of its deviations. As Money and Ehrhardt (1972) comment, 'The programming of psychosexual differentiation is . . . a function of biographical history.' They add most significantly that 'there is a close parallel here with the progamming of language development'. It is no accident that coping with the linguistic aspects of the transsexual's presentation is in its way quite as important as the surgical in developing a survival strategy for the individual.

The sexuality of a developing fetus is initiated by the inherited sex chromosomes. This blue-print fixes the physical development of the sex organs, and the secretions of fetal hormones from the developing gonads then take over the wider expression of sexual differences. Money and Ehrhardt (1972) state that 'the testicular secretions account not only for the shape of the external genitals but also for certain patterns of organization of the brain . . . that will subsequently influence certain aspects of sexual behaviour'.

The differentiation of the sex organs seems to operate on a hormone-controlled pattern superimposed on a basically female programme. If no male hormone secretion makes its mark, the fetal differentiation follows a female path. How far the related aspects of brain development follow this pattern is less clear. It is not relevant to the present chapter to pursue further this matter of underlying clinical cause of transsexuality although it is very interesting to think broadly about the subject. The fact remains that most psychiatrists feel there are probably a number of causes for this condition and that some may be biological as well as psychological. At present there is no evidence of chromosomal or hormonal abnormality to explain the condition.

To return briefly to Money and Ehrhardt's analogy between gender identity and language, they make the interesting comparison between being bilingual from early exposure to two languages and the 'learning' of sexual identity, although some feel that this is not a valid comparison. Early exposure to conflicting language signals may occasionally result in a poor version of both languages; problems with gender identity may have similar causality. Further lessons relevant to transsexualism may yet be learnt from this significant parallel between language and gender imprinting.

One aspect of the condition that is universally accepted is that true transsexualism is a state of mind which has been with the individual all his life. Most transsexuals say that even in very early childhood they believed something was seriously wrong with the way they felt about their body, and that they did not fit the sexual pattern that was expected of them. Of course, like most other children, those with gender identity problems usually try to the best of their ability to satisfy adult expectations, and superficially many succeed well into adult life.

Medical intervention

The seeking of medical help will ultimately mean seeing a psychiatrist, for the transsexual condition will take many forms, and it often requires considerable courage. For some people the priorities of what they want from life are clear to them and they only want the doctor's help to fulfil their aims. They are sure of their own diagnosis and single-minded in organizing their life. Others are far less able to deal with either their emotional problems or to see a practical solution to the organization of their present life, but they know they need help. If to have the sex-reassignment operation is the ultimate goal for any particular individual he will have to undergo a rigorous long-term psychiatric assessment. If this is successfully completed referral will be made to a urologist or possibly a plastic surgeon.

The operation is a major one. The penis is modified to form an artificial vagina and the patient is castrated. The new vagina requires a considerable period of dilation after the patient leaves hospital. Hospitalization usually lasts about a week and there is usually a recuperation period of at least six weeks off work.

Some clients also select to have breast implantation either at the same time as original surgery or afterwards. Patients will sometimes also have extensive plastic surgery to reduce a male jaw and change the shape of the nose. Electrolysis is an ongoing part of a transsexual's life and a very expensive one. Most clients will have to have several years of treatment, usually once a week, at least initially. It can, in some cases, be very painful, but it is an essential part of the preparation for living as a convincing female.

OTHER GENDER IDENTITY PROBLEMS AND BEHAVIOUR

Reference was made earlier to the other problems of sexual identity and although most are clear, by definition, it may be useful to discuss this area briefly as it is often so closely linked, and indeed often inter-meshed with the 'true' transsexual condition. It is certainly possible to misdiagnose a client as transsexual, for true primary transsexualism is fairly rare, and indeed Shore (1984) describes just such an interesting case history. This study details the account of a client called Mickey who attempted to solve what ultimately turned out to be problems of personality by living for 2½ years as a woman. As the difficulties of personality were resolved in various ways so was the need to live in the female role. These, however, are questions for the medical profession to solve while the speech therapist need accept the premise that the whole area is often grey rather than black and white.

Inevitably, there is confusion between transsexuals and transvestites. Both cross-dress, but the latter do this for satisfaction – often resulting in sexual arousal, or as Dolan (1987) further elaborates, 'a fantasy they have when wearing the clothing'. The transvestite does not, however, actually want to be a woman. Although most transsexuals and transvestites deny this, there is often considerable overlap between the two conditions. It is not unusual for a transvestite to decide that he feels more fulfilled in the female role and to decide that he has misdiagnosed his original condition. It is also the case that many individuals with what might be termed antisocial sexual practices are extremely disturbed by their own behaviour whether it be homosexualism, transvestism, bisexuality or forms of fetishism. In some cases to be able to give themselves the label of transsexual gives a degree of respectability to their behaviour and lifts some of the guilt feelings.

There is often the question as to whether there is a homosexual quality in the transsexual's desire to change sex. Most transsexuals also deny this although in the same breath some may express the desire for a male partner after the operation. In an interesting study on *Prediction of Regrets in Postoperative Transsexuals* by Blanchard *et al.* (1987), there seems to be an indication that the homosexual transsexual clients have fewer regrets post-operatively than their heterosexual counter-parts. It has also been suggested that one major factor lying behind many transsexuals' unhappiness in the male role is the fact that they may desire a male relationship even if not a physically homosexual one.

There are also many transsexuals who claim to have no interest in the sexual side of any relationship. As with other aspects of this complex situation there are many permutations and one should not be judgemental. The fact is clear, however, that the search for sexual identity has led many of these individuals to seek fulfilment of their sexual needs by indulging in a variety of sexual experimentation.

The effeminate homosexual may also cross-dress, adopt feminine mannerisms and use an affected voice, often referred to as 'camp'. In these cases there is no sense of sexual arousal obtained from their wearing of female clothes. As with the transvestite population some of these effeminate individuals decide that they would be happier as women, but although some eventually go forward for the operation and often pass quite well physically as females they do not actually qualify for the label of a true transsexual.

THE DEVELOPMENT OF THE TRANSSEXUAL PATTERN

Almost all transsexuals say that the feeling of being born into the body of the wrong sex was an integral part of their perception of the world from very early childhood, with its attendant sense of being different from their peers of the same sex. This repetition of the theme of early awareness of this puzzling, confusing and often distressing mental phenomenon is part of almost every transsexual case history. Identification, in almost all cases, was directed towards feminine, rather than masculine attitudes, activities and attire. Adopting the dress of the opposite sex is extremely important to the transsexual as an establishing factor of visual sexual identity.

In a great number of cases patterns of guilt and anxiety were laid down at an early age, and a sense that what was being experienced was 'wrong', even if they did not understand why this should be so. These very young children with their inability to articulate their sense of differentness inevitably found childhood confusing and unhappy.

SOCIAL AND PSYCHOLOGICAL EFFECTS OF TRANSSEXUALISM

The psychological and emotional reaction to this conviction of being transsexual will vary according to the degree with which any individual is able to tolerate other problems in his life. It may seem obvious, but like everyone else the transsexual is the product of heredity and environment. These are the factors that make individual personalities what they are. For this reason while some of these clients will suffer periods of such intolerable stress that it will upset their whole mental equilibrium, others will appear much more able to manage what they

225

claim is an equally frustrating situation. A very illuminating book on the subject of the personal transsexual experience was written in 1974 by one of Britain's most distinguished travel writers, James – later Jan – Morris. The book, *Conundrum* (1974), describes in detail the psychological distress that eventually resulted in a sexual reassignment operation. At the time of its publication far less was known by the general public about transsexualism than is the case today. The credibility of the author and the articulate way the condition was presented did much to lift some of the prejudice surrounding the subject.

The case histories set out in the Appendix illustrate the kind of pattern of development of the transsexual condition and the resulting social effects common to the majority. For example, both of these individuals had felt a sense of discomfort with their bodies since early childhood and believed that they should have been born women. Both had a compulsion to cross-dress and were happy posing as women even with the awareness that they may never appear totally convincing in that role.

In spite of all efforts neither was able to justify or totally rationalize their behaviour, but both felt convinced that a female psyche was trapped in a male body. There are few other common features, which is in itself interesting and immediately evident to anyone having much involvement with the transsexual population. There appears to be no common thread linking their individual obsessions that they have been born into the body of the opposite sex.

THE ROLE OF PSYCHIATRY

A psychiatrist's role is to treat the mentally ill. Most transsexuals do not come into this category. They do not want to change the conviction that they have a feminine psyche in their male body. They can talk rationally about their gender identity problem and have no difficulty relating to reality. It is true that many pre-operative transsexuals have an unrealistic view both of their ability to organize their lives during the probationary period leading up to the actual sex-change operation, and to envision what their lives will actually be like post-operatively. However, this is not, of course, an indication of mental illness. Also the fact that many transsexuals have what is considered to be a high level of neurosis does not in itself mean that they are necessarily any more ill than many individuals without gender problems, but only that in these cases their particular obsession about gender identity is the principal cause of their high degree of anxiety or depression.

A study of these neurotic tendencies was presented by psychologist

Dr Charles Mate-Kole at the International Conference on Gender Identity at Charing Cross in December 1986 (Mate-Kole, Freschi and Robin, 1986). The object of this study involved evaluation of several groups of transsexuals at various stages of their treatment to try to determine whether evident neurotic behaviour became less following gender reassignment surgery. It was found that there was a significant reduction of neurosis following the operation, a fact used by some members of the clinic to argue the justification of using public money for a non-medical problem.

The psychiatrist and others on his or her team will assess the progress of patients who are there at their own request or by GP referral. The object is not to try to effect a 'cure' for the condition, but rather to ascertain whether the individual has a realistic chance of being accepted as a woman after the operation, and appears mentally stable enough to cope with all the difficulties involved in making the transition. Both 'primary' and other gender dysphoric clients may eventually be put forward for surgery, if the latter have been able to prove convincingly enough that they have consolidated their gender identity feelings into the female mode. Psychotherapy and counselling should be part of the gender identity reassignment programme.

In the past, when far fewer people came forward with this problem, and it was considered quite a new and extraordinary phenomenon, more effort was made both to find the underlying cause and bring about a change of attitude. Experimentation was done with psychoanalysis, hypnosis and even electric shock aversion therapy on cross-dressed clients. There is no record of any of these treatments being successful.

It is important to differentiate between psychiatric treatment and psychiatric monitoring. Many transsexuals have had psychiatric help and counselling. It is obvious that in any group of people differing in sexual thoughts and habits from what is considered 'normal' behaviour some will experience mental distress of various types and degrees. The permutations are endless, ranging from simple anxiety, and feelings of guilt, to incapacitating depression. Possibly during the course of whatever treatment is considered appropriate, the reasons for the gender dysphoria may be discussed and speculated on. For the purpose of the treatment is not to 'cure' their gender identity dilemma, but rather to help the individual arrive at a stage of sufficient equilibrium to be able to take charge of his own life in whichever way he chooses.

In the process of monitoring the client's progress, the general attitude towards the clients is acceptance of the situation, but not overt encouragement, and the negative aspects are fully outlined. During this period suitable patients, without contraindicated medical problems, will be prescribed a course of hormone therapy to create breast development, soften body hair and sometimes alter the distribution of body fat. For those patients where the sex-reassignment surgery is envisioned in the relatively near future all clinics or private psychiatrists require the client to first undergo a trial period of at least a year, living and working full time as a female. Because one of the stipulations of surgical referral is that a client must be reasonably acceptable in the female role it is, as mentioned earlier, often during this probationary period that referral may be made to a speech therapist for help both with voice work and communication skills. Finally, when surgical referral is contemplated two psychiatrists must independently attest that in their judgements the client should be allowed to have gender reassignment.

The responsibility accorded to the psychiatrist's role is not enviable. He is put under great pressure by the client to make this referral for irrevocable surgery. It is undeniable that the client is an unhappy person, who is convinced that the sex-change operation will give him a chance for the physical and emotional fulfilment, which will enable him to lead a more satisfactory life. The doctor must be the judge of whether these expectations are realistic, often having only the reliance of the patient's own assurance that he is adequately managing his employment and domestic life, both practically and emotionally. The doctor is, of course, also well aware that the patient is often understandably reluctant to tell him about difficulties he may be experiencing in his new role. Self-doubts are unlikely to be freely expressed because of the realization that unless he appears reasonably mentally stable referral chances may be jeopardized.

In Britain two psychiatric opinions are required if surgery is contemplated, whether on a private basis or as a National Health patient referral. After mutual psychiatric agreement has been reached for the surgical referral, private patients undoubtedly have a shorter waiting time for surgery; although, of course, ability to pay should never be a consideration when considering the suitability of a candidate.

It is difficult to judge whether such an operation has benefited the client. For many life is enhanced considerably and a sense of contentment is achieved that was felt to be impossible. However, many realize that with the change of sex new, possibly unanticipated, problems have been created and in some cases these negative effects dilute the pleasure of the new life. For some the operation is not a success, and life becomes a half existence. Possibly these are people who never have been emotionally organized individuals, and are simply lacking the stability to cope with what is undoubtedly a tremendous emotional adjustment. It is for this very reason that the pre-operative assessment just discussed is of vital importance. Dolan (1987) discusses this issue when he remarks '. . . whereas sexual reassignment does relieve gender dysphoria, it does so without necessarily improving psychosocial adjustment and it does not have much effect on coincidental psychopathology'.

PRACTICAL CONSIDERATIONS, DISCUSSION OF ATTITUDES AND THE ROLE OF THE SPEECH THERAPIST

What aside from specific voice work (which will be discussed separately) should be done for these clients by the speech therapist? This is a complex question, as any speech therapist realizes from experience that clients are always more than a 'voice problem' or a 'dysphasic'. Whatever the reason for their referral, one is treating a whole communicating individual, not just the 'faulty element', and this philosophy extends equally to transsexual clients. If they are taken on for treatment the therapist should be prepared to treat not just the voice, but the whole person.

Expectations of treatment

The psychiatrist may refer suitable clients to the speech therapist for voice therapy, but there may not necessarily be any discussion of the candidate's suitability for surgery. From the doctor's viewpoint therapy results are the important factors resulting from the referral. The speech therapist's role does not necessarily include professional counselling, although without doubt some indirect counselling will inevitably occur with this client population. The knowledge that there is no constant feedback to a psychiatrist undoubtedly makes the speech therapy situation more relaxed for the client. However, in the rare case where the therapist is worried by what appears to be continuous and excessively unreasonable behaviour, such as undue lability or anger, he or she has a responsibility to seek a second opinion and report this to the psychiatrist. It must be strongly emphasized that working with these clients requires a wide range of management skills, and that in some instances voice therapy becomes secondary.

The common factor of their transsexualism tends to make the majority of these clients very obsessive in their feelings about everything relating to their sex-change, which includes help with their voice. The clients may very well expect more time than the therapist is able to devote to them, and they may also want and expect more counselling and psychological back-up than the therapist is qualified or wants to give.

It is important that the speech therapist realizes the limitations of his or her expertise in counselling these patients. The stability of these individuals will vary enormously, and not every transsexual referred to the therapist will necessarily prove suitable for treatment. The psychiatrist will not knowingly refer an unstable client, but it is not possible to anticipate all eventualities. A client should never be accepted without an official referral, and of course normal security measures should be observed.

It is useful to remember that although most situations are easily handled by an experienced therapist one should be alert to some recurring problems. As mentioned earlier, these clients may occasionally, because of their emotional vulnerability, exhibit some degree of unreasonable behaviour. Also sometimes a client's own self-image will be so inaccurate that he may interpret any suggestions about changing various aspects of this image as unreasonable criticism, and react accordingly. A client may, on occasion, even feel that the therapist is responsible for his voice failures. In addition many transsexuals will appear depressed; many have a history of suicide attempts. The therapy situation can expose the client's inadequacies in a way he often finds difficult to cope with.

General guidelines and attitudes

The following guidelines may be helpful. Only a short therapy contract should be given, which can be extended later if it seems appropriate. After assessment, it is often helpful to the client if the therapist gives him a written outline of the proposed therapy programme. This might take the form, for example, of fairly general explanations of facts concerning voice, and then specific exercises to follow. How this is presented will depend on the approach taken by individual therapists, and could perhaps include suggestions about relaxation techniques and breathing exercises as well as a discussion of the way voice is actually produced and why the male voice tends to differ from that of the female. In addition, practical guidelines about coping with criticism, and the general management of their new role might be indicated. Personal involvement and undertaking counselling at a level that one is not qualified to give, no matter how experienced the therapist, should be avoided.

The possible limitations of therapy should be explained. The therapist too should be aware of these limitations and not feel that therapy has necessarily been a failure if the voice continues to be a problem for the client. Often adequate voice results are achieved in the clinical situation, but will not be used outside that setting. The complex reasons for this may very well not be within the capacity of the speech therapist to solve, but knowing that this problem does occur is important. It is interesting to speculate that while the voice can still be seen to be such an important problem for the client that surgical referral is delayed, the client is spared having to take final decisions about his life.

Not every speech therapist wants to work with transsexual clients. The whole subject of treatment of these clients is an extremely controversial one. It is argued by many that public money should not be spent on people who are not 'ill'. It may be claimed that by giving treatment like speech therapy, for example, transsexuals are being encouraged to continue a lifestyle that is unwholesome and abnormal. In addition many feel that it is morally wrong to perform mutilating surgery on physically normal people, and also that by giving hospital space to these clients the waiting lists for other patients who they perceive as being in more urgent need of surgery by a urologist are lengthened.

In fact many transsexuals decide to pay for their operation, which cost in 1989 between £3000 and £5000 for private care. This does not address the moral issue of whether the operation should be performed at all, and many medically well-informed people feel that it should not. Individual therapists must decide this question for themselves. Transsexualism is undoubtedly a psychologically debilitating condition for a large number of people who need and deserve some sort of professional help if they are to function adequately in society. But degrees of misery are difficult to assess when debating whether one type of psychological disability is more deserving than another. There is no ideal solution for these people, not even surgery, although it does cosmetically alter the body so that the image is more acceptable to the client himself.

For people without experience of a sexual identity problem this whole question of surgery may raise moral and other questions which the speech therapist may be called to discuss. 'Few if any surgical procedures attract so much fear, misunderstanding and plain loathing as a sex-change' (Hodgkinson, 1988). Nevertheless, helping some of these extremely unhappy and emotionally frustrated people to masquerade as convincingly as possible as the opposite sex, does in a great many cases create enough stability in these individuals for them to become very much more effective, organized members of society than would otherwise have been possible. Therapists who feel that they do not agree with the rationale behind helping these people, or who feel that there is another solution in these cases, need make no apology for this attitude. It is a dilemma with no definite solution.

The male to female transsexual worried about aspects of his presentation will usually consider his voice to be his greatest problem. He may feel that he looks convincingly feminine when 'dressed', but worried that his voice sounds too male to allow him to speak confidently in public. He may, of course, also worry about facial hair, but this problem is one that is considered solvable by electrolysis if one can afford the long-term financial commitment.

Transsexual clients need to understand that the voice itself, although obviously very important, is only one aspect of the 'total package' that needs to be considered when trying to present a convincingly feminine image to the world. In addition to work on the voice the speech therapist often has involvement in helping the client with modification of his male to female social skills, which will be discussed, briefly, as a separate topic. For some transsexuals the importance of the impression that they make on those around them is relatively unimportant, while for others their whole existence is geared towards constantly polishing their appearance and vocal presentation. The individual needs and desires that motivate the actions of transsexuals are as varied and diverse as those of any group of people linked together only by a common interest. It is necessary for a speech therapist working with a client to find out what he actually expects from the voice therapy. This will cover an enormous range and is a vital factor in client assessment; it will give the therapist a guide to aspects of both the client's intelligence and personality. The therapy programme will then be planned on the basis of these expectations, and the therapist's evaluation of how realistic these aims are, after appraisal of the client's abilities so far as the therapy is concerned.

Although most transsexuals want the results of voice therapy, few actually like going through the discipline of manipulating the voice in order to produce these results. The act of dressing in female clothes requires no such effort, and has always been the pleasure that has satisfied certain obsessional feelings. However, work on the voice requires concentration on technique, and intellectual content of speech is often sacrificed. It may be fairly easy to say 'good morning' or order a pound of butter, using an acceptable voice. It is quite another matter to have a political argument, and the client should be helped to understand this.

Social skills

As mentioned, it may also necessary to help the client realize that aside from specific voice work he must take pains to develop certain feminine social skills if he is to pass in the role convincingly. The teaching of these techniques is an important part of the therapy programme, but one difficult to describe because each individual will present with different needs and abilities. There is no blanket formula to follow.

This is a delicate area because it infringes on the right of the individual to, as so many of them say, 'be myself', and to criticize often offends core sensitivities. To talk through the rationale behind the need to perfect the total presentation is the first step. One is not necessarily trying to create a female stereotype as much as a convincing image within the framework of the client's personality and ability.

The transsexual is often a very self-absorbed and egocentric individual who makes little effort to relate in any but the most superficial way to other people, and has failed to develop many social conversational skills. It is quite usual for a transsexual client to look and sound very convincing as a female, but fail to continue to project this image during his conversation. In these cases it may be useful to suggest exercises where the client has to make a deliberate effort to find out about other people's lives and interests and also to develop some of his own, not directly related to his gender identity problem. Role play is a helpful method to do this type of project, possibly using a video so that there is a means of self-monitoring as well as having a record of progress.

The overtly effeminate voice and manner of the homosexual should be eliminated. It should be emphasized that no female ever presents in this way. The inexperienced therapist may feel that this is a very delicate area to try to correct, but it is an essential part of the therapy. Attention should also be made both to overtly masculine language and those physical postures that call attention to themselves adversely.

Working on relaxation and eye contact exercises to help the client show a confident manner is very important. The ability to project an air of assured confidence will in a great many circumstances convince listeners that in spite of various masculine vocal qualities the speaker should be accepted as female with a rather idiosyncratic voice containing some masculine elements. Another skill is to learn and use personal management strategies, possibly suggested by the therapist, so that he can cope with critical scrutiny about his appearance or his voice. It must be accepted that it is not possible for every male transsexual to pass completely convincingly as a woman, and these limits which can be physical, emotional or intellectual have to be acknowledged by the individual concerned. If one had to make the choice between the importance of voice and appearance in judging a client's chance of passing well as a woman, appearance would be the more important aspect. The ability of the transsexual client to accept some unchangeable situations realistically as they are, and not as he wishes they were, will determine the success of his eventual adjustment to the new sex role.

To do this one should consider, as part of the social skills area, various outside influences that may affect the client's behaviour. Often transsexuals lead very solitary, isolated lives; many spend a large amount of their leisure with groups or in clubs that cater for people like themselves. In large cities throughout the world one is able to find venues that cater for sexual minorities, where their various preferences of partner can be indulged, and where they are free to dress as they wish. Transsexual and transvestite clubs are common and satisfy a social need because in this setting what is often considered by the outside world as decadent or bizarre becomes normality. These individuals often spend a great deal of time under stress. They are socially unacceptable to many people, and need a centre where no explanations for their looks or behaviour are necessary and where fear of detection is absent.

Unfortunately in the group setting there tends to be an element of mutual admiration which is neither genuine or realistic. For many transvestites this is relatively unimportant. To wear sexually explicit clothes is often part of the gratification they get from dressing like a woman, and most do not expect to pass as female all the time. However, for the transsexual the ultimate aim of cross-dressing should be to blend and fit in with a normal stratum of society.

To a limited extent guidance in this area can be attempted by the speech therapist. The therapist may in some cases be the first person to accept and relate to the transsexual in his new role. For this reason, and because of the fairly unique nature of the situation, the client occasionally becomes overly dependent on the therapist, and can sometimes be very demanding of time and attention. In some cases it would seem that the client feels that the fact therapy has been undertaken condones his actions, and to some degree this adds a reassuring sense of respectability to the situation. In these relaxed circumstances the therapy sessions can, unfortunately, sometimes become an arena for the patient to release many of his emotional feelings. Unless specifically working with transsexuals for a great deal of their time, speech therapists will rarely see many of these clients, and might not anticipate the occasional problems of management which can occur.

Teaching social skills to this client population may seem to some an infringement of the right of these individuals to simply move from the male to female role and be allowed to get on with their lives. However, some actively need some guidance in this area if they are to succeed in their new lives. Part of the general assessment of the client should include 'the social skills and competence as a communicator' (Elias, 1986). A well-motivated client should accept this as part of the whole therapy programme.

VOICE WORK

The weight of this chapter has been geared towards a theme of discussing various aspects of the transsexual condition. The aim has been to give speech therapists working with these clients a framework of knowledge to draw on regarding management of the patients when planning and carrying out therapy. The following outline of voice work with transsexuals is not a detailed explanation of specific therapy procedures. For those interested, a book on voice disorders edited by Margaret Fawcus (1986) contains a chapter concentrating almost entirely on specific voice work with these clients (Chaloner, 1986) where these techniques have been discussed individually and at length. In addition, for those wishing to pursue the subject of the acoustic and linguistic considerations of these clients, Oates and Dacakis (1983) discuss these aspects in depth.

This is only intended to be a practical guide, and specific therapy procedures will have to be varied to suit the different needs of the clients. It is assumed that anyone undertaking therapy with transsexuals will already have considerable experience with voice work and will simply apply this knowledge to the particular group of patients. It is worth mentioning that it is very useful to make a video, or at least a tape recording, of the initial assessment, and to make careful notes about the general first impression given by the client. As one becomes increasingly familiar with an individual the judgement of his performance quickly becomes less reliable.

The importance of fully exploring the client's, and not the therapist's, needs and expectations cannot be over-emphasized, and planning a realistic therapy programme cannot take place without it. As mentioned earlier some of these patients would like a more feminine voice as a result of therapy, but are simply not sufficiently motivated to do the specific voice work necessary to achieve very good results. Some clients plan after their sex-change to continue in their old jobs and in their same domestic routine, and have no genuine intention of trying to change their voice very much. They will already have adopted the philosophy that everyone knows their situation and have already built up a psychological barrier against trying to use a radically new voice.

There is also the feeling of some transsexuals that they actively dislike the pretence of voice alteration and the rest of society must take them as they are.

All of these situations are common. It must be remembered that a few transsexuals are referred to the speech therapist as part of the psychiatric assessment programme and not necessarily at the client's wish. Occasionally it is possible to help the clients to modify their thoughts about voice work, and to attempt compromises in the therapy programme. However, sometimes it is obviously unrealistic even to attempt this and quite inappropriate to try to effect a change in attitude; therapy in these cases is not indicated.

Voice work with these clients includes: resonance, pitch and intonation. It should be remembered that in the male voice the resonating area is almost always in the chest area, while in the female voice it is the head. The elimination of chest resonance is the single most important aspect of this type of voice work. It is useful to suggest to the client that he should try to imagine his body as a series of spaces or containers one on top of another. The therapist should explain that he must move sound up and down through these spaces until he has achieved the skill to do this easily. All the time that this exercise is taking place the therapist should encourage both auditory and kinaesthetic feedback; the client should not only hear the movement of the sound from space to space, but he should be able to feel the movement of vibrations in the different areas. Exercises can be given at this time to focus sound at the front of the face. It is also useful to suggest that the client try to retract the mouth corners. Ohala (1984) states that this will have the effect of shortening the mouth cavity, and that its resonances will therefore be raised.

It is interesting to note that the actual pitch of the voice will be perceived as higher when it is accompanied by head rather than chest resonance. When the technique of producing the voice with head resonance is achieved, then if necessary it can be suggested that the client try to raise the pitch very slightly; however, not too much emphasis should be directed towards this. It has frequently been noted that during voice therapy the client's voice pitch often becomes higher naturally, and as explained by Bryan-Smith (1986) this is probably because 'the client's ear became more acutely tuned to speech and voice patterns'. Gunzburger (1989) brings up a related point regarding voice presentation, suggesting that care should be taken 'to prevent adoption of an effeminate male quality resorted to by some transsexuals instead of the female quality that is desired'.

Intonation patterning is another aspect of therapy to be considered when working with these clients. The female voice has much more variation of pitch than the more monotone male voice. Using marked passages the therapist can encourage the male speaker to add variety to the voice. It should also be noted that the female voice usually has a rising intonation pattern at the end of sentences. The male voice usually has a falling intonation pattern. Emphasis should be on light delicate articulation, and again awareness of the front of the mouth should be encouraged. Slight rounding of the lips focuses the sound in the front of the face. With these aims in mind the therapist can achieve satisfactory results in any way that she finds most effective with her other voice patients. As with most voice work, good results depend on good breath support, achieved after mastering relaxation exercises (Greene, 1975). These are basic ideas familiar to all therapists.

In summary, the aim of the speech therapist is first to help the client achieve as good a voice as possible; second, to help him develop through the teaching of social skills a confident relaxed manner, so that he will appear at ease in the way that he looks and speaks; third, to teach a few basic strategies that the client can use to cope with the problems encountered if an occasion occurs when he has failed to pass convincingly as a female. To this end a realistic attitude should be instilled in the client so that should these problems occur he will be prepared to cope with it socially and emotionally. In addition, guiding a transsexual towards a change of attitude about the way he feels that society views his situation is often one of the greatest services a speech therapist can give the client. He should be made aware that while it may seem to him both unfair and unfortunate, it will probably never be possible to convince the entire world that what he is doing is 'right'. He must realize that not to accept this will have the effect of negating the satisfaction he hopes to achieve in his new life.

COUNSELLING

Brief reference has been made to counselling throughout this article as to a limited extent it is often an integral part of the therapist's involvement with these clients. If he or she undertakes work with transsexuals there will inevitably be occasions where help of this kind may be indicated. Some therapists will, of course, have more formal training qualifications in this area than others, and each must recognize the limits of his or her expertise.

Knowledge of background of the condition and an idea of some of possible problems facing the clients will form the basis of the therapist's baseline to work from. The techniques employed should be largely based on listening and helping the client to reflect back on what he has said. Direct advice about course of action should be avoided.

The therapist often has quite a valuable role to play in this area because just the opportunity to talk and possibly to clarify thoughts is in many cases a unique chance for these clients.

CONCLUSION

The intention of this chapter is to give an overview of the transsexual condition from the viewpoint of a speech therapist with experience of working in this field. It is a subject surrounded by controversy and speculation, even by those on the medical side working closely with these clients. It is a complex area, but by increasing the insight of speech therapists into various aspects of the subject it is hoped that a more effective service will become available to transsexual patients in the future.

REFERENCES

Benjamin, H. (1966) *The Transsexual Phenomenon*, New York.

Blanchard, R., Steiner, B. W., Clemmensen, L. H. and Dickey, R. (1987) Prediction of regrets in postoperative transsexuals, *Canadian Journal of Psychiatry*, **34**, 43–5.

Bryan-Smith, P. (1986) More than a matter of pitch, *Speech Therapy in Practice*, **2** (3), 28–9.

Chaloner, J. (1986) The voice of the transsexual, *Voice Disorders and their Management* (ed. M. Fawcus), Croom Helm, London, pp. 224–39.

Dolan, J. D. (1987) Transsexualism: syndrome or symptom? *Canadian Journal of Psychiatry*, **32**, 666–73.

Elias, A. (1986) Does the speech therapist have a role in the assessment and treatment of the male transsexual? (Abs.) *International Conference on Gender Identity*, London.

Greene, M. (1975) *The Voice and its Disorders*, Pitman Medical, London.

Gunzburger, D. (1989) Voice adaptations by transsexuals, *Clinical Linguistics and Phonetics*, **3** (2), 163–72.

Hodgkinson, L. (1988) Our money or their lives? *The Times*, London.

Mate-Kole, C., Freschi, M. and Robin, A. (1986) A controlled study of the effects of gender reassignment surgery on psychiatric symptomology, (Abs.) *International Conference on Gender Identity*, London.

Money, J. and Erhardt, A. (1972) *Man and Woman – Boy and Girl*, Johns Hopkins University Press, Baltimore.

Morris, J. (1974) *Conundrum*, Faber, London.

Oates, J. M. and Dacakis, G. (1983) Speech pathology considerations in the management of transsexuals: a review, *British Journal of Disorders of Communication*, **18** (3), 139–51.

Ohala, J. J. (1984) Ethological perspective on common cross-language utilization of FO of voice, *Phonetica*, **41**, 1–16.

Pauly, I. B. and Edgerton, M. T. (1986) The gender identity movement: a growing surgical-psychiatric liaison, *Archives of Sexual Behaviour*, **15** (4), 315–29.

Shore, E. R. (1984) The former transsexual: a case study, *Archives of Sexual Behaviour*, **13** (3), 277–85.

Wolff, C. (1979) *Bisexuality: A Study*, Quartet Books, London.

APPENDIX 9.1

Case history number 1

Paul appears to outsiders as a successful organized young businessman with a promising career ahead of him. At 32 he is well thought of in his firm, earns an excellent salary, frequently travels abroad and represents the firm at important foreign business meetings. He works in London but regularly travels home to see his family in Scotland; although he is well liked by business colleagues, he does not mix with any of them socially.

The reality of the situation is that when Paul arrives home at his flat each evening he changes his identity completely, assuming the role of a woman by putting on a wig, female clothes, and make-up. Until recently most of his female existence has been within his flat; however, during the last year he has become more adventurous, spending some evenings and weekends travelling about in crowded areas in London where he feels that Pauline can blend into the background without attracting attention. Visually Pauline is a convincing woman. Paul has been cultivating the art of conservative dressing and buys expensive well-cut clothes that fit well with the image he is trying to create.

This present lifestyle is the culmination of a lifetime of inner distress while outwardly appearing to have been successful in all the activities that he has undertaken. Paul is the third child of professional Scottish parents, and claims that from the earliest age that he can remember he felt unhappy with every aspect of his developing male body and identified emotionally and physically with his sister rather than his brother; cross-dressing began as an adolescent. Paul was a good student at both school and university, with a small circle of close male friends, none of whom knew anything of his transsexual feelings. He had a short-lived sexual relationship with a girl at university, but otherwise his female friendships were platonic, and there were no homosexual relationships.

While he was at university Paul told his parents that he wanted to have a sex-change operation, which evoked a reaction of total disbelief and extreme distress. Arrangements were made for him to have psychiatric help, and because his mother was so emotionally disturbed by his disclosure Paul felt that he was unable at the time to discuss it further with his family. The psychiatrist could find no apparent reason for the transsexual feelings and was able to do little to help his anxiety or confused state of mind. His brother and sister were not told of the situation and he did not confide in any of his friends.

During two of his university vacations Paul travelled alone in Europe and for the first time cross-dressed openly, and also for the first time felt the relief derived from being perceived as a female. The fact that all of these experiences were situations that involved being among foreign-speaking strangers did not detract from Paul's conviction that he could never be fulfilled emotionally until he had a sex-change. The suggestion that he might be able to live openly as a woman without surgery is abhorrent to him, and he wants the maleness of his body to be eliminated. As with most transsexuals, Paul is constantly afraid of the accidental detection of his physical sexuality when he is cross-dressed, which would result in public humiliation. This fear often involves the imagined situation of being, for example, knocked down in a street accident, being taken unconscious to hospital, and then examined by a doctor. This is a very real anxiety.

Paul's future plans are dependent on how well he is able to organize his life. His goal is to have a sex-change operation, but he is realistic enough to understand that his present career may be at risk if he does this. It may be possible for him to start again in similar work, but this cannot be guaranteed, and many business firms would naturally be reluctant to employ someone they might consider an emotional liability, when competition for high-level jobs is very great. Therefore at present he lives the lifestyle described, in an atmosphere of great social isolation outside the work environment. He has speech and grooming help, although the need for this is now minimal as he passes well as a female. He has regular electrolysis, is on a regime of hormone therapy, and sees the psychiatrist regularly for monitoring.

Paul remains unhappy and unfulfilled; he is very articulate in expressing his feelings, and has thought clearly and rationally about future plans and his present situation. He realizes that his is a selfish existence, and longs for human relationships involving the acceptance of him as a woman, but sees no resolution of the problem. He feels that to achieve peace of mind he must have the operation; yet he is unable to openly admit the situation, and to live full-time as a woman. His relationship with his family is very important to him. He perceives that this relationship and the whole future of his career would be jeopardized if he took this step; apparently at the moment he needs the stability which his family and his working environment give him, and is not able to risk sacrificing this.

It is interesting to look at this case study of a young man with an as yet unresolved gender identity problem, that is causing him the same discontent and obsessional feelings about cross-dressing described by most transsexuals. It is significant that it is often in these circumstances, when faced with such apparently insoluble dilemmas, that many trans-sexuals decide to marry and attempt a normal sexual relationship. Many even hope that marriage may help eradicate the problem. The reality of course is that the obsessional feelings about the gender identity continue, and the success or failure of the relationship depends on the ability of the partners to adjust to one another's needs. Some women are able to tolerate what others would find a completely unacceptable level of deviant behaviour in order to preserve what may otherwise be a rewarding relationship.

Case history number 2

Victoria is now 55 and a post-operative transsexual, having had the operation seven years ago. Her early background had a similar theme of discontentment about the male body. The home background was stable and Victor, as he was then known, was a good student at school and later worked as a successful salesman for a large company. Secret cross-dressing began in his teens, later doing this openly in the evenings when he was travelling away from home in connection with his job. He also visited clubs catering for transvestites and transsexuals whenever possible.

He married at 21, and over the next ten years his wife had six children; his wife had no knowledge of either his sexual identity feelings or his cross-dressing activities, finding out by accident after many years of marriage. Her reaction was of both shock and amazement that in such an apparently close relationship these feelings and this often bizarre double life had existed for such a long time.

Victor began to suffer from severe depression in his late thirties which he attributed to his lack of emotional and physical fulfilment; he asked his general practitioner for help, and was referred by him to a gender identity clinic. There he was told that he would have to live full time as a woman for at least a year before even being considered for surgical referral, and he decided to take this step. He approached his company, but in spite of the excellence of his previous work record, they would not even consider the idea of his continued employment with them in this new role. Sympathetic as many employers are to the situation on a personal level it is sometimes felt that the credibility of their firm will be questioned by employing a transsexual, particularly if there are face to face client relationships involved. However one feels about the morality of the situation it is, in the final analysis, the employer's decision.

With the need to earn money to support his family Victor took a local authority training course to teach him how to run a small business, which he bought with the proceeds of selling his house. This business was located several hundred miles away in a geographical area with which they had no previous connection. There were living quarters attached to the premises and as his wife was willing to support him throughout this upheaval it was decided to move the entire family. They were accepted into the community as a family consisting of his wife as a widowed mother living with a female relative. Future plans regarding their relationship were uncertain at that time, but it was felt that the children would be less disrupted by this situation than if their father left home. They did, however, divorce as this was a necessary stipulation at that time for anyone contemplating a sex-change oper- ation. Several of the children overtly suffered from the very consider- able stress of the situation and two of them required periods of psychi- atric counselling. Their standard of living also suffered badly during this time although Victor managed to build up the business gradually over the years.

After six years Victor finally got a referral to a surgeon, and had the sex-change operation, paid for by the National Health Service. Over the following two years Victoria, as she became, also had breast implant surgery, plastic surgery on her face and major cosmetic dental work.

It is significant to note that after the initial feeling of euphoria follow- ing the sex-change operation Victoria suffered from another period of depression. This is a common experience, and although almost all post- operative transsexuals express feelings of relief at achieving a long-term desire, they are sometimes surprised to find life itself with all its ongoing problems still has to be faced as before.

Victoria continued to live with her former wife, and they run a small successful business and the children, whom they see regularly, have left home. Victoria claims that family relationships are good, and that she feels she is a better parent as a female than a male.

Before surgery Victor had hoped to eventually find a male partner after the operation, although he did not classify himself as a homosexual and protested at any suggestion to this affect. However, it now seems evident that it is more important to Victoria to have the continued, and highly valued, support of his wife, than to seek a sexual partner.

Victoria passes well as a woman. She is small-boned, small featured and has a tanned weather-beaten complexion that complements her brisk countrywoman image. Her voice is light and acceptably female, and her manner is unself-conscious and confident. She wears little make-up, has a disregard for fashion and appears to have little regard for the kind of female image she presents. The inner contentment seems to be directly related to the altered body image. She relates well to other people, and appears to have a genuine interest in them, which is a quality noticeably lacking in many self-absorbed transsexuals. One feels at a surface level that Victoria's sex-change has been from her point of view a success.

10

Management and treatment techniques: a practical approach

Niki Muir, Pauline Tanner and Jenny France

INTRODUCTION

This chapter is based on the accumulated personal experiences and knowledge of those speech therapists who are working or have worked in formal psychiatric settings or with psychiatric patients in community speech therapy clinics. This specialism is still in the early years of development and so much of what is expressed here cannot as yet be corroborated by research. However, it is certainly known that many people with mental illness suffer some degree of communication dysfunction or inadequacy (see Chapter 1) and so the speech therapist's skills may therefore add a valuable contribution in the multidisciplinary psychiatric team. Speech therapists are increasingly aware of the need to evaluate their work and this is true in the field of psychiatry as in others.

It is hoped that this chapter will be of use and interest to other professionals such as psychiatric nurses, occupational therapists and clinical psychologists who, like speech therapists, have an interest in communication skills and remediation. The aim of this chapter is to describe a variety of approaches that speech therapists and others might use, with emphasis on the management of the patient in hospital settings. However, many of the therapies described would be suitable for patients living in the community, with some modification or adaptation. The approaches are not confined to any specific diagnostic group and will not deal with the management of elderly people as this is covered in Chapter 8.

REFERRALS

Referrals may come from many different agencies as in any other branch of the profession. Most tend to come via the medical profession. As latecomers and still newcomers to clinical teams in psychiatry, speech therapists may need to self-publicize. By familiarizing consultant psychiatrists and their colleagues with the skills particular to the speech therapist, referrals can be generated – often out of curiosity. It seems to the writers to be vital to see each patient who is referred even if later assessment proves them to be unsuitable for treatment. Written and verbal explanation of the reasons for unsuitability can often result in more appropriate referrals in the future.

As well as traditional medical referrals, patients can come via other disciplines such as speech therapy colleagues, nursing staff, occupational therapists, physiotherapists, psychologists and social workers, if there is an open referral system. In a close-knit institution, such as a psychiatric hospital with strong paramedical bonds and an open system, it is not unheard of for referrals to come via unlikely routes like the chiropodist, the pathology department or the chaplain!

Self-referrals are also quite common. The in-patient may drop into the department out of interest or even boredom. Many mentally ill patients may attribute their symptoms to a physical cause saying, for example, 'I can't breathe properly when I talk', 'My voice has gone funny', 'I can't find the right words when I speak', 'I can't talk to people any more'. All these difficulties, whether real or imagined, are worthy of investigation just as every patient is worthy of time and attention. Exploring the nature of the communication difficulties can often supply further pieces to the jigsaw puzzle presented by the person with a mental illness.

Whatever the source of the referral, it is important to inform the consultant and other doctors concerned with the patient's care. It is hoped they will be in agreement with the contact since medical support is as vital to those speech therapists who work in psychiatry as it is to those in a general setting or any other 'specialist' area. A fairly standard referral form is often all that is required and an example can be seen in Figure 10.1.

The addition of a space to record medication is important. The possible effects on speech of antipsychotic drugs are well documented, with evidence of extrapyramidal or cholinergic side-effects – such as dystonic reaction, tardive dyskinesia and bradykinesia – and are of obvious importance as has been discussed in Chapter 5. Certain drugs can lead to dysarthria, involuntary movements of the speech musculature and problems with initiating or maintaining breath control or vocalization. Also any movement disorder can prove distressing to the patient and impair concentration. It can also be helpful to include the heading 'specific difficulties' so that the speech therapist can be aware from the outset of any other medical conditions or major behavioural difficulties which may affect the approach on first meeting the patient.

BLANK HOSPITAL

REQUEST FOR SPEECH THERAPY

Name ....Date of birth ....Ward ....

Date of admission............................. Previous admissions.............................

Previous occupation.............................When last employed.............................

Unit No.............................Provisional diagnosis.............................

Medication.............................

This part to be completed by the doctor

Physical disabilities

Special difficulties (e.g. Absconds: Suicidal: Convulsive)

Problems needing attention

Date ....Doctor's signature ....

Speech Therapy Notes

Date	REMARKS	Signature

Figure 10.1   Example of request for speech therapy form (N. J. Muir, West Park Hospital, Surrey; P. Tanner, Horton Hospital, Surrey, 1989).

Examples of information that may be useful would be epilepsy, transient ischaemic attacks, violence, absconding and other physical or behavioural complications.

GENERAL APPROACH

The clinic

Accommodation can be a problem for speech therapists as a profession being fairly new to psychiatric settings. A general rule to follow is never to accept isolated treatment rooms as it is vital to have other personnel within call. In certain settings (e.g. secure units) a 'panic button' in the treatment room is essential. A treatment room large enough to create an informal and comfortable setting is likely to promote ease of communication and should have clear and easy access to the door. A patient may wish to leave quickly if the session becomes too stressful or their mood changes, and obviously if the patient should become aroused the therapist will need to be able to vacate the room quickly and with the minimum of confrontation. A telephone in the treatment room is important so that help can be sought in case of an emergency. It is pleasant to include coffee- and tea-making facilities to promote a social atmosphere, which can be of great benefit when establishing rapport.

Not all psychiatric settings are the large, cold, rather bleak hospitals that people tend to picture, but should they be so then it is often much appreciated by the patient if the clinical areas are a pleasant contrast. Date boards, clocks, pictures, pretty curtains, comfortable chairs, non-institutional crockery, some plants, good lighting and *plenty* of ashtrays are among the details worth attending to.

The therapist

Most speech therapists have gained skills from their training that would equip them well for work with the mentally ill. However, these skills, both broad based and specific, in the areas of speech, language and communication, are often unrecognized within the profession itself and outside. As skilled listeners, communicators and diagnosticians speech therapists have much to offer. Confidence, maturity of approach, adaptability and above all good self-monitoring skills are felt to be of great importance. Work with the mentally ill requires of the therapist the ability to think on his or her feet. Having assessed, set goals and planned therapy it may be necessary to change approach mid-session to fit the needs of the patient on that particular day or at that particular stage of their illness.

On a purely practical level the therapist would be well advised to follow a few basic hints with regard to appearance. In settings with severely behaviourally disturbed patients it is a sensible precaution for male therapists to wear detachable ties and for female therapists to avoid jewellery or scarves round the neck. Discussion with other staff is recommended to ensure appropriate choice of clothing, particularly when working with patients with a known history of violent behaviour or sexual disturbance.

Information gathering

On receiving a referral the therapist may first wish to meet the patient, to talk to other carers, or to read the full medical notes. Whichever approach to information gathering is taken it is very important not to have any preconceived ideas or expectations before meeting the patient. As in most other areas of speech therapy useful information to elicit would be a general history, medical history past and present, a social, family and cultural history and a general picture of present status. A knowledge of the patient's medication is felt to be essential, as has been stated.

The multidisciplinary team is an excellent way of eliciting information which will cover the many facets of difficulties experienced by patients. Liaison with, for example, occupational therapy, physiotherapy, psychology, social services, nursing and medical staff is essential.

First interview

The flexibility of approach that should run through all work in psychiatric settings also applies to the choice of location for a first meeting with the patient. It is often impossible to send an appointment card and rely on the patient arriving in the department. An escort may be necessary. It may be more appropriate to visit the patient on the ward or in the home and guidance may be sought as to whether this visit is better planned or unannounced. However the first interview comes about, a certain amount of informality is necessary. The therapist needs to appear relaxed, friendly and non-threatening. Choices of location and topic of conversation need in many cases to be dictated by the patient and directed by the therapist. All explanations of the reasons for the suggested contact and the role of the therapist need to be clear and simple, without any suggestion of condescension. A calm and soothing voice and general approach are also of great benefit. All the therapist's non-verbal behaviour needs to be carefully monitored and consistent with the situation – for example, over-direct eye contact can be threatening, as can sitting too close. Asking too many questions, use of touch, or direct attempts to confront delusional ideas may be inappropriate for a first meeting and subsequent ones too in some cases. Humour has been found to be of great use, when used sensitively, in establishing rapport and helping the patient to relax.

It is often underrated as to just how much 'gut reaction' can provide insights later borne out by formal assessment and the opinions of the patient's carers. Instinct can often guide thinking as to what will work for the therapist in any given situation and what it appears might work for a patient. It is very important to react instinctively in a first interview to any indication that the patient can no longer tolerate or cope with the topic or the situation. This demonstration of insight and flexibility may make the difference between attendance and non-attendance in the future. Experience has taught the writers that a short social meeting over a cup of coffee or in comfortable surroundings will accomplish much and also that to listen to the patient's own perceptions of their difficulties, no matter how bizarre, can be of significant value in indicating the line or lines of approach for later in therapy.

One thing well worth bearing constantly in mind when first meeting patients, especially those who are thought disordered or actively psychotic, is how complex and often misleading language can be. Vocabulary needs to be chosen carefully since words with alternative meanings can lead to errors and misinterpretations. There is a rather poor joke in which a therapist says to a neurotic patient with kleptomanic tendencies, 'just take things quietly'. The writers can quote an example of hearing a patient who was a long-term alcohol abuser with resultant Korsakoff's psychosis being asked 'How are you in your spirits?' On a more serious note there was some distress provoked but a good deal of insight gained in the following section of an interview which took place recently:

Therapist: 'What do you think triggers this off?'
Patient: 'That's it. I'm in the firing line. They've got me in their sights.
   They all want to kill me.'

ASSESSMENT

It is often imagined that assessment in psychiatry must be very complex and demanding, involving psychomotor testing, personality testing, neuropsychological testing, behavioural testing, and much else. There are no definitive formal assessments of speech, language and communication in mentally ill people – which has the effect at one and the same time of simplifying and confusing the issue. However, traditional speech therapy tests can be of use and will be discussed further. Access to other formal testing materials of the types listed above is beneficial, but these assessments may be better carried out by psychiatrists or psychologists who are likely to be more skilled in interpreting the results.

The mentally ill patient is likely to present with a wide range of signs and symptoms, and the greater the variety of assessment techniques employed the greater the likelihood of fitting the pieces of the jigsaw together.

Observations and informal assessment

The speech therapist naturally wishes to gain information on the patient's language skills (both receptive and expressive), on his or her speech (with regard to factors affecting intelligibility and general fluency, etc.) and on the patient's verbal and non-verbal communicative ability in many differing situations. Recording of observations is very important and can help the therapist gain great insight into many key areas. These would include comprehension at a simple social level as well as comprehension of complex ideational material and, on the expressive side, verbal output both semantically and syntactically, as well as at a simple pragmatic level, to establish if the patient can initiate and maintain discourse and interact in an appropriate way. It is also possible to begin to gauge concentration and attention span, and non-verbal behaviours such as personal care, mannerisms, tone, prosody, colour and affect of communicative behaviours. Evidence of concrete thinking, ideas of reference or of thought insertion, grandiose ideas or paranoia may be noted, as may any evidence of sensory impairment – for example, hearing loss or visual difficulty. Speech therapists may gain insight into the patient's motivation, memory skills and self-monitoring abilities or self-awareness. It may also be possible to begin to see any strategies the patient regularly uses either to cope, to mask or to avoid in any situation.

A skilled listener can begin to make some reasoned judgements in this very informal way. For example, is the patient using neologisms or is there evidence of paraphasia or of linguistic errors? It is possible to note if changes in vocabulary appear to reflect swings in mood, if speed of utterance or intelligibility vary with increasing mania or conversely with the onset of a depressive phase. In an informal setting it is also possible to pick up evidence of pre-morbid speech problems, for example articulation disorder or stutter, and in cases where English is not the first language to try and sort errors into those that are more obviously psychotic and those that are due to poor grasp of the language. Finally clues can be provided for future assessment and for management, particularly if certain behaviours appear to be regular, consistent and measurable.

Case history taking

When one works in any area of psychiatry the taking of a case history can prove difficult. If the patient is acutely ill they may at best only be able to give sporadic and ill-formed information and at worst be, for the time, inaccessible and therefore unable to give any information. This may, for example, occur in cases of elective mutism, severe depression and withdrawal. If the patient has been a long-stay resident in an institution the information on their past history that they are able to give may be very cloudy and many patients with chronic mental illness may have been in-patients for up to sixty years. The severity of the illness and the extent of the institutionalization will determine the amount of information that it is possible to elicit from the patient personally.

As in so many other areas of therapy, within a psychiatric setting a great deal of recourse needs to be made to the patient's support network. The family can obviously provide information but it may be only their very individual perceptions of the problem and therefore only one side of a many-sided coin. When working in a psychiatric hospital with long-stay patients access to the family may not be a possibility because the hospital is not local or because the family have dispersed or died. In these cases the history needs to be culled from medical notes and from nursing and other staff who may have known the patient for many years. However, it must be borne in mind that staff, like families, are vulnerable to personal prejudices.

Information needed on a case history is obviously fairly standard but there does need to be attention paid to certain areas. An example of a case history form can be seen in Figure 10.2.

All this information, gained from whatever source, can form part of a case history but it is again important not to be judgemental and not to use the information to form unshakeable opinions on the patient. Insights gained or descriptions recorded can be borne out by further assessment.

Checklists and formal assessment

Checklists can provide a valuable source of information if suitably devised. The speech therapist or a key worker can then record obser-

Speech Therapy Service – Case History Form

Name...Date of Birth...

Date of Admission to Hospital............................First Contact...........................

Ward..Key Worker...

Referred by..Date..

Medication.....................................Medical Diagnosis.......................................

Medical History

Family History (to include relationships with the family past or present)

Social History (to include preferences, abilities and psychosexual behaviour)

Educational History (to include standards attained)

General History (to include pre-morbid personality and present hobbies and interests)

Other Assessments (to include medical, e.g. CT scan, EEG, psychological, nursing)

Information from staff

Observations

Figure 10.2 Example of speech therapy case history form. (N.J. Muir, West Park Hospital, Surrey; P. Tanner, Horton Hospital, Surrey; 1989).

vations on various aspects of communicative behaviour. Examples of three checklists appear in the Appendix (Appendix 10.1, 10.2 and 10.3), one looking at general communicative behaviours and two at social skills, but the speech therapist may wish to devise checklists to record receptive or expressive skills, attention levels, memory or any other skill related to communication which can be measured objectively but informally. Due to the importance now given by all care staff to assessment of skills as the cornerstone for appropriate care planning, the speech therapist may be asked to devise the language and communication section of a broader-based checklist to be used by the whole team.

Language assessments

Various assessments more traditionally used with dysphasic patients can give accurate information on receptive and expressive language skills in mentally ill patients, including an Aphasia Screening Test (Whurr, 1974), the Minnesota Test of Differential Diagnosis of Aphasia (Schuell, 1965), and its Shortened Version (Schuell, 1973), the Boston Diagnostic Aphasic Examination (Goodglass and Kaplan, 1983), the Boston Naming Test (Kaplan, Goodglass and Weintraub, 1983), and the Token Test (De Renzi and Vignolo, 1972) or the Revised Token Test (McNeil and Prescott, 1978).

All these assessments can be used to measure change over time, which is particularly vital in the dementias and in degenerative disorders like Huntingdon's chorea. There can be difficulties in administering these tests given that patients may find the situation threatening and may have poor compliance and concentration. It may be that only certain sections of the tests are felt to be appropriate and this can lead to difficulty with obtaining valid scores. The tests mentioned were standardized on dysphasics, whose performance is likely to be less erratic than that of a psychiatric patient with communication difficulties. This all points to the need for the production of standardized tests of language ability for the psychiatric population and it is hoped that this will be a future development.

Speech assessment

The assessment of patients with symptoms of dysarthria is to some extent more traditional. The dysarthria may be due to the side-effects of drug therapy or to organic involvement. The therapist in psychiatry will require the same information on the mechanical breakdown of speech as the therapist in a general setting. The Frenchay Dysarthria

Assessment (Enderby, 1988), and the Dysarthria Profile (Robertson, 1982) are used a great deal, in the UK particularly, and provide vital information on the nature and extent of the dysarthria. In the assessment of voice the Victoria Infirmary Voice Questionnaire (Lockhart and Martin, 1987) is widely used.

Functional communication

Given that this is the area where patients with a mental illness are often experiencing the greatest difficulty, these tests can provide a greater range of information. Widely used is the Edinburgh Functional Communication Profile (Skinner *et al.*, 1984) and also the Functional Communication Profile (Sarno, 1963).

In the introduction to the Functional Communication Profile, which was developed at the New York University Medical Centre, the author equates the idea of measuring function in communication with tests measuring levels of disability and how it affects the patient's daily living skills. She points out that 'most tests have concerned themselves with identifying *what* the patient says and not *how* he communicated it'. All speech therapists recognize that analytical testing is fundamental to the understanding of language deficits and therapists are now aware of the difficulties in translating these findings into everyday terms and are therefore making efforts to look at the implications of the deficit in the widest sense, that is, can the patient cope with his life situation?

As has been stated elsewhere the psychiatric patient is often multiply handicapped in communication and functional communication profiles like those above look at a range of behaviours including those vital areas of gestures, body cues and visual cues.

Video and audio tape recording

Use of video and of audio tape recording can provide useful information when assessing a patient. Both can be very valuable in that when concentrating on formal testing it is often difficult to be aware of and record objectively all the patient's 'off-test' behaviours. Since both video and audio tape recording allows for play-back and for checking and rechecking feelings, reactions and findings objectively and with others in the team, they can serve as ongoing assessments and for treatment. Permission needs to be sought from the patient or the next of kin when making recordings. Failing that, agreement must be obtained from the patient's consultant. This is particularly important if the tapes are to be used for teaching or demonstration purposes.

Language analysis

Video and audio recordings provide the therapist with samples of speech, language and communicative behaviour that can be further analyzed. The tapes and/or transcripts can also be used for a comparison of pre/post-intervention levels of functioning.

The literature that has examined the characteristics of speech and language in psychiatric patients has confined itself mainly in two areas of abnormality – the language of dementia and schizophrenic language. The language of dementia is covered elsewhere in this book but it is relevent to mention some of the methods of 'analysis' that have been used in the study of schizophrenic language, with particular reference to methods which may be useful for speech therapists working in this field. There has been a considerable amount of literature on this subject. Techniques that have been used include word association tasks, Cloze procedure (Cheek and Amarel, 1968; Rutter *et al.*, 1978), reconstruction (Rutter, 1979) and linguistic analysis.

Word association tasks

This was one of the earliest techniques used and it focuses on the stimulus–response model of speech production and comprehension. The patient was given a word as a stimulus and his response was recorded. The results from these early experiments are unreliable because replication studies have failed to find comparable results.

Cloze procedure

This procedure is based on a journalism technique of readability. Speech samples are collected from schizophrenics (usually uninterrupted monologue) and are then transcribed with the fourth or fifth word deleted. A point is given for every word restored correctly and a Cloze Score is obtained. The Cloze Score is, in effect, a measure of the degree of redundancy in the text.

Reconstruction

In this method samples of schizophrenic language are transcribed and punctuated into sentences by a 'blind' assistant and the first ten sentences from each passage are typed onto separate strips of card, one sentence per card. 'Reconstructors' are then given the first sentence and are asked to put the rest of the jumbled sentences into their original order. A score is given for each sentence placed correctly after its immediate predecessor. This technique can be used by a variety of professions because it does not require a detailed knowledge of linguistics and it can be used to analyze both monologue and discourse.

Linguistic analysis of discourse

This has also been used by a number of researchers (Rochester and Martin, 1979; Rutter, 1985). The system has two parts, of which the first examines the number of cohesive ties in each sample and the frequency of each type; that is, lexical, reference, conjunction, substitution and ellipsis. The second analysis examines the reference network – phoric (i.e. reference back to previous text) and non-phoric – generally the presentation of new material, which may or may not be followed up by the patient in conversation. The unit of analysis is the nominal group, which corresponds approximately to the noun phrase in phrase structure grammar, and the first stage is to calculate the proportions of nominal groups which are phoric and non-phoric, respectively. Phoric units can then be broken down further. This system of analysis is only unlikely to be used when research is being carried out because it is time consuming and requires a trained linguist.

Linguistic profiles

In 1982 Crystal suggested a system of profiling linguistic disability which can be used in any case of abnormal language and could be useful to speech therapists in psychiatry. They are, in effect, gross simplifications of linguistic descriptions but they do require the therapist to have a knowledge of linguistic theory and technique. Crystal states that 'profiles try to focus attention on remedial paths in a systematic and theoretically motivated way'.

The profiling procedure involves obtaining a sample of patient data, transcribing it, analyzing the transcription, profiling the analysis on a summary chart, assessing the pattern on the profile chart and then interpreting the profile in remedial terms. Crystal has described four main profiles: LARSP, which is used to assess grammar; PROPH, which assesses segmental phonology; PROP, for non-segmental phonology (prosody); and PRISM, for assessing semantics in both the lexical and grammatical dimensions. Clinically, as part of assessment procedures, they have made a valuable contribution by adding clarification and detail of the language abnormality. The writers are not aware of any studies in psychiatry that have used Crystal's linguistic profiles as yet but they would be worth considering as assessment tools for research because they describe language in a systematic, theoretical way.

Reading tests

Testing reading skills can be of great value in establishing the status of a patient's abilities in order to devise a wide-ranging therapy programme involving as many life skills as possible. In a paper by Nelson and McKenna (1975) it was established that word-reading ability was less affected than other language-processing skills by dementing processes and it therefore follows that word-reading ability tests can provide useful indicators of the pre-morbid level of intellectual functioning. Tests that may be useful include the New Adult Reading Test (Nelson, 1983) and the Neale Analysis of Reading Ability (revised, 1988) which are weighted to elicit word meanings via the direct graphemic–semantic route rather than the graphemic–phonemic route.

Memory tests

Memory problems represent one of the commonest complaints of patients who are brain damaged and a deterioration in memory can signal the onset of a dementing process in patients with a previous history of 'other' mental illness. Concentration can be affected by drug therapy and so too can memory – immediate, recent and long term – for both storing and retrieval of information. Assessment of memory is undertaken as part of testing by psychologists and there are many tests for measuring memory function. The most valuable are felt by the writers to be those which identify the occurrence of everyday memory problems and attempt to qualify the frequency and severity of such problems. Two such assessments are the Rivermead Behavioural Memory Test (Wilson *et al.*, 1985) and the National Hospital Memory Battery (Warrington, 1985). Speech therapists will assess memory in the context of how it affects the language breakdown, and establish which pathway (visual, auditory, kinaesthetic) is most intact and can therefore be used in retraining.

Social skills assessments

There are many social skills rating scales available; examples of these can be found in *The Social Skills Training Manual* (Wilkinson and Canter, 1982). Since social skills training developed from two main sources, namely assertion training initiated in America in the 1960s and interpersonal psychology discussed in relation to mental health by exponents such as Trower, Bryant and Argyle (1978), assessment materials tend to reflect this bias towards one or other source. From assertion training come measurements of social behaviours which can then be improved by the use of techniques such as modelling, shaping, feedback and role play. From interpersonal psychology come ideas for assessments which analyze various elements of social behaviour and non-verbal communication skills.

The development in this area has had impact on approaches to assessment and therapy in mental health. Many professions are involved in social skills assessment; this may be devised and carried out by psychologists, occupational therapists, psychiatric nurses and others, as well as by speech therapists. Each profession is likely to have its own bias towards assessment and will add a varied dimension to this complex area. Two examples can be found in the Appendix (Appendix 10.1 and 10.2) one devised by a speech therapist and the other by a clinical psychologist.

A speech therapist's assessments are likely to include most of the communicative aspects of social interaction. What may be required from social skills assessments is information on verbal, vocal and non-verbal behaviours. Speech therapists working in psychiatry also see the need for social skills assessments to include information demonstrating the patient's insight into social and communicative behaviours – both his own and those of others. This aspect is often overlooked and the speech therapist may need to stress the receptive component in this area of assessment, which often only considers expressive behaviours. Any checklist devised should aim to assess the presenting behaviour or deficit by looking at certain aspects of social interactions and specific skills. The speech therapist may include eye contact, posture, facial expression, gesture and listening skills, as well as the ability to initiate and maintain appropriate social contact and response needs to be rated. Three- to five-point rating scales are usually sufficient for measuring levels of behaviour response in their varying degrees.

Behavioural testing

This is very obviously a form of assessment used by clinical psychologists, but as part of a multidisciplinary team approach in some behavioural units the speech therapist needs to be aware of such tests and particularly of the section involving communication. Evaluation of social skills, as above, is measuring one major aspect of behaviour of which the speech therapist will be aware in treatment.

All assessment used in behavioural units measure behaviour across a range of situations. The measurements obtained may focus on behavioural excesses or deficits. Patients in a very acute phase of a neurotic or psychotic disorder are likely to present with excess of certain behaviours, among which may be communication. Pressure of speech, speed of utterance, multiplicity of expressed ideas, egocentricity, fixed or delusional ideas are all likely to be identified by assessment. Chronic patients are likely to present with behavioural deficits and in communication the assessment is likely to reveal paucity of speech and ideas, lowered rate and volume of utterance and difficulties with initiating and maintaining interaction.

Examples of current behavioural tests in use by psychologists, Nursing staff and other care staff working in rehabilitation settings are the Clifton Assessment Procedure for the Elderly (Pattie and Gilleard, 1979), which has a cognitive scale and a social evaluation scale. This has proved of value in assessing the level of dependency of long-stay patients. The Rehabilitation Evaluation (Hall and Baker, 1983) has two parts, the first concerned with deviant behaviours and the second with general social and everyday behaviours. The National Unit for Psychiatric Research and Development Questionnaires (Clifford, 1987) is another example. These questionnaires are available to assess three areas of functioning: firstly, levels attained for possible community placement; secondly, social functioning; and thirdly, psychological functioning and problems. Results of all behavioural assessments should provide integrated information to assist in drawing up individual care plans and in service planning. The Social Behaviour Assessment Schedule (Platt, Hirsch and Weyman, 1983) is also often used in behavioural units. It has six sections recording patients' behaviour, social performance, adverse effects of the behaviour on others, concurrent events, support to carers and housing situation and it rates the frequency of behaviours and the degree of distress on a five-point scale for patients and for others in the home situation or ward. Information gained from this assessment is suitable for transfer to a computer. The speech therapist's role in behavioural assessments is one of expanding on communication which is often an under-explored or simplistic section of many tests and checklists. The role of the speech therapist in care planning needs to be one of prioritizing communication skills on the hierachy of aims and goals set by the care team.

Personality appraisal

There are great difficulties encountered in assessment or appraisal of personality. There is an element of invasion of privacy and the self-disclosure called for can be at the very least uncomfortable. In this particular form of assessment there may be false responses in that patients could alter their reply out of embarrassment or anxiety so that the reply is perceived as more 'socially acceptable'. It is recommended that only speech therapists with relevant training in this area should attempt these assessments, which usually take the form of Inventories. Chapter 7 considers this area further.

Personality inventories

Among those used are the Minnesota Multiphasic Personality Inventory (Hathaway and McKinley, 1970), which has an empirical construction and was based on studies of monozygotic and dizygotic twins after the work of Gottesman (1963). It has 550 statements to which the patient needs to respond as being true or not true for them. A test like The Eysenck Personality Inventory (Eysenck and Eysenck, 1963) is designed according to theory with experimental validation.

Personal construct grids

When used with patients able to make rational subjective choices, personal construct grids can provide great insight into how that patient views himself or herself and applying the personal construct theory can be of significant use in the area of personality appraisal. Personal construct theory is discussed further in this and other chapters. Personality appraisal is a very complex area since personality is an integrated whole which can be viewed from different directions, such as attitudes, temperament, aptitudes, morphology, physiology, needs and interests.

Other assessment tools for personality appraisal

Personality may also be assessed via Cattell's 16 PF (personality factors) Questionnaire (Cattell and Ebel, 1968), which relies on factor analysis of source personality traits rather than surface ones. Source traits are found by factor analysis which shows that highly correlated traits belong together. Examples of source traits would be ego strength versus emotionality and neuroticism and dominance versus submissiveness (Cattell, 1965). Surface traits are found by raw analysis of data and are so called because their similarity lies on the surface and the uniformity is clearly apparent. Examples of surface traits would be integrity and altruism versus dishonesty and independability or heartiness versus shyness (Cattell, 1952). The questionnaire postulates that analysis of the main source traits, among them dominance and emotional stability, will lead to a representative picture of the whole personality sphere.

Personality can also be assessed in the form of personal preference scales, for example that of Edwards (1954). In this the patient has to make forced choices between statements, judged to be equally desirable or undesirable. This is felt to minimize the effect of 'social acceptability' which, as has been suggested earlier, can affect response. The items in the test were chosen to reflect basic motivational needs, among them achievement, abasement, dominance and autonomy.

Also available are projective tests like the Rorschach Inkblot Test (Rorschach, 1942) or thematic apperception tests (TAT) where pictures are used to provoke story telling. These presume that many comments made from the imagination when weaving a story will reveal certain 'themes' and these themes may be highly personalized and reflect the life experiences, thoughts and feelings of the story teller.

DIFFERENTIAL DIAGNOSIS

All formal assessment tools used in psychiatry should offer pointers to diagnosis. Very complex symptoms are present and can involve emotional, social, psychological, organic and behavioural deficits or, in some cases, excesses. It is therefore vital to be able to sort one from the other where possible, and the major diagnostic dilemmas faced by the speech therapist will be discussed below.

Dementia versus dysphasia

The debate with regard to terminology is considered in Chapter 8, which outlines the pattern of language breakdown in dementia. This is an area where there is a good deal of research and certain broad areas of difference have been highlighted, which it is important to note. The ten-point table (Table 10.1) illustrates some notable differences in behaviours affecting language and communication and is derived from some of the recent research and from the personal experience of the writers (Stevens, 1985b; Hodkinson *et al.*, 1984; Walker, 1982; Wertz, 1984).

The Dementia Check List (Stevens, 1985a) is valuable in that it looks at general and language signs in mild dementia, moderate dementia and severe dementia. Chapter 8 considers this area in more detail.

Dysarthria: neurological or drug-induced

Whether dysarthria is neurologically based or drug induced has great implications for treatment, particularly pharmacologically. The recent medical history of the patient may give clues to the reason for the onset of the dysarthria. Any deterioration in health, evidence of vascular involvement, episodes of weakness, tremor, fainting or transient ischae-

Table 10.1 Differential diagnosis pointers

	Dysphasia	Dementia
1 Social behaviour (social skills)	Tends to be appropriate	Tends to be inappropriate
2 Orientation (time, place, person)	Likely to be intact	Likely to be poor
3 Short-term (recent) memory	Relatively good	Likely to be poor
4 Affect (emotional responses)	Tends to be appropriate	Tends to be bizarre or absent
5 Personality	Tends to be fewer changes	Tends to be significant changes
6 Level of insight	More insight leading to more frustration	Less insight leading to less frustration
7 Activities (communicative and behavioural)	Tend to be more purposeful	Can be purposeless, e.g. shouting, screaming or fiddling with clothes or objects
8 General behaviour	Likely to be more consistent	Likely to be more inconsistent
9 Initiation of activities	Likely to initiate an activity	Rarely initiates an activity
10 Retention of information (ability to learn)	Remains relatively intact	Tends to be poor

After Stevens (1985)

mic attacks would obviously point to neurological causation. Recent alteration in medication with an increase or change in the prescription of neuroleptics, even a very slight increase or a relatively minor change, would point to drug-induced dysarthria. In this case the patient will often complain of, or show signs of having, a dry mouth. There may be tardive dyskinesia, that is, slowing and impairment of voluntary motion, and/or orofacial dyskinesia, characterized by uncontrolled chewing movements, grimaces and manneristic tics of which the patient may be unaware. The patient may complain of and demonstrate signs of extreme restlessness or akathisia, which means the patient feels compelled to move about or keep getting up. For the medical team the differential diagnosis would significantly alter the management. If the origin is neurological, then further medical investigations are indicated – for example, EEG, ECG or CT scan may be deemed necessary. If the origin is drug induced then a review of medication is indicated and there may be the need to reduce the neuroleptic or to add one of the anticholinergic drugs, which would reduce the extrapyramidal effects caused in part by the suppressed dopamine levels. The speech therapist must be prepared to accept the situation if the benefits of the drug therapy, in terms of a marked improvement in mental state, outweigh the side-effects on communication. Should this be the case then the speech therapist can reinforce explanations of the side-effects and offer support to the patient.

It is worth pointing out that there may very well be side-effects, as mentioned above, in patients who have been drug or substance abusers. In these cases the speech therapist may be asked to offer individual sessions to patients involved in ongoing group psychotherapy and counselling at drug or alcohol dependency units.

For the speech therapist, certainty of this differential diagnosis will also have some treatment implications. If the dysarthria is drug induced then the therapist would need to assess the patient's level of insight, their self-monitoring skills and their bio-feedback mechanisms. Improvement in these areas can, when combined with traditional techniques, help the patient regain some measure of voluntary control over their speech. If there is a neurological basis then techniques will be those traditionally associated with therapy for dysarthria and involve exercises for musculature, respiration, prosody, rate and so on (Robertson, 1982).

Paranoia and hearing impairment

At first sight this might appear to be a rather odd pairing for the purposes of differential diagnosis, but the writers have observed the two conditions in parallel and become aware that a great deal of confusion can result. Patients with paranoid delusions report hearing 'voices' and these auditory hallucinations may take the form of actual speech which may be amusing, pleasant, aggressive, threatening, frightening or directive. The hallucinations may be prompted by outside influences like the radio, television or background noise. Patients with paranoid symptoms of their psychosis often find it very hard to discard or filter any extraneous auditory stimuli and they will often personalize what is heard. Therefore if there is also a hearing loss (whether it be conductive or sensorineural) the patient is only going to receive part of the auditory information. The paranoia may be intensified by the feeling of being withdrawn or removed from situations and sounds may take on different meanings. Failure to hear properly may lead to the patient wrongly construing or interpreting what is said or what is taking place. In addition there may be tinnitus, which can be described as a subjective ringing, roaring or hissing sound, and if one picks out the word subjective from the definition the parallel becomes obvious. The noises described by tinnitus sufferers can, for those who also suffer from paranoid delusions and auditory hallucinations, become highly significant. One patient known to the writers was profoundly deaf and when very ill became severely paranoid. As she began to recover the threatening, directive voices became animal and traffic sounds and as her condition stabilized she was able to report only her tinnitus.

If a patient is suffering from paranoid delusions there are obvious implications for assessment of any hearing loss. The therapist cannot simply confront the patient with a screening audiometer, which could have many connotations. The patient is likely to have a deep-rooted suspicion of any machine and may feel the therapist is trying to read their thoughts, damage their brain, deliver some electroconvulsive therapy, or inflict any number of other distressing possibilities. Explanation of screening audiometry needs to be very clear and preparation for the test must be careful. Results of formal audiological testing with a patient experiencing paranoid feelings can be unreliable. It may therefore be necessary to resort to more informal assessment and observation. Whispered tests at varying decibel levels and at varying distances can be helpful, as can observation of the patient in group and other situations. Any attempt at assessing hearing when the patient is severely paranoid is going to have to be carefully handled and the speech therapist may take the role either of performing a screening assessment to prepare the patient for referral to an audiometric clinic or prepare the audiologist to receive the patient, should the audiologist have no psychiatric experience. If closed circuit audiometry is contra-indicated or unsuccessful then stimulus response testing or EEG may be necessary.

Language disorder or intellectual impairment

Close liaison with the psychologist is vital in this area. The test most often used by psychologists to determine IQ is the Wechsler Adult Intelligence Scale (Wechsler, 1981), which gives qualitative and quantitative information via verbal subtests. Several verbal fluency tests are in use but one that psychologists particularly commend is Miller's Verbal Fluency Test (1984), which makes an allowance for the effect of IQ level and assesses the verbal fluency function as a measure of verbal intelligence and in relation to different types of cerebral pathology.

IQ testing performed by clinical psychologists will give full-scale IQ measurements, as well as separate verbal and performance scores. If the verbal score is significantly lower than the performance score one would need to look to the patient's case history or to the family for further information. There may have been, for example, delayed language acquisition, interrupted or unsatisfactory education, delinquency problems in childhood, or evidence of early-onset (prodromal) psychotic illness. All these factors would influence the development of language skills independently of intellectual functioning.

In mental illness settings there are often mixed diagnoses and the combination most often highlighted is that of moderate learning disorder (MLD) and mental illness. It is of vital importance that speech therapists should try to make clear for others the distinction between a degree of educational subnormality and a specific language disorder. This task is not made easy by less than full records and case histories, poor contact with relations and often unreliable information from the patient. The differential diagnosis can be further complicated when English is the patient's second language, as with some in long-term institutional care; for example, there are many Polish ex-servicemen who broke down during the world wars now in UK hospitals. Formal and wide-ranging language assessments like the Schuell (1965, 1973) and the Boston (Goodglass and Kaplan, 1983) can give a clear breakdown of abilities in certain areas. The Illinois Test of Psycholinguistic Ability (Kirk *et al.*, 1968) although usually used with children can also give useful and relevant information, even though no fully reliable score can be obtained and validated.

Dementia and depression

It is not uncommon to have a patient referred to speech therapy because there is confusion about the diagnosis between dementia and depression. Lezak (1983) stated that 'probably the knottiest problem of differential diagnosis is that of separating depressed from demented patients who early in the course of their disease do not yet show the characteristic symptoms of dementia'. For example, a depressed withdrawn elderly patient can be easily confused with a demented patient because neither talks much, the language they use is limited and restricted in content and they often appear unable to understand fully what is said to them. Therefore the speech therapist may be requested to carry out an assessment to help determine whether the problem is an organic or a functional one.

The Test for the Reception of Grammar (TROG) (Bishop, 1983) is designed to assess the understanding of grammatical contrasts in English and although it was not intended or standardized for this patient population (this test has been standardized for children but not with an adult population) it has been found to be useful because it shows a difference in performance levels between demented and depressed patients. As has been stated elsewhere, demented patients have difficulty in many areas of cognitive functioning including receptive language skills, but depressed patients can usually manage the TROG with no obvious problems.

Another reliable method of discriminating dementia from depression is to use verbal fluency tasks, which require the patient, in a fixed period of time, to name as many words as he can beginning with a particular letter, or to name individual items within a certain category. Depressed patients show relatively normal verbal fluency (Kronfol et al., 1978) whilst demented patients show poorer function (Miller and Hague, 1975).

Clinically it is important to determine the differential diagnosis between dementia and depression because obviously it has direct implications for the management of the patient and his illness. It may be possible that depressed patients will benefit from medication, counselling or changes in their social situation (e.g. by attendance at a day centre). Patients in the early stages of dementia and their families can be supported and encouraged to adopt coping strategies; for example, impaired memory function can sometimes be improved or at least maintained with the use of external aids like a portable notebook in which the patient can make a note of appointments and messages, and he can then refer to the book again whenever he needs to remember things (Wilson and Moffat, 1984).

Schizophrenia and dysphasia

It seems unlikely that an experienced speech therapist would have much difficulty differentiating between these two conditions. However, it should not be presumed that other disciplines have the same knowledge and skills as speech therapists. In fact, an article by Faber et al. (1983) demonstrates that both psychiatrists and neurologists have difficulty differentiating schizophrenic patients from dysphasic ones. Taped samples were taken from two groups of subjects: 13 aphasic and 14 thought-disordered schizophrenic patients. The tapes were then transcribed and presented to a speech pathologist, two neurologists and two psychiatrists for blind classification as either aphasic or schizophrenic. In addition, the speech pathologist categorized the specific type of language disorder seen in each patient (e.g. neologisms, paraphasias).

The proportion correctly identified by the specialists ranged from 66.7% to 92.6%. In the identification of the 27 subjects, correct classifications were made 25 times by the speech pathologist, 22 times by psychiatrist 1, 20 times by psychiatrist 2, and 18 times by each neurologist. Only the speech pathologist achieved a kappa value of 0.86, indicative of high discriminating ability.

There are no formal standardized tests that are likely to help differentiate schizophrenic language from aphasic disorder. For example, in 1972 Horsfall was unable to differentiate the performance of these two groups of patients using the Porch Index of Communicative Abilities (Porch, 1973). It is more helpful to look closely at the language abnormalities present in these disorders. Both the study by Gerson et al. (1977) and Faber et al. (1983) found it possible to distinguish the diagnosis on the basis of verbal production. For example, word approximations or a private use of words and derailment or tangentiality were seen significantly more often among schizophrenics than aphasic patients. Aphasics more frequently exhibited poverty of speech content, reduced auditory comprehension and word-finding problems. In addition, in Faber's study, complex word usage (not an abnormality) was observed in 79% of the schizophrenic patients but in only 8% of the aphasic patients. However, there is also substantial evidence to support the suggestion that there is considerable overlap of language dysfunction in both these groups. Faber et al. found an equal incidence of neologisms and paraphasias in both groups and specific language dysfunction in schizophrenic patients has been reported previously in studies by Di Simoni et al. (1977), Andreasen and Grove (1979) and Faber and Reichstein (1981). Most of the above studies do not discuss the paralinguistic features of the disorders but their contribution to the assessment process should not be underestimated. For example, the hesitancy and slow rate of utterance of some aphasic patients contrasts with the rapid, frenetic utterances of the acute schizophrenic. The two disorders use the paralinguistic features of volume, pitch and stress in different ways as well as an assessment of these features can help in the differential diagnosis.

Another discriminating feature of schizophrenia that is not usually present in dysphasia involves a disturbance affecting sentence to sentence sequencing and cohesion in monologue and discourse. Reconstruction studies by Rutter in 1979 and 1985 illustrated this feature very well. He did not find any linguistic abnormality at the sentence level where syntactic and lexical rules were used appropriately but the breakdown involved the connection of sentence to sentence. There is some

267

suggestion that a language abnormality of this kind could be classified as a pragmatic disorder (Ostwald, 1978).

It is critical that a correct diagnosis is made between dysphasia and schizophrenia because the management of the two disorders is so different. For example, an aphasic patient often requires speech therapy, at least for assessment purposes, whereas this may not always be appropriate for the schizophrenic patient. The priority for an acutely ill schizophrenic patient, who is using bizarre and disordered language, is probably to stabilize his mental state with medication so that he can then make full use of any 'therapy' offered to him.

Clearly assessment is the cornerstone to patient-oriented work in all areas of speech therapy. From the assessment comes insight into the patient's difficulties, measurement of those difficulties and the information with which to set achievable goals and plan therapy programmes. In mental health the illness itself can be all pervasive. It therefore follows that the effects of that illness on communication, itself an all-encompassing skill, can be dramatic and of infinite variety. It has often been said that the dividing line between 'sanity' and 'insanity' is very thin, with socially acceptable eccentricity being very little removed from 'madness'. Most people who are lucky enough to be thought of as 'normal' are aware of changes in mood which affect communication. If a person is tired, a little unwell or emotionally low then output is less, whereas if the person is in good form physically and emotionally and on a 'high' then output increases. Mood can be affected by others, by situations and even by the weather, and communication output swings with mood. If this is recognized personally it helps in grasping some of the facts about communication in mental illness. It will help therapists to remain aware of the importance of assessment, whether they be carried out by speech therapists or other team members, both informal and formal. In psychiatry, assessment is ongoing and information about the patient should constantly be added to. It is vital to observe and record communicating behaviours in as many different situations and emotional states as possible. Treatment itself forms part of this continuous assessment.

INDIVIDUAL PROGRAMME PLANNING

Individual programme planning (IPP) is a system of individual care planning and care delivery which originated in the USA and has been introduced in the UK with the mentally handicapped and more recently with the elderly mentally ill (Blunden, 1980). It is an exciting, innovative alternative to the traditional nursing process and it results in a more cohesive, less fragmented approach to patient care since it is applied within a multidisciplinary framework. The key points of the IPP system are that all disciplines are involved in the assessment and management planning procedures, it closely involves patients and their relatives or carers, it identifies an individual's strengths and needs on a continuing basis, and it identifies specific management goals and which team members are responsible for working towards these goals. Each patient is allocated a key worker, who in most cases is a nurse but can be from any discipline. It is the key worker's responsibility to coordinate and deal with all issues relating to the patient. For example, they need to ensure that all the assessments and the strengths/needs list are completed before the IPP meeting. They also send out letters to the next of kin and all other agencies involved in the patient's care, explaining the purpose of the IPP meeting and inviting them to attend.

Strengths/needs

Once their individual assessments are complete, each discipline contributes to the strengths/needs list. A strength can be defined as what someone can do for themselves, what they like or used to like doing, people or facilities which are of value to them or anything positive in their environment. A need is a problem that a person faces restated in positive terms.

Compiling a strengths/needs list is a most enlightening, rewarding and sometimes surprising experience because there is a distinct shift in emphasis from the usual, negative list of things the patient cannot do, to the more positive list of what he needs to do, how he is going to do it and what strengths he possesses to achieve his goal. This shift in emphasis helps lead to changes in staff attitudes, resulting in a more positive approach. The strengths/needs list is often modified or expanded at the IPP meeting.

IPP meetings

Each discipline is present at the initial IPP meeting, as well as a chairman, relatives and the patient/client himself, if he is capable of participating. The purpose of the meeting is to present the assessment findings to the client and/or their advocate, to give them the opportunity of adding to the strengths/needs list, to select appropriate needs to work on, and to identify core staff to be involved. Implementation of IPP has to be realistic and so the needs are prioritized at the meeting and the key needs, usually three or four, are selected to concentrate on initially. The criteria for selection are that it is something the patient values, that there is a realistic chance of success and that it can be achieved over a reasonable period of time. At this stage a core group of staff is selected – usually the key worker and any discipline that is directly involved in achieving the key need (e.g. a physiotherapist in the case of a patient with a mobility problem). Relatives and friends are encouraged to be involved in the implementation of the programme planning if they wish to be. At the end of the meeting a date is set for a review.

Goals

Consistency is required with programme planning of this kind and therefore 'needs' have to be converted into 'goals' which should be stated in clear behavioural terms. For example, a need stated as 'needs to improve personal hygiene skills' can be broken down into a goal: 'Mrs Smith should be encouraged to wash her hands and face in the morning'. Some goals are relatively simple but more complex areas will need to be broken down further into attainable steps. Evaluation dates are set so that the team can monitor the patient's progress and evaluate whether the steps on the goal plan are being achieved. All the IPP assessments, forms and records are kept centrally in the office so that they are accessible to all staff at all times and great care is taken to ensure that the goal plans are written in such a way that they can be carried out by any team member.

IPPs are a new development in the care and management of the elderly mentally ill in the UK and their value has yet to be scientifically proven. However, Warren (1988) discusses the system in use in one health authority in the UK, describing it as 'truly multidisciplinary, it is positive and takes into account a person's strengths regardless of their disabilities'.

This system could be usefully applied to the care and management of other long-stay groups of psychiatric patients, for example chronic schizophrenics, because it encourages the care team to focus its direction in a positive way and break down goals into achievable steps.

FACTORS INFLUENCING THERAPY

Before a speech therapist can decide what approach or therapy she is going to embark upon with a patient she needs to take into account several factors: those which are related directly to the patient (e.g. his age, level of motivation); those which relate to the therapist and other staff (e.g. any special skills or training which are required to carry out the therapy, such as signing skills); and practical considerations (e.g.

the distance of the clinic from the patient's ward). Clearly these factors would influence the choice of approach/therapy with any patient, no matter what the medical diagnosis, and they do not just pertain to psychiatric patients. However, because of the many variables involved in the management of mentally ill patients and the complexity of these cases, particular attention often needs to be given to these additional factors.

The patient

Many of these factors (such as age, sex, sensory impairment) are familiar to therapists and will not be covered in detail. However, there are a number of factors which relate directly to the patient and which, in the case of a psychiatric patient, need to be looked at in more detail because they will have a marked effect on the actual choice of approach and on its outcome.

Medication

It has been mentioned before that patients with a psychiatric illness are often receiving medication, sometimes in combination and often in quite high doses. The side-effects of medication are variable – for example, it can cause impairment of cognitive function and lead to reduced concentration and attention levels, or it can cause a dry mouth and make articulation difficult. These factors will have to be taken into account by the therapist.

Illness fluctuations

It is not uncommon to notice dramatic changes in a patient's level of functioning on a day-to-day basis or, in some cases, over a period of hours. For example, a manic-depressive patient may show fluctuations in his behaviour and performance as his illness itself fluctuates. It is important to take this into account when planning and carrying out the therapy because it will be necessary to adopt a flexible approach and change the tasks and material in relation to changes in the illness pattern.

Motivation and mental state

For management to be successful, the patient needs to be sufficiently motivated. This means that the therapy must be relevant to the patient, it must be functional and it must focus on the strengths and needs. The patient's mental state will influence the choice of therapy too – for example, an aggressive patient who is deliberately unsociable may not function well in a group situation while, conversely, a withdrawn institutionalized patient may need to be given the experience of communicating within a small group to 'draw him out' of himself. The mood swings which are often seen in psychiatric patients must not be overlooked if therapy is to attain its maximum effect and they may need to be 'incorporated' into therapy and used positively wherever possible.

Pre-morbid levels of functioning and education

It is sometimes difficult to obtain information about a patient's pre-morbid intelligence and educational attainments because there is little contact with the family and the patient's report is sometimes unreliable and incomplete. However, it is useful to have this information because it does help the therapist to choose an appropriate approach. For example, it can be difficult to run a communication group involving reading and writing tasks if the group is made up of both highly literate and illiterate members. It may be easier to 'grade' the groups according to ability.

Institutionalization

Many mentally ill patients have spent a great deal of their lives living in institutions of one kind or another. If you accept Lubinski *et al.*'s (1981) definition of institutional living as an 'encompassing, restrictive, artificial lifestyle – in which people who are not related, nor have first established a close relationship, are required to live together in close proximity', it is not difficult to imagine what the long-term effects of this way of life are on patients. They may become passive, dependent, withdrawn, bound by routine or even depressed. All of these changes will be reflected in the patient's communication, or lack of it. Therefore, any therapy that aims to improve the way that individuals in long-stay institutions communicate with each other and staff may have wide-ranging effects. However, it would be unrealistic to expect a patient who has suffered the damaging effects of institutionalization for a considerable number of years to change dramatically with therapy. There may be small improvements and a general increase in communicative awareness but not necessarily an increase in 'output'. It would also be foolish to expect these patients to participate fully in groups discussing current affairs or the price of foodstuffs. They will obviously be constrained by their restricted life experiences. Therapy needs to be functional and adapted to meet their requirements for daily living.

Reinforcement

Any form of therapeutic intervention has more chance of success if it is reinforced by other people in the patient's immediate environment such as friends, relatives and carers. In the case of long-stay psychiatric patients the levels of support and reinforcement available to them at the ward level can often be sadly lacking. It is important to remember this when planning therapy because it would be unrealistic, for example, to include an elderly confused patient in a reality orientation programme in the clinic unless it had the full support and involvement of the rest of the staff on a 24-hour basis. It needs to be stated once more that many mentally ill patients have little contact with their families and so this source of support and reinforcement is not available to them. It also means that the therapist is unable to benefit from the support of her patient's relatives.

Therapists and other staff

The attitudes and abilities of the speech therapist and other staff are factors which can influence the choice and outcome of therapy. For example, a project which requires reinforcement from nursing staff to achieve results is not likely to succeed unless they are committed to it. Past experience indicates that the necessary support is usually available in the cases where the initial referral to speech therapy was made by the nursing staff. In other cases, it is vitally important to involve the nursing staff from the beginning to capture their interest and encourage them to participate in the therapy. An effective way of achieving this aim is to set up therapy groups which involve speech therapy, nursing staff and other disciplines from the outset at the planning stage and during assessment and therapy.

Another factor which may influence therapy is the recognition that it is necessary to see results if intervention is to be valued. Therefore, it is important for speech therapists to encourage positive attitudes amongst staff by ensuring that the aims and goals for therapy are set at a realistic, attainable level.

Support/supervision

Speech therapists may be good at encouraging and supporting other disciplines but they often fail to recognize their own need for support and supervision. Special interest groups can help by giving their members an opportunity to meet on a regular basis to exchange ideas and experiences and share information. However, these groups are only able to meet a couple of times a year and it is important that more regular support and supervision is available to therapists working in this challenging field, especially since they often work in isolation. Rose (1989), a speech therapist working in psychiatry, illustrates well the value of supervision, stating 'it was very useful to have regular contact with someone who acted as a sounding board for ideas, who noted and reminded you of your achievements, understood the obstacles and was able to offer support and a fresh perspective'. She also makes the point that regular structured contact with staff can alert managers to early signs of 'burnout'. This is obviously an area of concern for all speech therapy managers but the additional pressures of working in psychiatry can make early 'burnout' a very real possibility and anything which may help prevent this is welcome.

Practical considerations

Sometimes there is a practical reason for avoiding a particular approach or therapy. For example, many long-stay psychiatric hospitals have wards which are a long way from the clinical areas and it involves the therapist and patient in a lengthy walk, often out of doors. If the patient is elderly and in poor health it is impractical to consider a daily 'trek' from the ward to speech therapy for a 'stimulation' group. An alternative would be to see the patient on the ward and involve the care staff in the programme. In some hospitals this is seen as the ideal way of working. Another consideration concerns security and safety. A female therapist should not embark on an individual therapy programme in the clinic with a patient from the secure unit unless she is confident that there are other staff in the near vicinity. It may be impossible to run a group for hard of hearing patients on the ward because of the noise from the television, other patients and so on. There may be little or no privacy on the ward, which does not encourage the patients to share their feelings and experiences in a relaxed way in group therapy. In these situations the choice of approach (i.e. clinic- or ward-based therapy) is dictated by the environment and other practical considerations. Many of these considerations can be overcome with initiative and good planning on the part of the therapist or acceptable, alternative methods of working can be found.

THERAPY PROGRAMMES

The type of approach taken by the individual therapist will be determined by just that – the individuality of that therapist – for example, if the therapist has counselling or psychotherapy training their approach will be along these lines. There are no set procedures for therapy laid down and the therapeutic approach will be governed by the therapist's personality, beliefs, training and personal skills. Providing the therapist and the patient feel comfortable with the therapy and can fully justify the approach to the satisfaction of all concerned, then it is felt by the writers that there is likely to be some measurable progress due to the well-reasoned commitment. Any therapy programme must be based on the patient's needs and on their present situation and possible future. In psychiatry, therapy programmes must have a great deal of in-built flexibility to allow for possible rapid deterioration or improvement in the mental state of the patient. Adaptability, both in the therapist and the therapy, is essential and cannot be over-emphasized. Since communication is infinitely variable it is felt communication therapy must therefore have variety built into its structure. With appropriate adaptation many different kinds of therapeutic approach can be employed to great effect, often within a single session.

Patient needs

Information on the perceived needs of the patient will obviously come from the assessments carried out by the other carers involved and often from the patients themselves; however, there is often a lack of unanimity in this information. Again the therapist needs to look at the total picture – past, present and future. Therapy needs to be planned firstly around things that the patient feels will improve their quality of life and secondly in terms of what other carers (e.g. family and nursing staff) feel will improve the patient's or their own quality of life. There can also be a divergence of ideas and aspirations here and the therapist may need to mediate or even to compromise initially.

If in the past the patient has clearly never been outgoing or eager to socialize it is unlikely that therapy will do much to change that. Indeed, should it make the attempt? To illustrate, this is the case of a long-stay patient referred because of a cerebrovascular accident (CVA). Assessment was completed and therapy undertaken with vigour but no success. A chance meeting with a nurse who had previously known the patient for many years provided the opportunity to fill in the gaps in the patient's records with regard to their communicative history. Apparently the patient had always been withdrawn and uncommunicative and what should have been a good prognosis for recovery of expressive function after the CVA became an impossible task with that particular patient, who had no wish to communicate and few needs to communicate due to the mental illness and the effects of long-term institutionalization.

Institutional care can have devastating effects on communication. Needs are met often without the patient having to ask, settings are often unconducive to communication, activities are directed and there is little freedom of choice, privacy and opportunity. When planning for the needs of patients within an institution the therapist often has to look at the institution itself. The size of the place, number of patients per ward, number of staff, facilities available on the site and the proximity to local amenities, family and friends can all have a bearing on relevant planning. Even in 'mini-institutions' or in hostels there has to be some structure and the patient's needs are conditioned to some extent by the environment.

Planning therapy programmes to be in line with individual patient's needs will also involve understanding the patient's personal preferences and interests. These preferences and interests can be affected by the environment and the length of stay in that environment. There is likely to be less choice of reading material and other leisure activities like television and sport. This decreased choice coupled with the effects of the illness and with shortage of money (social security payments are very restrictive) can lead to inactivity, boredom and lack of motivation. This will set in motion a vicious circle which only very careful and appropriate therapy planning can break.

Therapy programmes as planned by different disciplines within mental health can have very different priorities. A speech therapist's priorities are those of improved attention, self-monitoring, understanding and expressive skills and the maintenance and improvement of communication skills in all their great variety. It is very much the opinion of the writers that improved levels of communication which bring the patient greater pleasure and insight can actually bring about improvement in other skills. Greater interest in self and others can promote better personal care and hygiene. Greater knowledge of self and improved feelings of self-worth can raise levels of motivation and compliance. The rewards of communication, if the patient can perceive them, can have all-round effect, helping the patient to question, assert and interact.

Goals need to be graded and to be perceived by all involved as being achievable. The patient in particular may find it very difficult to see a goal as being achievable. It may be necessary to break down each goal into a set of smaller targets and it may be that even each of these targets takes much time to achieve. It may also be that some patients need to go up every step of the ladder towards the goal before the skill becomes fixed and even then it may take a lot longer before that skill becomes generalized to include a range of other parallel situations. The therapist therefore needs a great variety of approaches and angles to any particular target, so that neither client nor therapist becomes discouraged. It may be in planning treatment that the therapist chooses to use parts of many techniques at his or her disposal. This points to the need to gain information and in some cases formal training across a range of therapies, and also again highlights the need for a truly multi-disciplinary approach to therapy.

Therapy types

There are many differing types of therapy which have a place and a relevance for the speech therapist working in psychiatry, many of which can be translated between the varied client groups. Some therapy can be seen as being more traditional, in that it is standard speech therapy practice. Other techniques come from the speech therapist's unique knowledge of communication in its many forms as applied to a psychiatric setting. Other techniques, for example the various differing styles of psychotherapy, require new learning. Whatever type of therapy is selected it must be totally based on the needs of the particular patient, within their particular situation and in line with any other treatment being received.

Given that the patient may find it very difficult to relate to others because of the nature or the longevity of their illness or because other contacts have proved unsatisfactory, a good deal of time needs to be spent in building rapport. If the patient has lowered insight or self-esteem or if they have lost sight of the benefits and rewards that improved communication can bring, then the therapist will need to work hard to establish rapport and make the purpose of the proposed therapy clear and meaningful. If the initial stages of the contact are unsatisfactory then there will be little progress. Much of the success of the therapy relies on the motivation of the patient, and the therapist can initially be the 'motivator' until other, more beneficial and objective rewards take over. If the patient at first only wishes to attend because of a good rapport with the therapist this is no bad thing, so long as this is specified as a communication goal and boundaries are clearly set and certain fairly informal 'contracts' are made, for example regular dates and times of attendance, duration and content of the session.

Individual treatment involving standard speech therapy approaches

At first most contacts between the speech therapist and the patient are going to be on an individual basis, unless the therapist is going into an already established group at the request of other professionals. Assessment, whether formal or informal, is best done on an individual basis so the needs of the patient can be clearly established and discussed. Assessment is obviously the precursor to therapy and the results of the assessment form and shape the future sessions. Some individual clients may progress from one-to-one sessions into group sessions or may received both individual and group therapy. There are certain patients who because of the specific nature of their difficulties can only benefit from individual therapy. For example, organic conditions, like Huntingdon's chorea, present unique problems which can differ hugely between sufferers. The extent of the deterioration and the rate of deterioration mean that the needs of the particular patient can only be met through individual therapy. The therapist needs to take into account the physical handicap as well as the cognitive deterioration, both of which can vary considerably between patients.

Patients with a hearing loss for which a hearing aid has been issued may also benefit from individual therapy. They will need to be taught strategies to cope with the loss and manage the aid in line with their own personal needs. As hearing aids are now small and quite sophisticated some patients, particularly if elderly or with fine motor coordination problems, can find regulating the aid difficult. Many patients find amplification intrusive and need individual help to derive the best possible benefit from their hearing aid in their various daily living situations. Being aware that the battery needs charging, how to change the battery, how to fit the aid comfortably and correctly and how to avoid feedback, all need to be addressed for the individual patient and the carers involved, and given that many psychiatric facilities do not have established audiology services this task may need to be undertaken by the speech therapist until more satisfactory arrangements can be made. Useful handouts can be obtained from organizations like the Royal National Institute for the Deaf and from local organizations. The speech therapist can often be instrumental in referral onto more appropriate agencies.

Patients suffering from dysarthria, whether drug-induced or due to organic conditions, often have very distinct needs which are best dealt with through individual therapy sessions. Therapy will involve proven techniques like breathing exercises, tongue, lip and palate exercises and vocal training. Patients may experience any one of the accepted types of dysarthria – flaccid, spastic, ataxic, hypokinetic, hyperkinetic or mixed (Darley *et al.*, 1975) – and establishing the differential diagnosis is the first role of the speech therapist. Treatment techniques aimed at improvement of respiration, phonation, resonance, articulation and prosody will vary with diagnosis, and implementation will be dependent on those influencing factors of insight, motivation and potential for sustaining progress. A useful compendium of proven techniques and exercises can be found in *Working with Dysarthrics* (Robertson and Thomson, 1982). Rosenbek and La Pointe (1978) outlined specific goals for therapy, namely modification of posture, muscle tone and strength, modification of respiration, phonation, resonance, articulation and of suprasegmentals and prosody, and the two central goals of helping the patient become productive and also providing alternative modes of communication, discussed later in this chapter. Therapy will also be aimed at improving self-monitoring skills and bio-feedback mechanisms, so tape recording, video sessions and mirror work can be of great benefit, and to avoid being too confrontational and distressing for the patient this type of therapy is often best on a one-to-one basis.

Voice work, specific articulation work and stuttering therapy, all of which are required by some patients in mental illness settings, are also likely cases for individual therapy. It may be felt that to treat the symptom is less valuable than to treat the underlying cause but it is the experience of the writers that some patients become so distressed by a voice, articulation or fluency problem that they need the reassurance of direct therapy. Relaxation techniques and counselling will obviously form part of the therapy sessions and in the long term are likely to provide the greatest benefit, but direct work by the speech therapist on the symptom can be invaluable as part of a total treatment 'package' undertaken by the team of carers.

Therapy for stutterers has changed greatly over the years. Historical and current approaches are discussed in detail in Van Riper (1973). It is reasonable to suppose that in a higher proportion of patients with a mental illness a stutter is more symptomatic of the deeper disorder of personality or thought than it is likely to be in clients without identified mental health problems. Therefore psychotherapy, such as that outlined by Barbara (1962), personal construct psychotherapy as discussed by Hayhow and Levy (1989) or even a psychoanalytic approach (Glauber, 1958) may be the most relevant type of treatment. These approaches to therapy are discussed more fully in the next section of this chapter. Traditional techniques commonly used would be 'prolonged speech' (Ryan and Van Kirk, 1974), which evolved from experiments with delayed auditory feedback, 'easy stuttering' (Irwin, 1972) which involves replacing all stutterers with stutters without tension, and 'modification' bound on the principle of stopping, releasing tension and using light contact to restart the utterance (Van Riper, 1973).

Full explanation of technique to all concerned, support, feedback and opportunity for 'assignments' must be built into the programme in the same way as for patients outside a psychiatric setting. A recent compilation edited by Rustin *et al.* (1987) is most informative about both theory and current treatment practices.

Therapy for patients with voice disorders has also changed over the years (Boone, 1983). It has long been recognized that there are both organic (English, 1976) and functional disorders (Murphy, 1964) and it would be wrong to assume that all psychiatric patients fall into the latter category. Investigation of possible organic causes needs to take place. An excellent practical guide for exercises is available by Martin (1987) outlining relaxation, respiration and phonation techniques. Vocal abuse is often a problem for patients in large institutions; many smoke, or need to shout to express feelings, gain attention, combat the size of the wards, etc. Johnson (1985) uses a structured programme for the reduction of vocal abuse which can be helpful to these patients. Support and counselling as discussed in the useful practical book by Brumfitt (1986) are likely to form a part of speech therapy sessions.

If a patient has had a CVA or there is the onset of a dementia with resultant language difficulties, individual therapy is often indicated. The needs of that patient are likely to be very personal, conditioned by their history, their present and future needs and their underlying mental illness. It is unlikely that there will be many patients with uncluttered symptoms and much of the remedial therapy aimed at re-establishing both receptive and expressive skills can often best be undertaken via mainly individual work. Again aims of therapy must be clearly defined for both patient and other carers involved so that it can become an accepted and widely used part of that patient's general management.

There has not been much evidence from formal research, until recently, to support the idea that specific treatment methods were effective in improving specific deficits experienced by those with dysphasia. Recent evidence as in Weniger *et al.* (1980) is showing that improvements achieved in therapy can generalize into real life. Therapy for patients with dysphasic difficulties needs to be aimed at certain key areas, namely understanding, both written and oral; expressive skills, both written and oral; and non-verbal skills, both the ability to recognize and use them appropriately. The neuropsychological approach to assessment and therapy for dysphasia has been influential (Lezak, 1983).

In this area of therapy, as in all others, the aim is to maximize the patient's present abilities and where possible extend them both in terms of decoding skills and encoding skills and to maintain those levels in a range of situations, thus improving the quality of life. A useful manual outlining proven strategies and techniques is *Working with Dysphasics* (Fawcus *et al.*, 1986) and much that is included in this manual of treatment procedures for dysphasia will be of value in planning appropriate activities for psychiatric patients with acquired dysphasia.

It is important to note that for many patients, particularly those in group homes or large wards in an institution, there is often very little opportunity for one to one contact. The place of individual therapy therefore assumes a greater importance and its role needs to be stressed and preserved.

Group treatment involving standard speech therapy approaches

Many emotional problems are caused by an individual's difficulties relating to his peers. Patients with a mental illness may find it very difficult to establish meaningful friendships or to form interpersonal relationships, and interactions across a range of situations may be very unsatisfactory. Group therapy can provide tremendous support and help relieve some of the feelings of isolation, of being 'the only one'. It can help deal with anxieties and conflicts by having responses from many different people. Although the speech therapist may be the group leader it is important that the aims of the group are clear and acceptable to all members and that, where possible, the therapist becomes much more of a 'facilitator' than a 'director'.

Depending on the setting, the speech therapist working in psychiatry can expect to be involved in many different kinds of group therapy, alone or with other professionals. Groups for the hard of hearing, listening and attention training groups and language groups (along similar lines to more traditional stroke groups) may be undertaken, as well as those discussed in more detail below . The aim of any group therapy is to provide information as well as support and to improve abilities to interact. Numbers – if a group is to be effective – need to be limited to between two and ten depending on levels, needs and the staff/patient ratio. As with any group therapy, patients with a mental illness need to be fairly carefully selected so that the group will remain reasonably cohesive.

Reality orientation groups

Reality orientation was first developed in the 1950s in the USA. It became more widely researched in the 1960s (Folsom, 1968). This approach to therapy has often been considered to be purely of value in the treatment of elderly people. However, confusion and disorientation are features of many mental illnesses and can further be complicated by the effects of drugs and long-term institutional care, Reality orientation has its place for many patients regardless of age. It is to be hoped that reality orientation is no longer considered merely a matter of day, date and weather board, but is considered in the light of the wider reality involving people, locations and the general environment. The work done on reality orientation stresses the need for it to be a 24-hour approach, as in Holden and Woods (1982) and Hanley and Gilhooly (1986). These publications and others show reality orientation as a consistent technique providing methods of stimulation which will hopefully help combat confusion, disorientation and memory loss. This approach is also helpful for staff and carers as it gives a structured approach for working with patients and relatives and can help to maintain levels of interest and motivation. Many patients with mental illness have lost touch with reality and many can no longer select and process external cues and clues which will help them regain a measure of touch with reality. In the community it is now accepted that there are certain multinational signs and symbols which are interpretable to all, which help people to find their way round and locate their needs. A full awareness of the principles of reality orientation will allow carers to plan the environment in wards, hostels and other environments, and thus help patients relearn basic facts about themselves and their environment and discover compensatory ways of functioning through the retraining. Written and pictorial signs on doors can help considerably, as can colour coded doors, as in one long-stay elderly ward known to the writers when continence was improved merely by painting the toilet door red. Clocks need to be large and prominently placed. Maps need to be large and clear to aid direction finding. Hospital shops and banks need to be central and clearly signposted. Many suggestions can be found in the booklet *24-hour Approach to the Problems of Confusion in Elderly People* (Holden *et al.*, 1982).

Reality orientation therapy can be very varied and many different materials and techniques can be used (Rimmer, 1982). Large photographs of staff and locations can be valuable. Being able to go outside and experience the weather being talked about or see the seasonal flowers is of great importance to a large majority of patients. Obviously a great deal of repetition and reinforcement is needed and the structure of reality orientation techniques may not suit all carers, but it can be very effective in maintaining links with reality for many patients who would otherwise lose touch completely. The behavioural approach of reality orientation offers rewards of praise and a sense of achievement.

Reminiscence therapy

Reminiscence therapy, particularly in groups, is also effective for a range of patients and not merely the elderly population. There is a great deal of pleasure to be derived from the past and reminiscence therapy can be a starting point for much valuable interaction. The work of Holden *et al.* (1982) which has been mentioned in the preceding section on reality orientation also discusses reminiscence as therapy. It is felt that evoking memories of the past can encourage people to recall, share and reflect on their own experiences. It provides stimulus for group discussions and informal conversation. Holden suggests that 'reminiscence in itself is thought to be therapeutic in that it arouses people's interest and attention and calls upon their store of knowledge and experience, and this in turn facilitates communication'. This statement was made in relation to the elderly with dementia but in the experience of those working in psychiatry it is equally true for other mentally ill patients, particularly those who have been in hospital for some time. People often have shared memories which can bring them together to interact and communicate in the same way that shared problems and interests in the present can. Listening to or performing music of the past whether it be old-time music hall or the Beatles can be a relaxing and sharing activity. If the therapy also consists of comparisons between past and present it can help to reinforce reality and can be a good adjunct to reality orientation. There is quite a lot of material available for use in reminiscence, for example pictures and articles showing famous faces and events which were prominent in the past. Slides are also very useful. Much of the material has an emphasis on 'then and now', which again serves to update the individual or the group; the nostalgia series (Holden, 1984) is widely used.

Both reality orientation and reminiscence therapies are further discussed in relation to their value with older people in Chapter 8. Amongst other groups which benefit from the involvement of a speech therapist are social skills and communication groups. The purposes of these types of therapy are many and various and are discussed in more detail in the following section.

Psychotherapeutic approaches to treatment

For years speech therapists have been reluctant to discuss patients' emotional problems for fear of causing distress. Attitudes are now changing, as Brumfitt (1986) points out. It is known that speech is very much a part of personality and that expressing feelings is good and so therapy becomes more rewarding and satisfying. Brumfitt goes on to say that communicatively impaired people need help in coming to terms with and understanding the nature of their disorder, and speech therapists may go some way to doing this. Some patients may have communication problems that are a direct result of emotional stress, so that time and security to explore feelings will help them to find a new perception of themselves and so deal with life more positively. Parker (1983) draws attention to speech therapists having a wide variety of skills and highlights their training as providing a detailed understanding of language and its many facets, structure and content. Parker goes on to state that the ability to listen as well as talk is as much a part of a speech therapist's skill as is the work towards the patient's intelligibility.

It is known that there are considerable benefits from encouraging the patient to talk. The opportunity to speak to a receptive, professionally trained listener is known to be therapeutic and frequently the patient feels an improvement in his symptoms or an alleviation of distress following such an interview. But how many professionals are really trained to listen and, if they are, actually put into practice those trained listening skills? Many psychiatric patients have reported that their greatest need is a chance to talk with someone who has the time and interest to listen to them and to believe their discourse. In the experience of the writers, a number of fit ex-psychiatric patients encourage speech therapists to continue the battle to set up speech therapy services in psychiatry. It is appreciated that a speech therapist's training leads them to share sensitive listening skills without having the authority/responsibility to threaten the patient's future well-being by prescribing drugs or increasing medication for passionately expressed feelings or by taking punitive measures. The overall aim is to encourage patients to talk about the present, that is, 'the here and now'; to talk about the past, as there is a need to be able to re-experience feelings and understand significant events from the past; and to be able to identify change in order to work back to the present and so progress to the future. This last step is often spontaneously taken by the patient, when ready. When considering the future, formal rehabilitation programmes can be planned. It is often the case that these three areas – the present, past and future – go along side by side in therapy.

Speech therapists may feel that to step into psychotherapy and concentrate more on what is said than how it is said is professionally beyond their capacity and control. Further specialist training is essential and it is advisable to accept any in-service experience working in different areas of psychotherapy. It helps to develop confidence in new settings and provides a choice of approaches to treatment from the repertoire of psychotherapy techniques, thereby enhancing the patient's treatment. It is also a fascinating area of work and complements the speech therapist's more traditional role. Good communication can prevent socialization from developing into isolation and independence from becoming dependence. It is the vehicle for expressing feelings of frustration which show in touchiness, depression and anxiety. An early sign of developing mental illness is the change in the pattern of non-verbal and verbal communciation. Communication skills therefore are vital to mental health and well-being.

Wolberg (1977) groups the psychotherapies into those which aim to dismantle and rebuild new personality (the reconstructive psychotherapies), those therapies which attempt to teach new patterns of behaviour and social functioning (the re-eductional psychotherapies), and finally those therapies which provide support, guidance, advice and reassurance (the supportive psychotherapies). Wolberg lists the reconstructive psychotherapies as Freudian analysis, Kleinian analysis, ego analysis, neo-Freudian therapy, Adlerian therapy, Reichian analysis and brief dynamic therapy. The re-educative therapies include behaviour therapy, cognitive therapy, client-centred therapy, gestalt therapy, emotive release, psychodrama, transactional analysis, and it might also be appropriate to include personal construct psychotherapy. The supportive psychotherapies are milieu therapy, occupational therapy, music therapy, reassurance and ventilation.

Harrington (1988) draws attention to the theoretical differences between psychotherapy and counselling, but their boundaries are becoming increasingly blurred and boundaries between different schools of therapy are constantly being breached. Kleinians and Jungians have joined together, behavioural and dynamic therapists are coming closer together and similarities between Adlerian and cognitive therapists are acknowledged. Harrington goes on to give support for therapists selecting treatment modes that suit their personalities and states that flexibility goes with an eclectic approach to treatment as it allows therapists to integrate what is best from a variety of approaches and allows for change.

A primary goal of psychotherapy is to increase the patient's ability to handle his own problems and to take responsibility for his own actions. Ruesch (1987) explains that successful living is an art which is not mastered by all, and those who fail – the patients – seek improvement while those who believe that they know about failure – the therapists – attempt to induce improvement. A give and take develops when patient and therapist meet – this is called psychotherapy. In his invaluable small manual Cox (1988) describes dynamic psychotherapy as a process in which a professional relationship enables the patient to do for himself what he cannot do on his own. The therapist does not do it for him, although he cannot do it without the therapist.

Recording group sessions

Problems recording the complexity of the group's activity, non-verbal and verbal communciations and the interactions within the group are daunting, however many therapists (often of mixed disciplines) are present in a group setting, and the pooling of observations of the group as a whole and each personal contribution within the session is an ongoing task. A completed group therapy interaction chronogram (GTIC) is a heuristic device for rapidly recording sequential group therapy sessions (see Figure 10.3). It demonstrates the progressive phases within each session and exhibits dynamic patterns in successive sessions. It is particularly useful where other methods such as audio tape recording and use of one-way screens are not appropriate (Cox, 1988).

The GTIC is a simple record of the number of patients and therapists present, represented by the appropriate number of individual circles so that it is possible to record events of the various interactive phenomena which occur in every group. The GTIC form is completed as soon as possible after the termination of the group session. It is also a suitable means of recording any external factors which influence the group session as well as providing an indication of the content of the session and any particular event which might have occurred. There is no standard form of notation which should be universally applied, as this would be restrictive and reduce the interdisciplinary scope. Indications for using the GTIC are varied as the therapists' theoretical backgrounds and clinical foci differ. The GTIC may be used by therapists whose experience varies from full analytical training to that of social workers, counsellors, nursing staff and other medical staff, as well as psychiatrists. It is useful when the established means of recording are contraindicated and can also be a method of comparing the dynamics of two sessions that may be some months apart, as well as convey information to a co-therapist colleague who has been absent from the

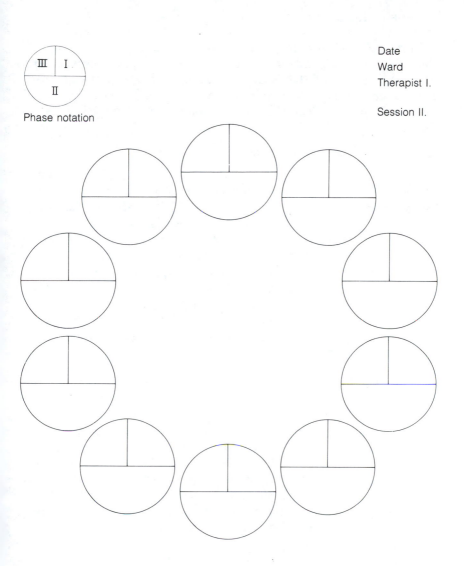

Date
Ward
Therapist I.

Session II.

Phase notation

Figure 10.3 Group therapy interaction chronogram.

group. The GTIC also provides flexibility which may be necessary if a therapist is working with groups in several different settings. Cox goes on to state that it can be used as a teaching aid as well as being used by different specialized disciplines who will see different uses and will adopt their own particular styles of notation relevant to their work.

Dynamic reconstructive therapies

Traditionally Freud is looked upon as the father of modern psycho-therapy and psychoanalysis is frequently referred to as the talking cure. It was treatment devised by Freud in the 1890s based on free association, interpretation and transference. The basis of analytic psycho-therapy is the therapeutic relationship, where the therapist works actively to develop a trusting relationship in which the patient can feel accepted and understood, even when he is expressing or talking about his less pleasant characteristics (Hobbs, 1988). Hobbs goes on to state that the patient is helped to disclose intimate and painful aspects of himself and his experience; this process of self-disclosure is accompanied by the expression of associated feelings, this combination often proving therapeutic in itself.

These forms of therapy are very time consuming and demanding financially and so are not well represented in centrally funded systems of health. Therapy in a hospital setting is more likely to be in groups rather than individual therapy and may well include patients suffering from neurotic, psychotic and personality disorders. In the case of psychotic patients it is unwise to include them in this type of group if their symptoms are acute; ideally they should be stable, with careful observation to ensure that psychotic symptoms are not re-emerging, as stresses within these types of group are quite capable of precipitating a relapse. Patients with poor concentration, memory problems and exhibiting disinhibited behaviour would not be considered suitable for this treatment.

A speech therapist's role, unless specially trained, will not be in individual work but they can quite appropriately be included in group therapy, provided a trained psychotherapist is coordinator of the group. With careful tuition a speech therapist can have a lot to offer in this type of treatment and can learn, both at an experiential level about himself or herself and use the therapy as a training for the acceptance of patients' histories, particularly those which include violence and abuse of all kinds. These groups are predominantlly dependent upon the use of language – its limitations for some patients, and a means of development for others. A speech therapist's particular skills are useful in observing vocal changes and the re-emergence of dormant accents which may occur transiently and become subtly re-established; their significance is important in personal change and development. Further recommended reading includes *Issues and Approaches in the Psychological Therapies* (Bannister, 1975), *An Introduction to the Psychotherapies* (Bloch, 1986) and *Psychotherapy: A Dynamic Approach* (Dewald, 1969).

Behavioural psychotherapy and other re-educative therapies

As behavioural therapy is symptom oriented the therapist is interested in the present and gives less weight to the underlying factors and aetiology of the condition. Changes can be effected without focusing upon causes of the symptoms; by treating the problem there may be beneficial wider changes too. This type of approach to treatment relies upon detailed assessments and the problem should be current, repetitive and measurable. Ideally the therapist needs to observe the patient whilst symptoms are evident.

Many professionals other than clinical psychologists are now trained to include behavioural techniques within their treatment programmes. In some settings treatment is planned, organized and carried out by clinical psychologists with other members of the team. There are now increasing opportunities for speech therapists to train in a number of behavioural methods and so enhance and augment their skills, as well as learn to appreciate the advantages of working closely with other professionals and sharing responsibility for treatment. In turn, speech therapists are able to share and impart their particular skills and expertise to others.

Behavioural methods may be helpful in the treatment of some depressive states, the rehabilitation of chronic schizophrenics and, combined within treatment plans, for some personality disorders. This type of treatment has been effective, for example, with such cases as agoraphobia, simple phobias, social phobias and social skills deficits.

Marzilier (1978) emphasizes the strength, power and efficiency of words and states that verbal methods of analysis and treatment need not undermine the basic principles of behavioural orientation. He then goes on to point out that verbal therapies can be a means of effecting behavioural change as behaviour therapy draws heavily on words in treatments while many verbal psychotherapies are often very active or behavioural in their work. This knowledge may help to endorse the speech therapist's input to these types of treatment. Recommended further reading is *Behavior Modification: A Handbook of Assessment, Intervention and Evaluation* (Gambrill, 1977).

Anxiety management training

Anxiety management training might well be part of, or a prelude to, many treatment programmes as anxiety states are common in areas of mental illness as well as in the general public. There are three components of anxiety management, the first being learning to control the symptoms by relaxation, distraction and controlling thoughts (speech therapists are generally familiar with relaxation techniques and further details are provided in this chapter under the heading 'Relaxation and hypnosis'). The second component deals with avoidance by encouraging the patient to gradually increase his exposure to anxiety-provoking situations or sensations, and the last component is increasing the patient's confidence.

During an anxiety attack patients can be taught to occupy themselves by employing mental tasks, such as counting objects in order to distract attention away from the anxiety attack. Patients can be helped to control their thoughts by recognizing that frightening thoughts are usually illogical and exaggerated ways of perceiving the situation and that frightening thoughts can be replaced by more logical ones.

Social and communication skills training

This treatment is helpful for those who have difficulty approaching others and so forming and maintaining relationships; at the same time it can be used to encourage patients to express their feelings (Hooker, 1989). The types of patient who might well benefit from this treatment are those who experience interpersonal difficulties but are not actively psychotic, such as the personality disordered; some adolescents who are in need of psychiatric support and treatment; patients who have at some earlier time used appropriate skills but may have lost them due to mental illness; and the long-term or chronic psychiatric patient.

Social skills training highlights the importance of non-verbal communication. This includes focusing on eye contact, facial expression, body posture, gestures, proximity in interpersonal communication and physical appearance. It also involves vocal skills and may include attention to vocal pitch, vocal volume and quality of voice, speed of utterance and intonation of vocal production. Verbal skills emphasize the appropriate use of language and the way in which it is produced, including both the rhythm and inflection of speech. Training includes the development of conversational skills such as how to begin, maintain and close a conversation. Topics can range from different styles of speech used in different circumstances (for example, informal and personal levels of communication) to personal disclosures.

Perhaps one of the most important areas to highlight is that of listening skills. Although apparently passive, listening involves hearing and remembering what has been heard; non-verbal actions and verbal prompts supported by questions demonstrate that the listener is attending and supporting the communication act. If active listening skills are employed other benefits accrue, in particular the continued development and expansion of linguistic skills. Social skills training is usually performed in a group setting and one of the many advantages of being a member of a group is the opportunity to observe, use and develop newly acquired language skills, for which listening skills are a prerequisite. Groups provide opportunities to role-play the difficult social situations.

The programme should be planned and organized around the individual members and the group to suit their particular problems and needs rather than fitting the group or individual into a set treatment package. The group, through formal instruction (for example, handout information sheets), modelling, role play and discussion allows patients the opportunity to rehearse social tasks, particularly speaking skills, with other group members. This is probably difficult and a cause of some anxiety to most patients in the group. Here the inclusion of anxiety management may be necessary, with emphasis on exposure, habituation and relaxation techniques. The programme should be organized to run slowly and comfortably so that the group generates its own style and leaves space for self-help, reinforcement, spontaneity and the development of increasing communication throughout the sessions. The therapy will offer not just rehearsal of a variety of situations and the spoken communication that goes with them but also a better understanding of what is implicit in those situations.

The length of the treatment will vary depending upon the skills of the members and topics will be expanded or simplified to an appropriate level – as will the methods of practice. A typical ten-session course of training might be as shown in Table 10.2, although many social skills programmes may well take longer than ten sessions.

The role of the therapist will vary considerably with the level of the group; for example, with withdrawn, institutionalized chronic patients there obviously will have to be a lot more modelling, shaping and prompting. The input from the therapist needs to be more and the sessions need to be shorter, more frequent and spread over a longer period of time for there to be any effect. With younger, more verbal and

Table 10.2 Social skills group plan

SESSION ONE:	Non-verbal expression (posture, relaxation, etc.)
SESSION TWO:	Non-verbal expression (gaze, touch, appearance, gesture)
SESSION THREE:	Vocal expression (voice control, style, emotional overtones)
SESSION FOUR:	Simple verbal expression (greetings, introductions, chatting, etc.)
SESSION FIVE:	Work, home or hospital-based situations
SESSION SIX:	Expressing feelings
SESSION SEVEN:	Group interaction
SESSION EIGHT:	Initiating friendships
SESSION NINE:	Developing or maintaining stronger bonds (e.g. family, partners)
SESSION TEN:	Revision

N. J. Muir, West Park Hospital, Surrey (1989)

active patients who are likely to have greater motivation and insight, the therapist will still need to model, shape and prompt but there is likely to be more interaction between the group members and topics can be more fully explored.

Role play is an important part of social skills and communication group work. In itself it can be very stressful and is therefore best left until later sessions when the group members know each other better and feel more comfortable in the group situation. Role-play topics can cover meeting people, ice-breaking techniques, saying no, complaining, expressing anger, handling compliments, coping with rejection, asking for things, and all manner of topics which may be shared experiences for group members. Diaries, so that the patient can record their activities, feelings and progress, can be valuable. Handouts on the particular session can provide good reinforcement and appropriate assignments can also be of great benefit.

The therapist needs to be very aware of his or her own social and communication skills, and videoing can help the self-monitoring skills of all participants in the group. Appropriate use of humour, approval and constructive criticism can all be of great value if used at an accessible level for the group members. A good deal of revision and recapping is recommended to make sure that ideas and techniques have been understood and can be used personally by each group member to the best of his or her ability.

There are no hard and fast rules for the running of a social or communication skills group. Interaction without variety, change and flexibility will be sterile and the purpose of such groups is to provide stimulation and make interaction behaviours more manageable and rewarding. *Social Skills and the Speech Impaired* (Rustin and Kuhr, 1989) is an extremely useful manual, providing theoretical background and much needed innovative and practical help and ideas for treatment.

Assertiveness training

As a continuation of a social skills programme assertiveness training might be added to encourage the socially appropriate expression of thoughts and feelings. This training can be approached in two ways: in order to help those who display a lack of appropriate assertion, and others who display over-assertiveness or aggression.

The treatment is carried out by using role play, modelling and coaching. Video cameras are particularly helpful if used throughout training for self and group criticism and appraisal. Once again non-verbal and verbal skills are an integral part of the training; those more fluent and competent in self-expression are more likely to achieve satisfactory results.

Behaviour modification groups

Behaviour modification groups and individual programmes can also benefit from the input of the speech therapist – particularly if the behaviour in question may be used for communication. On assessment the patients may present with many frequent and inappropriate behaviours which the team may consider need modifying – for example, constant monologue, shouting, swearing or standing too close. Conversely, the problems may be associated with infrequent but desired behaviours – for example, lack of response, inability to ask for things, or no eye contact.

In some mental illness hospitals reinforcement techniques are used in the form of token economy (Elliot *et al.*, 1977). Immediate reinforcers will be determined by the team and may be praise, sweets, cigarettes or other appropriate tangible rewards for the patient. Tokens are less immediate but of greater long-term value in that like a currency they can later be exchanged for food, cigarettes or 'privileges'.

This type of therapy can be difficult for speech therapists to become fully involved in since speech therapy requires the growth of insight in a patient and behavioural techniques are not necessarily dependent on developing insight but on modifying aberrant behaviours, by the presentation of reward. However, much speech therapy can be considered loosely behavioural in approach and there is much that can be learnt from behavioural therapy and applied by speech therapists in psychiatry – in particular, the use of positive and negative reinforcement techniques, desensitization techniques and the modelling techniques that will lead to effective counter-conditioning (Paul and Lentz, 1977).

It is not recommended that the speech therapist becomes involved exclusively in behaviour therapy without proper training and even then the need for team support and close liaison with the psychiatrist, psychologist, psychotherapist or behaviourally trained nurse is stressed. As with many therapies it is incumbent on the speech therapist to be aware of the principles of the behavioural approach and how to apply them when appropriate and in conjunction with others.

Anger control management

This particular approach to treatment might only be needed in certain settings – for example, in forensic or adolescent units, with individuals who have specific anger problems or behaviour problems associated with brain damage, or in the case of family problems including child abuse. Once again an ideal setting for the training is within a group. It is known that anger can serve as an important expressive or communicative function in that it provides expression of negative feelings. Healthy relationships depend upon people being able to express their anger and give negative feedback. Most structured treatment programmes are based on the work on *Anger Control* (Novaco, 1975). His book gives clear detail on how to go about planning and organizing treatment. Experience working in anger control groups points to two opposing groups of angry people: the 'exploders' – the uncontrolled, outgoing aggressively eruptive people who externalize their anger; and the 'bottlers' – the over-controlled, apparently placid people who internalize their anger. The 'exploders' are usually verbally fluent, loud and expressive but not necessarily imaginative, accurate or sensible in their expression, and so are frustrated by their limitations and obvious verbal failure. The 'bottlers' have usually always had communication problems, they cannot say what they want to say and tend to add to angry memories until eventually some small unrelated incident or irritation provokes a major physical eruption. It is thought that providing a more colourful and extensive vocabulary is a necessary part of treatment!

People who feel threatened and insecure often become angry. Sometimes things are personalized unnecessarily, resulting in an angry situation. As alternative ways of coping with provocation are learned, there will be less angry reactions and less impulsive behaviour.

Treatment is aimed at using anger to work to the patient's advantage and therefore to help the patient learn to be able to manage anger and be in control of a situation. Understanding the function of anger is helped by keeping a diary of experiences and monitoring self statements during anger together with the discussion of its functions. Relaxation training is used extensively as anger involves tension. Group work involves continuous communicative involvement, sharing, assessment and criticism, as well as gentle teaching and reinforcement to promote progress.

Cognitive therapy

It is known that treatment directed to behaviour and mood changes also produces changes in cognitions (that is, people think differently when they feel and behave differently) and that personal assumptions are fashioned and maintained by experience; assumptions may give rise to maladaptive patterns of thinking which generate anxiety or mood disturbance. Beck *et al.* (1979) state that patients have mental constructs and this concerns the way they perceive their present personalities, their past and their future. Techniques of cognitive therapy are now applied increasingly by a number of disciplines in a variety of therapeutic settings. Increasing numbers of speech therapists are also following an interest in the cognitive neuropsychological approach in order to study the performance of people who have lost the ability to speak, move, remember and see due to brain damage, in order to find out what has gone wrong and what is still intact. The aim is to be able to devise rehabilitation programmes based on a theoretical analysis of the disorder to be treated.

Treatment by cognitive methods is an effective method of treatment for depression and some anxiety states and is achieved by the patient being encouraged to analyse the frequency, precipitants and consequences of natural thoughts and to then assess their validity. The patient is helped to think more positively about himself and therefore feel better about himself (Hobbs, 1988). Patients may keep a diary of mood states, and are encouraged to modify their 'inner speech' to become more positive.

This style of therapy can also invade other treatment programmes rather than being used as a direct approach, particularly where programmes are being designed to fill specific treatment needs. Much of what happens in group work and individual sessions could well include a cognitive approach. Programmes for developing interpersonal relationships, self-awareness, communicative skills and anger control, for example, will rely to some degree on cognitive therapy. Further recommended reading is *Cognitive Behaviour Therapy for Psychiatric Problems: A Practical Guide* (Hawton *et al.*, 1989).

Personal construct psychotherapy

This is based on a theory by Kelly (1955) which is concerned with the personal use and meaning of concepts or constructs and the emphasis is placed on a person's need to anticipate, for example, feelings and events. Human lives are seen as constructed and reconstructed on the basis of people's anticipations of what might follow (Button, 1986). Kelly's theory was that man continually attempts to predict and control his world and to do this he invents 'constructs' which are bipolar and it is through these constructs that he perceives events. Personal construct theory is presented as a complete formally stated theory: it accounts for all human behaviour, it makes philosophical assumptions explicit and it is concerned primarily with 'the person'. It is of course dependent upon language and therefore offers an extremely useful method of assessment of how the patient perceives his world and his place in it. His linguistic limits are exposed and grids can therefore be used as ongoing assessments and as a basis for treatment. Grids or 'repertory grids' are used as a means of measuring the interrelationships between a person's constructs, and the term is used to describe a methodology which derives a mathematical representation of part of a person's construct system. There are many varied forms of grids which can be completed during assessment and treatment, but in order to use this technique knowledge and access to an appropriate computer is necessary. This emphasizes once more the need for specialized training. Structured techniques such as self-characterizations and essays are also most useful, and they can all be studied within a group or with individuals, on one occasion or successively over time. For further information about grids and their use Fransella and Banister's *A Manual for Repertory Grid Technique* (1977) is a useful reference.

It is a particularly attractive form of treatment for use by speech therapists with the mentally ill as it is a method of sharing treatment and its responsibility, and it offers the patient some control over the direction of treatment and in negotiating where to begin. The patient can easily witness progress and movement to subsequent grids. Perhaps one of the most valuable aspects of this method is the monitoring of development of language and its use as a means of augmenting language skills. The use of the grid can indicate developing language use through the way constructs are used. The patient's increasing development and choice of constructs demonstrates the expansion of his language skills. Personal construct therapy can be used equally effectively in individual and group work.

The book *Personal Construct Theory and Mental Health* edited by Button (1986) gives detailed consideration of the practical implications and intricacies of a personal construct approach to mental health and provides a useful introduction to those uninitiated in personal construct theory. It also fills a gap for those working in mental health and already converted to this style of treatment.

Supportive psychotherapies

Supportive psychotherapy can be practised in a number of settings and on an individual or group basis with patients or with their family and friends. Speech therapists are most likely to work in this way in a formal group setting in a psychiatric unit, ward or day centre.

Many chronic mentally ill people can only survive with constant support in order to prevent social isolation. This is necessary even in a large and busy psychiatric ward where support is also needed to help those upon whom the patient may depend and thus exhaust. Psychotherapy in these cases is not always aimed at psychological change but the maintenance of emotional stability, as many of these people lack the capacity for understanding their psychological difficulties.

Supportive psychotherapy provides empathy, encouragement, guidance and practical support. In a group setting it offers a chance for patients to learn to redefine their own means of communication so that they can adapt to changing situations and learn to inter-communicate. The group offers contrasts which are particularly important in institutional life and this might lead to liberation and the feeling of being a real person again.

In some settings individual changes may occur – there might be a developing need to talk and to develop tentative relationships and begin to see that life has something extra to offer and to explore the possibility of making progress and risking a change. The therapist(s) and group help to reassure and support this progress and ensure that any change is well prepared for and further support is at hand. Conversely, when the problem is insoluble or the illness chronic, support may help the patient accept his present position and live as well as possible despite it.

Groups for severely disturbed patients provide evidence that they have a marked affect on adjustment. The primary goal of this type of psychotherapy is to increase the patient's ability to handle his own problems and to take responsibility for his own actions. The main task is to stimulate the psychotherapeutic dialogue through which some patients may gain courage to go out and put what they have learnt into practice. The important fact is that patients may attempt new things or attempt again previously used skills or behaviours. Some of the results observed in these groups by the authors have been that some chronic schizophrenics are more likely to be transferred to less disturbed wards and maintain improved behaviour and that, together with medication, delusional thinking lessens, which helps towards discharge.

Family therapy

Family therapy is a recently developed form of treatment arising from two main approaches: the psychodynamic and the communication systems methods (Gelder *et al.*, 1986). The psychodynamic method uses concepts from psychoanalytical treatment and assumes that family problems originate in the separate past experiences of the individual members, particularly the parents. This is a non-directive form of treatment. The communication systems method does not attempt to explore the past so much as attempt to change the present. It is assumed that family problems can be traced to unspoken rules of behaviour, disagreements or rule making within the family and that this may lead to distorted communication. The therapist helps to expose the rules and work with the family to modify them and to improve communication by varying ways of communicating with each other and helping the family set goals.

The indications for family therapy are judged on clinical grounds and one of the most common areas of application is with adolescents and children. This could be treatment where the speech therapist has an important role to play, but it is important to draw attention to the need for specialized training. Working with families either on a regular basis or doing brief sessional therapy is particularly helpful for those speech therapists working with communication problems in mental health. It helps to trace some of the communication patterns used by the patient back to the family setting and to identify the origins of the problem. Another advantage of this type of work is that many families, particularly of institutionalized patients, like to feel included in treatment and are happy to establish a communicative link with the clinical team. Much useful background information is gathered during these sessions and often an improvement in patient and family relationships develops by encouraging more open and freer communication. It is an opportunity to support and assist families to come to terms with their relation's illness and past problems and build towards a more positive future. Recommended further reading is *Basic Family Therapy* (Barker, 1986).

Counselling

Counselling is a form of psychotherapy in which a person who faces a specific challenge is helped to clarify and find solutions to the problem, which may involve making an important life decision or coming to terms with a significant life event (Hobbs, 1988). Counselling may enable a person to overcome a problem before it generates psychological crisis and the need for crisis therapy. It involves cooperation from the patient rather than dependence or regression and aims to reduce emotional tension by encouraging free expression. The patient can begin to think more clearly and achieve a better understanding of his problem. Often counselling is an integral part of the overall treatment plan for the patient – this might mean that one therapist is wearing two therapists' hats, for example, as a speech therapist working with the communication problem and as a counsellor helping adjust to the difficulties and feelings arising from the disability. Training in the use of counselling methods is considered essential in order to develop the qualities that determine a counselling relationship, including genuineness, non-possessive warmth, accurate empathy, unconditional acceptance and respect for the client, permissiveness, caring and the communication of these attitudes to the client (Rogers, 1951). For further reading see *Practical Counselling and Helping Skills* (Nelson-Jones, 1988) and *Your Patient may need Counselling* (Brumfitt, 1986).

Relaxation and hypnosis

The teaching of relaxation skills is a technique used by speech therapists in the treatment and management of a variety of speech disorders, including stammering and voice dysfunction. It can be helpful too when working with psychiatric patients who have no obvious speech or language pathology; for example, it can be a good idea to start off a social skills group with some gentle relaxation practice to give the patients a feeling of calmness and confidence. An extension of this simple procedure is to use hypnosis (Marcuse, 1959).

Hypnosis can be used in a number of ways: as induction without suggestion, which is similar in effect to deep relaxation because it involves using induction techniques to arrive at a state of light hypnosis; in direct therapy to elicit relevant facts, for example, recall of a traumatic incident in childhood which 'triggered' a stammering response; as an indirect therapy in conjunction with other therapeutic procedures (for example, psychotherapy or personal construct therapy) or to eliminate symptoms such as anxiety associated with phobias (symptom therapy). Obviously these procedures may be combined at any one time. It has been demonstrated that hypnosis can be a powerful adjunct to conventional speech therapy teaching as in the treatment of, for example, voice disorders (Lucas and Levy, 1984) but the degree of success is often dependent on the competence and experience of the therapist. Roet (1986) says 'hypnosis is a tool in the hands of the therapist, not a treatment'. Clearly the speech therapist who is considering using hypnosis with mentally ill patients should only attempt to deal with problems with which she feels competent. In particular, the beginner should avoid treating psychotic or severely disturbed individuals. There is the theoretical danger that these patients may prefer the fantasy of hypnosis to the real world and, as a result, may cause difficulty for the therapist in terminating the hypnotic state. For further information on hypnosis and speech therapy, the British Society of Hypnosis can be contacted via the College of Speech Therapists, who also have guidelines on the use of hypnosis in speech therapy.

Augmentative/alternative communication

As in any other speech therapy clinic there will be some psychiatric patients who will be unable to depend on the use of speech and language to fulfil all their communicative needs because, for example, they have impaired language function as a result of a cerebrovascular accident or disturbance to the coordination of the fine oral/facial motor movements required for speech, as a result of an illness like multiple sclerosis. For these patients a communication aid or a gestural system *may* be an acceptable augmentative or alternative form of communication.

Computers

Use of computers is gathering popularity in many areas of mental health as they can be used as a communication tool between people. There is a need to work together jointly in order to learn how to use a computer, and so therapist and patient are likely to increase rather than decrease their communication together, thereby reducing social isolation.

The three main functions of a computer for the mentally ill patient are treatment, education and entertainment. Computers used in mental health have been known to generate formation of spontaneous small groups. Curiosity about what others are doing around the screen and keyboard can lead to tentative approaches and eventual participation in this new and fascinating occupation. They may therefore be a valuable aid to the improvement of communication competence as well as being used as a method of assessment and treatment in a number of ways. As part of treatment, programmes can be designed to be used in memory work, and this can be an additional help towards accurate diagnosis. They can also be used as an assessment to establish a baseline for cognitive ability. By dealing with a number of levels of ability and graduating in difficulty, they help to increase dexterity, concentration and overall performance. Computers can also be used in reality work, reminiscence and problem-solving therapy, all of which necessitate the patient's involvement and interaction with others.

Communication aids

A communication aid can be described as an assistive device which provides an augmentative or alternative means of communication for the speech impaired (Enderby, 1987). There is an extensive range of devices available, from simple communication charts to complex computerized equipment. In the UK there are a number of communication aids centres which provide an evaluation and demonstration service. The speech therapist in psychiatry may come across patients who would benefit from an assistive device. It is necessary to assess the patient's strengths and needs thoroughly in order to try and match these with a suitable aid, and it is recommended that advice be sought from specialists in the area of assistive communication and, where possible, the patient should be referred to a communication aids centre. Once a suitable aid has been identified the speech therapist is often involved in finding the funds to purchase it, 'teaching' the use of the aid to the patient and staff and finally the 'maintenance' of the aid and liaison with the manufacturing company. It is the experience of the writers that a communication aid can be used successfully by some psychiatric patients, even long-stay chronic patients, and it can both enrich and expand their life experiences.

Gestural systems

It is an asset for any speech therapist in a psychiatric setting to have a working knowledge of a gestural system. The preferred system for use with adult psychiatric patients is Amer-Ind, which is based on the ancient hand talk of the American Indians and has been adapted for use with the speechless by Skelly (1979). Its advantage over the other systems such as Makaton and Deaf Signing is that it can be taught quite easily at the simplest functional level to patients with impaired speech and language, thereby providing them with a means of communication, albeit limited. In addition, it can help the therapist to convey messages to patients with impaired comprehension, for example to patients in the advanced stages of dementia or patients with severe hearing impairment. In this way a gestural system which is easily understood by the untrained viewer can greatly facilitate communication between staff and patients.

In the case of patients with concomitant mental handicap it may be more appropriate to consider the Makaton Language Programme (Walker, 1979) because this is the one most commonly used with mentally handicapped people in the UK. Obviously this will be inappropriate if other countries or districts adopt different systems.

Congenitally deaf patients may wish to use or be taught one of the deaf signing systems such as British Sign Language (BSL) or Paget-Gorman (Brennan et al., 1980). BSL is currently the preferred system in the regional deaf units for the mentally ill in the UK.

Feeding therapy

Another area of therapy that the speech therapist is likely to be involved in is feeding and general mealtime behaviour. There are many practical and ethical considerations to be taken into account and this is a very difficult and potentially very worrying area. Patients may be having feeding difficulties for many different reasons; for example, there may be a breakdown in the feeding mechanism due to a degenerative disorder like Huntingdon's chorea or vascular (multi-infarct) dementia, or there may be pseudo-bulbar palsy, increased extrapyramidal (Parkinsonian) involvement or even tumour. None of these feeding problems can be diagnosed without further investigation and this is often not made easily available to mentally ill patients. Scans and videofluoroscopy are expensive and often only available at major hospitals, which may be some distance away. Should there be errors in diagnosis or misjudgements made in advice or therapy, then the speech therapist could be held accountable and may face litigation.

Unless the speech therapist in psychiatry has particular training in or accredited experience of working with feeding problems it is recommended that advice should be confined to what can be observed to be going wrong. It may be that head and neck posture is poor or that the patient is uncomfortable and unsupported in the chair or too much food or fluid may be being taken into the mouth and to the back of the tongue without preparation for the swallow. To discuss with the care staff the importance of good posture, small amounts and much reinforcement of cues like 'chew', 'swallow', 'slowly' etc. can provide them with much needed support. The preservation of the cough reflex needs to be emphasized as does the need *not* to mix textures too much and *not* to encourage the patient to 'wash it down with a drink' but rather to dry swallow several times or to cough.

Specific advice on how to approach the patient with feeding/swallowing difficulties may be found in Logemann (1983). If there was a recognized dysphagia team within the locality, then referral to the speech therapist in that team would be strongly indicated. Failing that, advice could be sought from a speech therapist colleague with dysphagia training.

Many long-stay patients have very poor and often antisocial mealtime behaviour. This may consist of gorging food, taking from other people's plates, or simply slurping, dribbling and being generally messy and unpleasant. For many of these patients rewards are rare and food or drink provide one of the few chances of self-gratification. It is as if behaviour has regressed to the level where they can only be sure the food or drink is theirs when it has been consumed and that basic needs have to be fulfilled immediately. Behavioural techniques can prove very useful in modifying these acquired mealtime habits. Altering the surroundings to lessen the temptation to take from another patient's plate, serving two small portions instead of one large one so that the second will act as a reward, as well as repeated verbal cues and modelling and shaping techniques can all produce results. Social skills sessions at mealtimes can also prove effective. It is often because awareness of the social aspect of mealtimes has been lost that patients display obsessional or gorging behaviour. Reintroducing the social aspect in gradual stages can reintroduce the idea that mealtimes are not purely for physical gratification but can be interactive and relaxing.

Challenging psychotic behaviours

A type of therapy that may seem like a contradiction in terms is that of dealing with the 'schizophrenic behaviour' as a therapy. It involves techniques like confrontation, distraction and redirection. The therapist may agree with the patient or disagree in order to make them aware that there are other ideas and beliefs than their own and that their own ideas are not easily understood by others.

The therapist needs to have established a good rapport with the patient and to be accurate in gauging the mood of the patient before confronting the delusional system. Delusional beliefs are often of long standing and can be supported by a whole range of quite reasoned arguments which fit in exactly with that fixed idea. For example, one patient known to the writers was, when very ill, convinced that he was on earth at the behest of the Inter Galactic Federation. Money, knowledge, strength and power were unlimited so any challenge to his delusions was easily responded to with 'I don't have to because . . .'. His history was well documented so his former employment was known and could be used to challenge him in very grandiose moments – for example by saying 'I know you believe that you can earn £50 000 an hour but how much did you earn when you worked for . . . ?' As this patient became more stable and began to gain some insight he even began to see some amusement in a comparison of his imagined earnings with his previous hourly rate.

It may be necessary to ask a patient to stop if they are becoming too unrealistic. The therapist can agree to listen for a specified length of time later but request that for the present they return to the topic under discussion. This may need to be done many times in a session. There may be the need to reintroduce the topic several times in one session, for example by saying 'that is very interesting but we were talking about X'. If this kind of redirection is done in a pleasant, non-threatening way then the patient is likely to cooperate and may even be able to learn from the redirection.

Some patients will use their illness as a crutch and as a means of getting out of situations. A 53-year-old male schizophrenic who had been in and out of hospital for many years had perfected a nice line in avoidance tactics. When asked to partake in a cookery group in the occupational therapy department because it was hoped he could join a pre-discharge group, his response was 'I can't do that, I'm a mental defective, and it's your job to look after me'. He was immediately complimented on his impeccable powers of reasoning and similar logic was used to prove the need for the group.

There is always the concern that confronting a patient and challenging in any way the delusional beliefs will provoke anger and aggression. This is seldom the case if the situation is handled with tact and insight. If the therapist is aware that the patient has resorted to psychotic behaviours to avoid a threatening situation or an anxiety-provoking topic then merely by changing the situation or pursuing another topic there can be a re-establishment of the status quo. It is important to be aware of boundaries and to work within them and only push them forward at an appropriate and jointly determined rate.

Unsettled, inappropriate and violent behaviour

Some of the reluctance about working in mental health is due to continuing lack of knowledge about the unusual behaviour exhibited by some of those people suffering from mental illness. Much information is based on myth, mystery and misinformation and the subsequent fear or horror surrounding the stories heard or read.

The major fear is that of being involved in, or the recipient of, a violent incident. Inappropriate, unpredictable, aggressive, abusive and antisocial behaviour is encountered from time to time and may demonstrate the recurrence of symptoms of mental illness or a prelude to the initial diagnosis. Even when in hospital or on regularly monitored medication, control of symptoms can break down and the patient become so disturbed that he is difficult to nurse on a large ward or might even need temporary isolation until he feels safe and well enough to rejoin the ward setting. In a very few cases this state could go on for some considerable time.

Occurrence of an aggressive incident should not necessarily mean never working with those people who have had a previous history of unpredictable behaviour. Careful management, organization and treatment planning will make it possible to include such patients in various therapies as well as maintaining confidence, calmness and a positive approach to treatment by the therapist.

If as a therapist one is fearful, agitated, anxious or unsure these feelings are quickly transmitted to the patient who, if he was not feeling uncertain at the beginning of the session, will quickly respond to these feelings of discomfort during the course of the session, enough perhaps to precipitate a premature conclusion to the treatment session. This will not augur well for future therapy. Individual therapy for some of these patients is often stressful and inadvisable as stress is likely to precipitate impulsive aggressive behaviour, particularly if the patient should feel trapped within the therapeutic setting and, added to this, if he is with a person who he does not know as well as he does his regular nurses. If individual work is possible it is wise to include a nurse in the therapy programme, particularly during the early sessions, and this has many additional therapeutic benefits too.

Therapy sessions should be structured to ensure that they are held regularly on the same day at the same time and place and that the session does not last too long. It is better to finish whilst the patient is still interested as this encourages positive feelings towards future sessions. Interruptions once the session has begun are to be avoided wherever possible. In fact there are bonus points for the therapist if, for instance, called to the telephone she refuses to go and asks that a message is taken. This helps engender feelings of importance and commitment to therapy and so helps cement the therapeutic alliance.

Overall therapeutic goals should be kept straightforward, should be understood wherever possible by the patient and naturally must be within the patient's ability to accomplish. As many of these patients will be on some form of medication which could affect both memory and concentration it is essential to explain clearly about changes or cancellation of therapy and to check that the patient has fully understood the message. Even so those suffering from thought disorder and poor memory or concentration can still be muddled in spite of constant reminding by nurses and are likely to have forgotten and misinterpreted the message between sessions. Misunderstandings are unlikely to occur if explanations are satisfactory initially.

As previously mentioned it is important that both patient and therapist feel safe throughout their sessions together. Therefore, the same rules should be noted as those used when working with other psychiatric patients. In addition to keeping the treatment room door freely accessible to both patient and therapist there should also be an emergency bell at arm's length and there should be no furniture between them. If a table is needed, rather than sit opposite each other, it is best to sit at right angles so that neither therapist nor patient is trapped.

During the course of therapy the patient might want to talk about himself, his illness and his past violence. This latter subject does not suggest that he is feeling violent at the moment – quite the opposite, he is in fact possibly feeling safe enough to talk about his violence. Therefore, the therapist needs to feel able to accept this subject and respond accordingly. If, for example, a patient should become agitated or disturbed by responding to his hallucinations, by defending his delusions or denying his mental illness, in order to help keep him calm gently direct the focus of the conversation away from the source of trouble by responding sympathetically and introducing a new topic.

For those patients recovering from an unsettled time, small or large group meetings for communication and discussion or support can provide opportunities for observation and assessment of the patient in a formal therapeutic session as well as encourage the patient to express how he feels, how he felt previously, and what his hopes are for the future. This might well be the first experience of formal group therapy where there is a chance to talk about the illness; to share symptoms and problems; to demonstrate a continuing lack of or the returning of insight into the illness; to debate the value of medication; share previous experiences and history; express anger, disappointment, sorrow, happiness, friendship; and perhaps have a good laugh. The format of the group needs to be carefully planned, ideally two patients sitting alternately between the therapists in a circle. This does of course mean a much higher ratio of staff to patients than is usual. If patients should then become unsettled the situation can be diffused with the minimum of disturbance within the group. Occasionally a patient will wish to leave the session; his exit should be mentioned at the time and an invitation offered to join the next group session. The nurses who care for these patients know the signs of developing unrest, they can anticipate difficulties and identify situations and subjects that are likely to cause problems in each of their patients and it is this knowledge that makes it possible to organize successful groups even with the most disturbed mentally ill patients. The need to maintain good communication links with the multidisciplinary team and in particular those nurses who work closely with the individual patients and who are regularly in the group is paramount to the continuation of successful therapy.

It is good practice to arrive well before therapy sessions to discuss the previous week's progress, to learn about the patient's present state and to plan the following session. A post-session talk is equally necessary to share thoughts of the past session, to identify the patient's immediate needs and to report progress or concern and to renegotiate any relevant changes. Experiences working in such groups and with very many disturbed patients have proved to be worthwhile even if the progress is limited or transient. Some patients do make recognizable progress, move to less secure settings and maintain this progress, as well as give hope to others not yet ready to move on. For further reading on this subject *Clinical Approaches to Violence* (Howells and Hollin, 1989) is suggested.

RESETTLEMENT

Given that many psychiatric hospitals were built away from the parent community in the belief that 'fresh air would be good' for patients, resettlement can prove problematic. Many patients from inner city areas no longer have any links with their place of origin. Communities which have become accustomed to an institution on their doorstep, where problems are seen as being contained, are going to be understandably resistant to large numbers of patients being resettled locally.

It is only comparatively recently that the damaging effects of long-term institutional care have been studied and the research has brought about therapeutic changes. It is now known that avoiding admission, early discharge and combined behavioural, social and domestic rehabilitation in open hospitals may be a better practice and may prevent the accumulation of long-stay institutionalized patients, allowing them to return to participate in community life. This is certainly true of those patients who are least impaired and who have been most responsive to drug and social therapies; although, as was stated in Chapter one there will be those who continue to need long-term care and whose behaviours would set them apart in a community setting (Curson *et al.*, 1988).

Role in the community

Increasingly now the input of a speech therapist to community care teams is being either offered or sought. The role in these teams is as varied as in all other areas of psychiatry. Assessments of communicative abilities and needs can provide information for care groupings, and can be of value in selection of patients for pre-discharge groups in hospital. Speech therapy skills can help a team in drawing up a philosophy of care for a hostel ward or group home. Laying emphasis on communication as the major social skill can help maintain all therapy programmes on as broad a base as possible, so that resettlement is not just a matter of independent living but of development and integration.

The educational role of the speech therapist is obvious with community care staff. There is a need to be sure that everyone is aware of the communicative needs of individual residents and of the group as a whole. The educational role of the speech therapist with the community itself is perhaps less obvious but as 'public relations officers' and speakers on the needs of the mentally ill speech therapists can be equally as effective as any other profession. Church groups, schools, local council committees and any other local community groups may welcome extra information and the greater awareness of need that it brings. This may help allay some of their fears when faced with the problems that providing local care can bring.

Follow-up is very important in resettlement. It can prove difficult in that some patients may be discharged to accommodation at some distance. However, it is important to remember that simply because the goal of community care has been reached, this does not mean complete success. The stresses and strains of moving are familiar to most. It is known that there are difficulties in adjusting to new surroundings and in establishing new routines and new contacts. For patients discharged from hospital the task of adjustment can be formidable and therefore maximum support is called for. Many patients who are otherwise fairly stable find the idea of leaving 'asylum' intolerable. One patient known to the writers is a 44-year-old woman with schizophrenia. She is well motivated within the hospital, cares for herself and manages her money and her social life. Her illness is well controlled by medication and her insight is good. In every way this lady is an ideal candidate for a hostel. However, when faced with this plan for discharge several times in the last few years, symptoms have recurred. She becomes depressed, develops phobias about travelling or going out and has even suffered a return of auditory, visual and somatic hallucinations. It is hoped that a hospital hostel on the site and eventual local placement with other residents in a group home may provide the answer.

The speech therapist's role in community care is one of assessment, education, planning, providing therapy in the home environment or day centre and maintenance of skills. This role will be a common one for all team members and will hopefully be effective and enable the patient to feel supported, encouraged and able to develop links within the community. The hope for the future is that there will be more multidisciplinary community care teams coming into existence with the resources to meet the needs of this group of patients.

DISCHARGE FROM SPEECH THERAPY

Many patients seen by the speech therapist working in psychiatry are likely to need to be 'on the books' for some time. Progress may be very slow and the outcome of therapy, aimed at improving the quality of life, difficult to measure. Recent work by Ponton (1989) demonstrates an innovative way of looking at case-loads and takes into account not only the level of clinical need but also positive and negative factors which will influence the outcome of therapy. Discharge from speech therapy may be due to the influencing factors of poor motivation and support which contraindicates continuation of therapy. In a psychiatric setting, as in many other settings, speech therapy will only be successful in helping the patient achieve the aims and goals set if there is a carry-over outside the clinic so that skills can be generalized.

Discharge may also come about because the patient has reached the targets agreed at the commencement of therapy. It is possible to discharge a patient because there has been maximum improvement but there should be a recommended period of review which could be gradually lengthened, i.e. one month, then three months, then six months. This is because complete withdrawal of an important relationship could prove upsetting to some patients who may not see discharge as an achievement but a loss of one or many mechanisms for support. A structured and graded approach is as appropriate to discharge as it is to therapy.

In some cases discharge may have to take place as the patient has moved from the hospital, group home or hostel to the community too far away for full follow-up by a specialist speech therapist. As stated, community care is in its infancy and care teams, with speech therapy representations, are as yet not numerous. Before a patient is discharged from speech therapy the local mechanisms and opportunities for follow-up and support must be investigated fully, explained to the patient, and if indicated contact made with a local speech therapist who will be prepared, if fully briefed, to maintain links as part of a wider team-based support network.

STAFF/CARER-ORIENTED WORK

Therapists working in psychiatry divide their time between direct patient contact and working with staff and carers. This is an important component of the job and should not be undervalued. A public relations job is vital to establish the department and encourage appropriate referrals. Educational aspects of the work are ongoing and may be formal and informal.

Formal education

The 'formal' area of work with staff and carers involves a great deal of structured teaching which might be in the form of workshops, lecturing and demonstrations. The teaching does not usually relate to any particular patient and is of general interest. It is usually to groups of people and the speech therapy input may be just a small section in a multidisciplinary programme, for example as part of a course in the care of elderly people for nursing assistants. Another example would be feeding workshops run by the speech therapy, physiotherapy and dietetics departments, designed to be of general application to qualified nurses, who want to update and expand their skills even if they are not caring for any patients with feeding problems at that time.

Formal teaching is with both students and qualified staff of all disciplines. Most of it takes place within the hospital, in the school or nursing or within the speech therapy department. However, there may also be opportunity for some teaching outside the hospital to speech therapy training establishments, to meetings of speech therapists and other disciplines or special interest groups. It is impossible to say which of these teaching situations has the most application, albeit indirectly, to patient care but it is important to remember that any contact with student nurses and doctors is valuable because they will be the ward managers of the future and their attitudes and behaviour will have a direct effect on the rehabilitation of our patients.

In some settings, the speech therapist will also be involved in some formal teaching of relatives and carers. This can be a rewarding and enlightening experience for therapists and it can be quite challenging as well because one has to 'pitch' the information at the right level to be both interesting and meaningful to them.

Problems and solutions

It is useful to look at some of the problems associated with formal teaching programmes because in this way it may be possible to avoid the pitfalls – for example, the initial stages of setting up a workshop are vital. Proper negotiations with managers are important as workshops take a lot of preparation and time on the part of the facilitators and the workshop leaders need assurance that enough staff will be released from duties and allowed to leave the ward or departments in order to participate. It is especially important that nursing managers make a commitment in advance, to allow their staff to attend because they obviously have to find alternative means of staffing the wards during this time. Often the teaching is to a group of mixed disciplines and the need is to keep everyone's concentration and interest. This means that there should be plenty of audience participation with shared anecdotes, examples and role-playing. Humour is a useful means of keeping the group's attention and there needs to be a varied approach to teaching, with the use of aids such as overheads, slides, video and handouts. An informal atmosphere can help to relax participants and make them more willing to be involved. Finally, it is helpful for the organizers to have some written feedback at the end of a course or workshop so that they can evaluate its achievements objectively.

Informal education

It is possible to teach a great deal to staff and carers in an informal way. For example, if the therapist has a patient to whom she is teaching Amer-Ind signals, she will be feeding back the patient's progress to the ward staff and relatives, if appropriate, and teaching them the same

311

signals so that they can recognize and respond to them when the patient uses them. In this way, they will be able to reinforce the programme at every opportunity. In other cases it may be necessary for the therapist to demonstrate good practices to the carers – such as the use and maintenance of a patient's hearing aid or communication aid, or the best position in which to feed a patient and the most suitable food textures to give.

Counselling staff/carers

The close working involvement of therapists and carers may lead to situations where the therapist is required to take a counselling role. In many cases this is an entirely appropriate use of therapist's time. However, the therapist may sometimes find herself required to counsel in an area with which she is unfamiliar or uncomfortable. In this instance, she should refer the carer on to someone who has the appropriate skills. Often there is another team member who can take the case on, but occasionally the need arises to use another agency (for example, a marriage guidance counsellor). It is becoming more common for speech therapists to embark on extensive counselling courses to enable them to deal more effectively with this area of their work.

Another way of supporting carers is to set up carer support groups. These are usually started by a couple of disciplines, perhaps a community psychiatric nurse and a speech therapist, and are structured to allow time for informal discussion and mutual support, as well as allowing for some formal presentation of material from an invited speaker (for example, a social worker talking about benefits). It has been stated before that any group of this kind needs very careful planning and organization if it is to be effective (Penner, 1989; Hepburn and Wasaw, 1986).

Changing staff behaviours

It is the speech therapist's responsibility to encourage good communication practices amongst staff and carers and this will inevitably involve some teaching, either formal or informal, to help them achieve an understanding of the processes involved in effective communication (for example listening skills and clear, comprehensive speech). The carers need to be aware of the importance of using non-ambiguous language themselves if they are to expect appropriate responses from patients. They need to be taught to listen more carefully to what patients are saying because with careful listening it is often possible to make sense, for example, of the utterances of schizophrenic patients and make correct interpretations of their references. It must not be assumed that all staff have good listening skills intuitively – they do not. One good way of teaching good communication practices is by demonstrations within interview situations. The speech therapist can show the carers what strategies to employ to talk to confused patients or the hard of hearing, for example by sitting the patient in a good position where he can see the speaker's face clearly, by using gestures to reinforce the speech, by repeating the main features of the message, by using simple, non-ambiguous language, by giving the patient plenty of time to make a response, and by breaking his response down and repeating it back to him in question form to make sure it has been correctly interpreted. These are relatively simple skills to acquire but they do need to be taught to carers.

One final point about changing staff behaviour concerns the indirect benefits of therapy programmes. There is evidence in the literature to state that the attitudes and behaviour of staff often change in a positive way when they are involved in specific therapy programmes with patients. For example, some of the early research into reality orientation programmes in the 1970s discovered an unexpected benefit in that the programme gave a focus for the staff working in the notoriously stressful area of the care of elderly confused people and the increase in their involvement and interest led to a reduction in absenteeism and sickness and to better time-keeping and more fulfilled staff (Powell-Proctor and Millar, 1982). Further evidence of this benefit on a smaller scale can be seen with individual members of staff who take particular interest in speech therapy programmes with individual patients – they report that their involvement makes their job more meaningful and satisfying.

Speech therapists will always be thin on the ground in psychiatry and therefore there will only be a relatively small number of patients who will benefit from direct contact with a speech therapist. However, it is possible to reach a much larger population of patients through teaching large numbers of staff and carers the best ways to encourage and facilitate communication with and between their patients.

CONCLUSION

Speech therapy is a comparatively new profession and it is still in the process of evaluating the service it provides. Psychiatry is probably the newest field within speech therapy and, as stated in the introduction to this chapter, it is an exciting and challenging area in which to work. The therapists currently working in psychiatry appear to be moving away from traditional therapy by developing innovative approaches to the management of communication disorder in mentally ill people. It could be argued that they are also moving away from the traditional role of the speech therapist in the multidisciplinary team, but the writers prefer to view the change as an extension and expansion of their traditional role. The speech therapist's role in psychiatry is somewhat unique and it needs to be evaluated with carefully planned and conducted research. At the same time there is a need for detailed guidelines on quality assurance so that standards for intervention and therapy can be both described and maintained. This is an ideal time for speech therapists to demonstrate their value and make an important contribution to the care of communicatively-impaired people.

REFERENCES

Andreasen, N. G. and Grove, W. M. (1979) The relationship between schizophrenic language, manic language and aphasia, in *Hemisphere Asymmetries of Function in Psychopathology* (eds J. Gruzelier and P. Flore-Henry), Elsevier, New York.

Bannister, D. (ed.) (1975) *Issues and Approaches in the Psychological Therapies*, Wiley, Chichester.

Barbara, D. A. (1962) *The Psychotherapy of Stuttering*, Charles and Thomas, Springfield, Illinois.

Barker, P. (1986) *Basic Family Therapy*, 2nd edn, Collins, London.

Beck, A. T., Shaw, A. J. Rush, B. F. and Emery, G. (1979) *Cognitive Therapy of Depression*, Wiley, Chichester.

Bishop, D. (1983) *Test for the Reception of Grammar*, University of Manchester.

Bloch, S. (ed.) (1986) *An Introduction to the Psychotherapies*, 2nd edn, Oxford University Press, Oxford.

Blunden, R. (1980) *Individual Plans for Mentally Handicapped People: A Draft Procedural Guide*, Mental Handicap in Wales, Applied Research Unit, Cardiff.

Boone, D. R. (1983) *The Voice and Voice Therapy*, 3rd edn, Prentice-Hall, Englewood Cliffs, New Jersey.

Brennan, M., Colville, M. and Lawson, L. (1980) *Words in Hand: A Structural Analysis of the Signs of British Sign Language*, The BSL Research Project, Moray House, Edinburgh.

British Society of Hypnosis in the Practice of Speech Therapy. *Guidelines held by The College of Speech Therapists*, Harold Poster House, London.

Brumfitt, S. (1986) *Your Patient May Need Counselling*, Winslow Press, Bicester, Oxon.

Button, E. (1986) *Personal Construct Theory and Mental Health*, Croom Helm, London.

Cattell, R. B. (1952) *Factor Analysis*, Harper and Row, New York.

Cattell, R. B. (1965) *The Scientific Analysis of Personality*, Penguin Books, Harmondsworth, Middlesex.

Cattell, R. B. and Ebel, H. W. (revised 1968) *Sixteen Personality Factor Questionnaire*, NFER Nelson, Windsor.

Cheek, F. and Amarel, M. (1968) Studies in the sources of variation in Cloze Scores: II, the verbal passages . *Journal of Abnormal Psychology*, **73**, 424–30.

Clare, A. W. (1988) Individual psychotherapies, in *Companion Guide to Psychiatric Studies*, 4th edn (eds R. E. Kendell and A. K. Zealley), Churchill Livingstone, Edinburgh, pp. 726–42.

Clifford, P. I. (1987) *The National Unit for Psychiatric Research and Development Questionnaire*, available from Lewisham Hospital, London SE13 6LH.

Cox, M. (1988) *Coding the Therapeutic Process: Emblems of Encounter*, Jessica Kingsley, London.

Crystal, D. (1982) *Profiling Linguistic Disability*, Edward Arnold, London.

Curson, D., Liddle, P., Patel, M. and Barnes, T. (1988) Psychiatric morbidity of a long-stay hospital population with chronic schizophrenia and implications for future community care. *British Medical Journal*, **197**, 819–22.

Darley, F. L., Aronson, E. E. and Brown, J. R. (1975) *Motor Speech Disorders*, Saunders, Philadelphia.

De Renzi, E. and Vignolo, L. A. (1972) The token test: A sensitive test to detect receptive disturbances in aphasics. *Brain*, **85**, 665–78.

Dewald, P. A. (1969) *Psychotherapy: A Dynamic Approach*, Blackwell Scientific Publications, Oxford.

Di Simoni, F. B., Farley, F. L. and Aronson, A. E. (1977) Patterns of dysfunction in schizophrenic patients on an asphasic test battery. *Journal of Speech and Hearing Disorders*, **41**, 494–513.

Edwards, A. L. (1954) *Edwards Personal Preference Schedule*, New York Psychological Corporation.

Elliot, P., Barlow, F., Hooper, A. and Kingerlee, P. E. (1977) Maintaining patients improvement on a token economy, in *Behaviour Research and Therapy*, **17**, 333–6.

Enderby, P. (1987) *Assistive Communication Aids for the Speech Impaired*, Churchill Livingstone, Edinburgh.

Enderby, P. (1988) *The Frenchay Dysarthria Assessment*. NFER Nelson, Windsor.

English, G. M. (1976) *Otolaryngology: A Textbook*, Harper & Row, New York.

Eysenck, H. J. and Eysenck, S. B. G. (1963) *Eysenck Personality Inventory*, NFER-Nelson, Windsor.

Faber, R. and Reichstein, M. B. (1981) Language dysfunction in schizophrenia *British Journal of Psychiatry*, **139**, 519–22.

Faber, R., Abrams, R., Taylor, M., *et al.* (1983) Comparison of schizophrenic patients with formal thought disorder and neurologically impaired patients with aphasia. *American Journal of Psychiatry*, **140**, 1348–51.

Fawcus, M., Robinson, M., Williams, J and Williams, R. (1986) *Working with Dysphasics*, Winslow Press, Bicester, Oxon.

Folsom, J. C. (1968) Reality orientation for the elderly mental patient. *Journal of Geriatric Psychiatry*, **1**, 291–307.

Fransella, F. and Bannister, D. (1977) *A Manual for Repertory Grid Technique*, Academy Press, London.

Gambrill, E. D. (1977) *Behaviour Modification*, Jossey-Bass, London.

Gelder, M., Gath, D. and Mayou, R. (1986) *Oxford Textbook of Psychiatry*. Oxford University Press, Oxford.

Gerson, S. N., Benson, D. F. and Frazier, S. (1977) Diagnosis: schizophrenia versus posteria aphasia. *American Journal of Psychiatry*, **134**, 966–9.

Glauber, I. P. (1958) The psychoanalysis of stuttering, in *Stuttering: A symposium* (ed. J. Eisenson), Harper & Row, New York, pp. 71–119.

Goodglass, H. and Kaplan, E. (1983) *The Boston Diagnostic Aphasic Examination*, Lea and Febiger, Beckenham, Kent.

Gottesman, I. I. (1963) Heritability of personality: a demonstration. *Psychological Monographs* **77**, whole no. 572.

Greer, R. (1989) Hypnosis is no last resort. *Speech Therapy in Practice*, **4**, 9.

Hall, J. and Baker, R. (1983) *Rehabilitation Evaluation*, Vine Publishing, Aberdeen.

Hanley, I. and Gilhooly, M. (1986) *Psychological Therapies for the Elderly*, Croom Helm, London.

Harrington, J. A. (1988) Contemporary issues in psychotherapy, in *Perspectives in Psychotherapy* (eds P. Hall and P. D. Stonier), Wiley, Chichester.

Hathaway, S. and McKinley, J. (1970) *Minnesota Multiphasic Personality Inventory*, NFER Nelson, Windsor.

Hawton, K., Salkovskis, P. M., Kirk, J. and Clark, M. (eds) (1989) *Cognitive Behaviour Therapy for Psychiatric Problems: A Practical Guide*. Oxford Medical Publications, Oxford.

Hayhow, R. and Levy C. (1989) *Working with Stuttering: A Personal Construct Approach*, Winslow Press, Bicester, Oxon.

Hepburn, K. and Wasaw, M. (1986) *Support Groups for Family Care Givers of Dementia Victims: Questions, Directions and Further Research*. (*New Directions for Mental Health Services*, Vol. 29), Jossey-Bass, San Francisco.

Hobbs, M. (1988) The psychological treatments, in *Essential Psychiatry* (ed. N. Rose), Blackwell Scientific Publications, Oxford.

Hodkinson, H. M., Stevens, S. J. and Kenny, R. A., (1984) Is dysphasia a feature of speech in senile dementia of Alzheimer's type? *Journal of Clincial and Experimental Gerontology*, **6**, 261–7.

Holden, U. P. (ed.) (1984) Nostalgia Series, Winslow Press, Bicester, Oxon.

Holden, U. P. and Woods, R. T. (1982) *Reality Orientation: Psychological Approaches to the 'Confused' Elderly*, Churchill Livingstone, Edinburgh.

Holden, U., Martin, C. and White, M. (1982) *Twenty Four Hour Approach to the Problems of Confusion in the Elderly*, Winslow Press, Bicester, Oxon.

Hooker, D. (1989) Personal communication.

Horsfall, G. H. (1972) An investigation of selected language performance in adult schizophrenic subjects. *Dissertion Abstracts International*, **34**, 425B–53B.

Howells, K. and Hollin, C. R. (1989) *Clinical Approaches to Violence*, Wiley, Chichester.

Irwin, A. (1972) The treatment and results of 'easy stammering'. *British Journal of Disorders of Communication*, **7**, 151–6.

Johnson, T. S. (1985) *V.A.R.P. Vocal Abuse Reduction Program*, Taylor and Francis, London.

Kaplan, E., Goodglass, H. and Weintraub, S. (1983) *The Boston Naming Test*, Lea and Febiger, Beckenham, Kent.

Kelly, G. A. (1955) *The Psychology of Personal Constructs*, Norton, New York.

Kirk, S., McCarthy, J. and Kirk, W. (revised 1968) *The Illinois Test of Psycholinguistic Ability*, NFER Nelson, Windsor.

Kronfol, Z., Hamsher, K., Digre, K. and Wazir, R. (1978) Depression and hemispheric functions: changes associated with unilateral ECT. *British Journal of Psychiatry*, **132**, 560–7.

Lezak, M. D. (1983) *Neuropsychological Assessment*, 2nd edn., Oxford University Press, Oxford.

Lockhart, M. and Martin, S. (1987) The Victoria Infirmary Voice Questionnaire, in *Working with Dysphasics* (ed. S. Martin) Winslow Press, Bicester, Oxon.

Logemann, J. (1983) *Evaluation and Treatment of Swallowing Disorders*, College Hill Press, San Diego, Calif.

Lubinski, R., Morrison, E. and Rigrodsky, S. (1981) Perception of spoken communication by elderly chronically ill patients in an institutional setting. *Asha*, **46**, 405–12.

Lucas, H. and Levy, M. (1984) The use of hypnosis in an unusual voice disorder: a combined clinical psychology and speech therapy approach. *Bulletin of the College of Speech Therapists*, **383**, 1–2.

Marcuse, F. L. (1959) *Hypnosis, Fact and Fiction*, Pelican, London.

Martin, S. (1987) *Working with Dysphasics*, Winslow Press, Bicester, Oxon.

Marzillier, J. S. (1978) Verbal methods of behaviour change. *Behavioural Psychotherapy*, **6**, 85–90.

McNeil, M. and Prescott, T. (1978) *The Revised Token Test*, Pro-ed, Austin, Texas.

McNeil, M., Rosenbeck, J. C. and Aronson, A. E. (1984) *The Dysarthrias: Physiology, Acoustics, Perception, Management*, College Hill Press, San Diego, Calif.

Miller, E. (1984) Verbal fluency test. *British Journal of Clinical Psychology*, **23**, 53–7.

Miller, E. and Hague, F. (1975) Some characteristics of verbal behaviour in pre-senile dementia. *Psychological Medicine*, **5**, 255–9.

Murphy, A. T. (1964) *Functional Voice Disorders*, Prentice-Hall, Englewood Cliffs, New Jersey.

Neale, D. (revised 1988) *Analysis of Reading Ability*, NFER Nelson.

Nelson, H. E. (1983) *The Nelson Adult Reading Test*, NFER Nelson, Bicester, Oxon.

Nelson, H. E. and McKenna, P. (1975) Use of current reading abilities in the assessment of dementia. *British Journal of Social and Clinical Psychology*, **14**, 259–67.

Nelson-Jones, R. (1988) *Practical Counselling and Helping Skills*, 2nd edn, Cassell Educational, London.

Novaco, R. W. (1975) *Anger Control*, Lexington Books, London.

Ostwald, P. F. (1978) Language and communication problems with schizophrenic patients: a review, commentary and sythesis, in *Phenomenology and Treatment of Schizophrenia*, (eds W. E. Fann, I. Karacen, A. D. Pokorny and R. L. Williams), Spectrum, New York.

Parker, M. (1983) Sharing special skills. *Remedial Therapist*, **5** (21), 12.

Pattie, A. H. and Gilleard, C. J. (1979) *The Clifton Assessment Procedure for the Elderly*, NFER Nelson, Bicester, Oxon.

Paul, G. and Lentz, R. J. (1977) *Psycho-Social Treatment of Chronic Mental Patients*, Harvard University Press, Cambridge, Massachusetts.

Penner, S. (1989) A beginner's guide to setting up a relatives' support group for carers of elderly people with a mental illness. *British Journal of Occupational Therapy*, **52** (3), 3.

Platt, S., Hirsh, S. and Weyman, A. (1983) *The Social Behaviour Assessment Schedule*, NFER Nelson, Bicester, Oxon.

Ponton, C. (1989) District Speech Therapist, N. W. Surrey Health Authority, Goldsworth Park Health Centre, Woking, Surrey (personal communication).

Porch, B. (1973) *The Porch Index of Communicative Abilities*, NFER Nelson, Windsor.

Powell-Proctor, L. and Millar, E. (1982) Reality orientation: a critical appraisal. *British Journal of Psychiatry*, **140**, 457–63.

Rimmer, L. (1982) *Reality Orientation Principles and Practice*, Winslow Press, Bicester, Oxon.

Robertson, S. J. (1982) *Dysarthria Profile*, Winslow Press, Bicester, Oxon.

Robertson, S. J. and Thomson, F. (1982) *Working with Dysarthrics*, Winslow Press, Bicester, Oxon.

Rochester, S. R. and Martin, J. R. (1979) *Crazy Talk: A Study of the Discourse of Schizophrenic Speakers*, Plenum Press, New York.

Roet, B. (1986) *Hypnosis, A Gateway to Better Health*. Weidenfeld & Nicholson, London.

Rogers, C. (1951) *Client Centred Therapy*, Houghton Mifflin, Boston.

Rorschach, H. (1942) *Rorschach Inkblot Test Psychodiagnostics*, Hans Huber, Berne.

Rose, G. (1989) All speech therapists need some supervision. *Therapy Weekly*, February 23, 10.

Rosenbeck, J. C. and La Pointe, L. L. (1978) The dysarthrias, description, diagnosis and treatment, in *Clinical Management of Neurogenic Communicative Disorders* (ed. D. F. John), Little, Brown & Co., Boston.

Ruesch, J. (1987) Communication and mental illness, in *Communication: The Social Matrix of Psychiatry* (eds J. Ruesch and G. Bateson), Norton, New York, pp. 50–93.

Rustin, L. and Kuhr, A. (1989) *Social Skills and the Speech Impaired*, Taylor and Francis, London.

Rustin, L., Purser, H. and Rowley, D. (1987) *Progress in the Treatment of Fluency Disorders*, Taylor and Francis, London.

Rutter, D. R. (1979) The reconstruction of schizophrenic speech. *British Journal of Psychiatry*, **134**, 356–9.

Rutter, D. R. (1985) Language in schizophrenia: the structure of monologues and conversations. *British Journal of Psychiatry*, **146**, 399–404.

Rutter, D. R., Wistner, J., Kopytynska, K. and Button, M. (1978) The predictability of speech in schizophrenic patients. *British Journal of Psychiatry*, **132**, 228–32.

Ryan, P. B. and Van Kirk, B. (1974) The establishment, transfer and maintenance of fluent speech in fifty stutterers using delayed auditory feedback and operant procedures. *Journal of Speech and Hearing Disorders*, **39**, 3–10.

Sarno, M. T. (1963) *The Functional Communication Profile*, University Medical Centre, New York.

Schuell, H. (1965) *The Minnesota Test of Differential Diagnosis of Aphasia*, University of Minnesota Press.

Schuell, H. (1973) *The Shortened Schuell Test*, University of Minnesota Press.

Skelly, M. (1979) *Amer Ind Gestural Code Based on Universal American Indian Hand Talk*, Elsevier, New York.

Skinner, C., Wirz, M., Thompson, I. and Davidson, J. (1984) *The Edinburgh Functional Communication Profile*. Winslow Press, Bicester, Oxon.

Stevens, S. J. (1985a) *Dementia Checklist*, Hammersmith Hospital.

Stevens, S. J. (1985b) The language of dementia in the elderly: a pilot study. *British Journal of Disorders of Communication*, **20**, 181–90.

Trower, P., Bryant, B. and Argyle, M. (1978) *Social Skills and Mental Health*. Methuen, London.

Van Riper, C. (1973) *The Treatment of Stuttering*, Prentice-Hall, Englewood Cliffs, New Jersey.

Walker, M. (1979) The Makaton: in perspective, *Apex*, **7**, 12–14.

Walker, S. A. (1982) Communication as a changing function of age, in *Communication Changes in Elderly People* (ed. M. E. Edwards), College of Speech Therapists, London, pp. 31–8.

Warren, J. (1988) All change at Chiswick. *Geriatric Nursing and Home Care*, 10–12.

Warrington, E. K. (1985) *Recognition Memory Test*, NFER Nelson, Bicester, Oxon.

Wechsler, D. (1981) *The Wechsler Adult Intelligence Scale*, Psychological Corporation, Sidcup, Kent.

Weniger, D., Hube, W. R., Stachowiak, F. J. and Poeck, K. (1980) Treatment of aphasia on a linguistic basis, in *Aphasia: Assessment and Treatment* (eds M. T. Sarno and O. Hook), Almquist and Wiksell, Stockholm.

Wertz, R. T. (1984) Language deficit in aphasia and dementia. *Clinical Aphasiology Conference Proceedings*, BRK, Minneapolis, pp. 350–9.

Whurr, R. (1974) *An Aphasia Screening Test*, available from R. Whurr, 2 Alwyne Road, London N1 2HH.

Wilkinson, J. and Canter, S. (1982) *Social Skills Training Manual*, Wiley, Chichester.

Wilson, B., Cockburn, J. and Baddeley, A. (1985) *The Rivermead Behavioural Memory Test*, Thames Valley Test Company, Reading.

Wilson, B. and Moffat, N. (1984) *Clinical Management of Memory Problems*, Croom Helm, London.

Wolberg, L. R. (1977) *The Techniques of Psychotherapy*, Grune and Stratton, New York.

APPENDIX 10.1: INFORMAL ASSESSMENT SHEET FOR SOCIAL/COMMUNICATION SKILLS

	1	2	3	4	5	Comments
EYE CONTACT Ability to look at others and to maintain this in an appropriate way	Very limited or excessive	Rather limited or tends to be excessive	Middle range	Virtually normal	Normal	
POSTURE Ability to sit/stand or present yourself in a relaxed and comfortable way open to communication/interaction	Withdrawn, hunched, distant from main group	Tends to be withdrawn	Variable	Reasonable	Normal Relaxed Open	
GESTURE/FACIAL EXPRESSION Using the body and face as an aid to communication – i.e. smiles, hand movements	Very limited or inappropriately excessive	Tends to be inappropriate	Some but not a lot	Fair	Used appropriately	
INITIATION Ability to start a conversation	Nil	Limited	Variable	Fair	Good ability	

	1	2	3	4	5	Comments
MAINTAINING Ability to carry on and sustain a conversation or a task	Not able	Sometimes appropriate	Variable but more appropriate	Fair	Good ability	
CONCENTRATION Ability to follow cues, topics, tasks with full attention	Very poor concentration	Erratic	Needs prompts	Fair	Good concentration	
GROUP AWARENESS AND PARTICIPATION Comfort in the group. Ability to interest with others. Turn taking. Listening to others	Very poor or disruptive	Limited or somewhat disruptive	Can be achieved with help or cues	Fair	Good	
MOTIVATION Desire to attend the group. Ability to make a contribution	Does not appear motivated	Tends not to wish to contribute	Variable	Tends towards wishing to contribute	Appears well motivated	

Appendix 10.1 (continued)

	1	2	3	4	5	Comments
SUBJECT MATTER						
Repetitive/Able to change/Delusional Stable/Personal/General	Fixed	Tends to be inflexible	Some ability to change	More able to change	Varied	
RELAXATION ANXIETY	1	2	3	4	5	
Feeling/State of mind projected in group situation	Very tense	Tends to be tense	Variable	Usually fairly relaxed	Relaxed and confident	

N. J. Muir, West Park Hospital, Surrey (1989)

APPENDIX 10.2

PATIENT'S NAME:

RATER'S NAME:

Please complete the following form concerning this patient's social behaviour during the past WEEK/GROUP MEETING. Use your observations of his behaviour in WARD/O.T./GROUP. Please restrict your rating to behaviour *during this time* and do not give your general impression. To make the rating, place a tick in the appropriate column.

	A applies	Tends more towards A	Between A & B	Tends more towards B	B applies	
Happy to be engaged in conversation						Tries to avoid being engaged in conversation
1. Very short answers to questions						Gives full answers in reply to questions
2. No delay in reply to questions						Very slow to reply to questions
3. Tries to terminate conversation as quickly as possible						Happy to continue conversation, even if unable to do more than answer questions
4. Speech very hesitant						Speech flows well

Appendix 10.2 (continued)

	A applies	Tends more towards A	Between A & B	Tends more towards B	B applies
5. Initiates conversation (as opposed to asking for something) with members of staff					Never initiates conversation (as opposed to asking for something) with members of staff
6. Initiates conversation (as opposed to asking for something) with other patients					Never initiates conversation (as opposed to asking for something) with other patients
7. Tries to avoid asking for something if he needs it					Will ask for something if he needs it
8. Avoids eye contact or eye contact inappropriate					Eye contact inappropriate

H. Nelson (1989) Horton Hospital, Epsom, Surrey (unpublished)

APPENDIX 10.3: LANGUAGE/SPEECH/COMMUNICATION CHECKLIST

Other languages used ....

Ability to understand ....

Does the client respond to	with a clue	without a clue
gesture	....	....
single words	....	....
short sentences	....	....
expanded sentences	....	....
written words	....	....
written phrases	....	....
written sentences	....	....

Comments ....

....

....

Ability to express:

(a) Verbal

Does the client use   words ....

phrases ....

expanded sentences ....

Comments ....

....

....

(b) Written

Does the client	write	dictation	copy	spontaneous
	words	....	......	....
	phrases	....	......	....

Comments ....

....

....

Note the clients preferred hand ....

Ability to read:

Does the client read and understand	a newspaper ....
	a simple story ....
	a letter ....

Comments ....

....

....

Note the client's preferred reading material ....

Ability to calculate

Does the client write numbers ....

Does the client carry out simple calculations

written .... in their head ....

Comments ....

....

....

N. J. Muir, West Park Hospital, Surrey; P. Tanner, Horton Hospital, Surrey (1989).

11

The multidisciplinary team

Rosemary Gravell

Much has been written over recent years about the need for a multidisciplinary approach to all aspects of health care. Such an approach is, perhaps, of particular value in the field of psychiatry where the most important resource is the staff and lay carers involved – that is, the human resource; and where communication is central to all intervention and rehabilitation efforts.

Team-work is defined as 'the coordination of several people in cooperation to strive for a common aim' (Pollock, 1986). In relation to health care it involves a group of people who are responsible for the care of the patients, their daily well-being and overall diagnosis, treatment and future management.

Much of the work of the team in psychiatry will have rehabilitation aims, that is, towards helping a person to adjust to the limitations of his or her disability/illness by regaining lost skills and/or developing coping strategies. The ultimate goal is to restore each individual to their maximum potential level of independence – psychologically, socially, physically and economically. The approach must focus on abilities rather than disabilities and must be multidisciplinary as no one profession has all the answers.

An effective system of communication is crucial to ensure that all involved have a clear understanding of the aims and methods to be used with a particular person, but beyond that there needs to be familiarity with the overall skills and procedures of each team member. This short chapter will discuss the value of adopting a team approach, how teams may function and the contributions of different disciplines to overall patient care.

WHY WORK AS A TEAM?

The main focus of this chapter is how the team functions, but the starting point is the question 'why have a team at all?' In some ways this can only be answered when the team approach has been properly evaluated, but the initial reason is to meet the needs of the patient – the team should be seen to offer more effective management working together than individuals working separately. As Squires and Wardle (1988) put it, 'Teams come together because they cannot fulfil an objective alone'. Historically it has evolved gradually through a recognition of the many and varied needs of most patients, an awareness of the need to meet these by using specialist knowledge and a movement away from the belief that only medical staff are crucial in the process of providing care. Teams function very differently in different settings and with different individual members but always with the one objective which is to improve the care that can be extended to patients. Of course this objective may or may not be achieved and some of the problems will be discussed in the following pages.

FUNCTIONS OF A TEAM

The multidisciplinary team (MDT) has a role to play in individual assessment and treatment, in group treatments and in working with or through families and informal carers. Decision making on a broader level, for example in formulating management policies, controlling the environment and establishing good practice standards from the point of referral to 'aftercare', is perhaps a neglected area. The MDT depends upon being given enough authority to carry out its terms of reference. A further role is in using the team to attempt to change attitudes of other staff and lay people in the surrounding area towards psychiatric patients. Existing stereotypes affect the way people approach those who are treated by the psychiatric services, and these stereotypes can affect the 'communicative balance' of interaction described by Shadden *et al.* (1983) in relation to work with elderly people.

While these functions seem to be generally accepted in theory, the MDT approach frequently falls short in practice. Pollock (1986) has outlined some of the main barriers to effective team-work. Firstly she suggests organizational factors, then role conflicts, gender issues, training and personality differences. As a recognition of why MDTs fail is a first step in making them work, these issues will be considered more fully.

Barriers to team-work

Organizational barriers may be due to intraprofessional differences or leadership issues. The former are exemplified by professional hierarchies, shift work, philosophical differences (e.g. cure versus care) and a failure for all professions to be seen as having equal importance, so that contributions from certain disciplines are valued more than others. Staff whose sole responsibility lies in one area or unit may not always understand the pressure on those with wider commitments. The issue of leadership is crucial and will be addressed later in this chapter, but it is often a trouble spot. There are many instances when the seemingly natural leader is least committed to the ideals of team-work and adopts an autocratic approach, 'representing' everyone without individuals being given the opportunity to voice their views, vetoing some suggestions and over- or under-valuing contributions from particular disciplines. Difficulties may also arise in team-work if the leader has poor organizational skills and lacks control over the group.

Role conflicts are not uncommon and the topical question of skill mix will also be considered later in this chapter. Confusion is more likely in certain 'grey areas' such as group work and social skills training, but may arise even in aspects of care apparently clearly falling into the specialist knowledge of one profession. There may be rivalry if approaches to work and theoretical backgrounds differ. The question is not as simple as determining professional boundaries; it is individuals who make up the team, and differences will result from basic training, professional experience, interest and further training. If some members are unable to attend regularly there is the risk of communication breakdown and ignorance leading to confusion.

Pollock also talks of gender conflicts as affecting the MDT approach. Sex stereotypes may be used to guide task allocation, to establish styles of work and leadership, and influence how contributions from individuals are received. Training differences and professional approaches to training will often create particular feelings in relation to the role of other professionals, and personality and attitude differences must not be underestimated in considering why teams fail to work effectively. Indeed teams are made or broken by the people involved.

There may be strains placed upon effective team-work if the team as a whole is not recognized by other specialisms, or if the field in which it functions is considered a second class area of care – something sadly still true in mainstream hospital services' attitudes to work with elderly people and psychiatric patients.

Effective team-work

If a multidisciplinary team works well there are great advantages to the individual patient and the overall service (and indeed to team members). Perhaps of greatest value is that a broader perspective is available, made up not just of professional differences, but as a result of the diversity of backgrounds, ages and experience involved. The MDT approach should allow more consistent intervention and better continuity of care. In psychiatry when the therapeutic relationship often extends over considerable time periods and when numerous staff may be implicated this is of particular importance.

Building a team will depend on the provision of opportunities for all members to meet and on the recognition of possible barriers. Each member should be prepared to contribute openly and thus each must respect the contributions of the other members as being of equal value to their own. Acknowledging different points of view is part of successful team-work. All members must accept that the starting point is for them to know what their role is and why, and to be prepared to explain this to the patient, their relatives and to other members of staff – without professional jargon.

Conflicts due to inappropriate leadership, roles and gender issues must be raised and discussed. Multidisciplinary training sessions can help to ensure each professional's role is understood and be a basis for discussing skills overlap, which is such a controversial issue. The team needs the opportunity to define professional boundaries and identities – for that particular team.

O'Sullivan (1988) states that 'effective team-work is dependent upon a good concept of self, a supportive and an empowering relationship with team members, and a sense of kinship with the affiliated organization'. Her workshop came to the agreement that the crucial elements were that all must understand and value the purposes of the group and components of communication (listening, meeting procedures, etc.) and that the organization, team and individuals must be *perceived* as being supportive of each other and of the programme. Inherent in this is that individuals in conflict with the team may have to withdraw.

There may be particular problems for those professions represented by only one or two people, and an effective MDT can help to reduce the isolation that can result. All members will benefit and the cohesion of the team be strengthened by using the team forum for positive feedback. This will reinforce the efforts and expertise of individuals. Undoubtedly a team approach can allow diversity and flexibility of work and combining and sharing treatment planning and responsibilities can lead to the development of new skills. Furthermore a harmonious MDT can be a powerful healing agent, enhancing the effects of formal therapies.

STYLES OF TEAM-WORK

How a team approaches its work will be a function of various factors, such as whether it is goal or mission oriented (O'Sullivan, 1988), whether it adopts a particular model (e.g. social, behavioural, organic, psychoanalytic), whether it is community or hospital/unit based, and whether it has a broad or narrow brief. For instance, to develop a general psychiatric service might be a broad task while to address issues of resettlement for particular patients is a narrower responsibility. The membership of a team will obviously affect its style, as will the leadership, the way in which individuals view their role being crucial. Some may adopt a 'territorial' approach, applying their skills and reporting back to other members; others may assume a 'permissive' stance, cutting across professional boundaries, while – as Gravell (1988) suggests – neither is necessarily better and a combined approach is often most practical.

There is no one answer to the question of what is the best style for a team to adopt, but it is important that members appreciate that 'unity does not preclude autonomy' (Gray, 1982) and that being a fully integrated team member should not diminish individual contributions but rather clarify the particular skills an individual has to offer.

Leadership

The quality and style of communication within the team may well depend upon the team leader. Pollock (1986) feels that ideally 'the most senior member of the profession most involved' should be the leader, and their status will therefore depend on the unit and the model adopted. Pollock does not define 'the most senior' which presumably may be either the most experienced or knowledgeable in a field, or the 'highest ranking' in hierarchical terms. In practice it must be said that hospital teams usually are medically led, and there may be legitimate legal reasons for this. The leader should be used not to provide an autocratic chair or to allocate tasks, but as a coordinator who will take on the roles of clarifying, guiding and supporting the team's work. He or she should ensure that all members have an opportunity to contribute and that their contribution is listened to, valued and when appropriate acted upon. Positive feedback such as reporting successes and progress is equally as important as negative feedback. Sadly the authoritarian style of leadership which was the norm for many years, under the medical model of intervention, is often still seen.

There may be value in using a key worker approach, whereby each patient's case is coordinated or 'led' by a named member of staff. It is important that 'difficult' patients are evenly distributed if such a system is to operate in a balanced way. A recognized leader would still offer overall guidance, as team meetings are not purely case discussions. All meetings should have 'a clearly defined purpose, time and duration' (Hume and Pullen, 1986) and the leader must ensure this is appreciated and understood by all members.

Community-based teams

The move to community care of mentally ill people has been seen as the third revolution in psychiatric care (after Pinel's unchaining of patients and Freud's psychoanalytic theory). It stresses the social environment as both an etiological factor and crucial to rehabilitation (although it should be recognized that there is the potential to recreate institutions in the community).

Team-work has been discussed and implemented with varying degrees of success in community settings, but teams inevitably seem to be less cohesive than those that are hospital or unit based. Members must be gathered together, which may be difficult because of geographical considerations, professional priorities and timetabling. Patients are dispersed over wide areas, and will rarely share the same permutations of services in their care programmes. Leadership is more difficult to assume – Fox (1985) makes this point that family doctors, who many would still see as the natural leader because of the carry-over from the medical model of thinking, often see the management of chronic illness as secondary to the curative role, yet it is in the former cases that the team approach in the community often has the most to offer.

Community teams may be based in a hospital or health centre (depending on service policies and availability of accommodation) and such teams tend to operate under the psychiatrist. Others are based on the existing primary care structures and thus attached to the general practitioner. There are a few somewhat experimental community mental health teams, which operate independently of the GP (although accepting referrals from primary care as well as other sources) in specifically allocated buildings.

Often community teams operate as a collection of case workers exchanging reports on current situations and delegating further responsibilities. Each team member's contact with the patient is likely to be independent of that of others and a 'case work' approach may be the best option, with a key worker for each person taking charge and ensuring the relevant personnel attend meetings and clarifying the distribution of tasks. All must be aware of others' roles and be prepared to ask for advice and support, to extend similar help to others and to report back if this approach is to be effective.

Hospital-based teams

Hospital teams are more likely to meet as a matter of routine, and therefore the chance of adequate communication is facilitated. Regular planned meetings may be for case conferences, ward discussions, policy planning and decision making. Hospital teams may involve the patient and/or informal carers, but it is probably true to say the latter are more likely to be involved in community-based teams. The make-up of the MDT will often be very different depending upon their base, but the leader will tend to be from the medical staff, usually the most senior member involved.

There may be problems in a hospital setting when certain professions overlap a number of medical specialisms, or when a discipline is only rarely involved with individual patients. In the latter instance there may be a role in terms of general advice and teaching, and to maintain links and maximize this role it can help if meetings are attended regularly, if not frequently. A further difficulty arising is the existence of competition of ill-feeling between teams from different specialisms, for example if one team is perceived to be getting more resources than another it may easily lead to a lowering of morale.

TEAM MEMBERSHIP

Team membership will vary depending upon whether the team is operating in the community or hospital/unit and depending upon a variety of factors stemming from the general philosophy and approach to care adopted in a particular region or unit. There are, however, certain core professions which will be represented in all psychiatric teams. These include medical staff, nurses, psychologists and occupational therapists. In different settings other disciplines will also be regarded as core members of a particular team, while others will form an extended team – perhaps being called upon in particular situations. Often discussion of the MDT is limited to those with a clinical role and skills, but it is important that managers and administrators are recognized as playing a central role. Without a commitment at this level the work of the MDT will be severely limited, and barriers may be created (such as over-accommodation issues, training needs, funding and so on) that disrupt or negate their work. Table 11.1 lists possible members of the MDT working in psychiatry, and new staff will need to familiarize themselves with the roles of each profession in order to operate effectively as a team member. It is worth, therefore, offering brief outlines of the most commonly represented disciplines.

Table 11.1 Membership of the MDT

The patient
Informal carers (family, friends)
Administrators
Psychiatrist/medical team/GP
Nursing staff (hospital, community psychiatric nurses)
Auxiliary nursing staff
Clinical psychologists
Residential/day care staff
Occupational therapists
Social workers
Speech therapists
Audiometrists
Physiotherapists
Therapy aides/assistants
Dietitians
Dentists
Chiropodists
Remedial gymnasts
Opticians
Art therapists
Music therapists
Drama therapists
Teachers
Volunteers and voluntary organizations
Caterers
Domestics
Chaplains

The administrator

The administrator is needed to assist in 'solving the organizational problems thrown up by trying to provide a comprehensive mental health service' (Downham and Walker, 1976). Managers of the service must be committed to development and aware of the needs and clinical priorities, while working within specified budgets and with finite resources. This will necessitate close liaison with the clinical team. Adminstrators within psychiatry particularly need an awareness of the fact that personnel factors are most critical. Hospital managers are viewed legally as the health authority's representative and must ensure that the service acts within the provisions of the 1983 Mental Health Act and other relevant legislation.

The psychiatrist

The role of the psychiatrist will vary depending upon the individual's approach and the model within which they work. It is important that the psychiatrist clarifies what approach they adopt, what they want for their patients and what they expect of their patients. Others are then in a better position to know what they can offer. Certain aspects of the psychiatrist's duties are unalterable – for example, he or she will be the team member responsible for prescribing and monitoring drug use and has certain legal responsibilities towards the patient. Medical staff are involved in compulsory admission and treatment procedures – in-patients may be held in hospital for up to 72 hours, for example, and one or two doctors (depending on whether it is an emergency) must recommend compulsory admission. Certain therapeutic procedures may require either the patient's consent or a second medical opinion (e.g. psychosurgery or ECT and medication if it is more than three months after they were first administered).

The nurse

Usually nursing staff form the largest single discipline, although this may not always be true for community teams, and there may be problems of continuity because of this and because of shift systems. The role of the nurse is diverse as duties are to the ward/unit, individual patients and to the team. He or she acts as a communicator and as such is central to the patient's well-being, by linking between self, patients, and the rest of the team.

In the UK many nurses follow the Nursing Process (Royal College of Nursing, 1981) and therefore are responsible for certain patients on the ward and will represent them at case conferences and other team meetings. It is valuable when nursing staff can be involved in therapies, but it is often impossible when units are poorly staffed and underfunded. Such stresses should be appreciated by other staff, keen to use nursing staff to ensure carry-over of their work.

Nursing auxiliaries often have little training, but given appropriate instruction and support can be active members of the clinical team. Such 'untrained' human resources must not be underestimated by professional members of the MDT.

Ramsden (1981) sees the role of the hospital-based nurse as threefold: as an observer, noting change and general condition; as a teacher; and as a supporter of the patient. She feels the nurse must be flexible and not 'inflict needless routines and standards' upon the patients. In the community the psychiatric nurse should be involved in discharge planning and act as a link between the consultant and general practitioner; he or she will visit regularly or at crisis and will offer counselling and support to individuals. The CPN is in the best position to monitor change and ensure a quick response to any worrying signs (Drake, 1981).

The occupational therapist

Finlay (1988) stresses that the value of occupational therapy often 'lies within aspects which are hard to quantify, such as the patient-therapist relationship or the satisfaction gained through activity'. Within psychiatry she highlights feelings, behaviour and skills as the areas to consider in assessment and therapy, towards developing the abilities to cope within work, social and domestic life.

The occupational therapist (OT) may work on the ward or unit, if hospital based, but often works in a department away from the ward, thus offering a different setting and a new group of people for the patient to meet. The aim of therapy is to use the personal relationship between therapist and patient to develop occupational (which includes leisure) activities, in a way that will help the patient to gain an understanding of their patterns of behaviour and, when necessary, learn to control or modify these patterns. The OT plays an important role with long-stay and newly admitted patients in the hospital, and in resettlement work and/or maintaining people in the community. In the latter case particularly individual work will need to be backed up by involvement with families and other carers, and the OT will also have a role in mobilizing social support (Finlay, 1988).

Willson (1981) summarizes the OT's role as being to 'provide opportunities for patients to practise skills which they may have lost or never have learned and also to develop roles other than those related to sickness and dependency'. This would involve creating the best environment and helping people cope within different settings; assessing abilities which are retained as well as which are lacking; setting realistic goals towards personal independence; and considering the impact of communication difficulties on everyday activities. This latter aspect should of course mean there is close liaison with speech therapy.

The social worker

In the UK social workers in hospitals are not employed by the National Health Service, but by the local authority – as are their community-based colleagues. Links both inside and outside the hospital are essential, allowing social workers to deal with day-to-day problems *in situ* (such as sorting out benefits and other finances) and also to liaise and maintain links between the patient and informal carers. The social worker may be a particularly critical team member if patients are regularly readmitted and discharged. Along with other disciplines there may also be a role in running psychotherapy groups and in counselling. The social worker has certain critical legal responsibilities, for example in making application for a person to be admitted against their will, following the recommendation of the psychiatrist, for assessment or treatment, under the relevant section of the Mental Health Act (1983). It is recognized that a level of experience and training is necessary to take on this aspect of the social worker's responsibilities, and in order to maintain standards that individual must be nominated as an Approved Social Worker by their local authority (Gostin, 1983). The 1983 Act means there is a duty, in taking the decision to make an application, to interview and to prepare a social report after the incident.

Davies (1981) suggests the role of the social worker, in summary, is in working within the team; planning discharge; organizing and liaising between agencies to mobilize resources; interpreting the client's needs to the community (and sometimes vice versa); and in personal casework or group work.

The clinical psychologist

The clinical psychologist administers psychological tests of intellectual function, other cognitive processes, attitudes and inner mental mechanisms to aid diagnostic appraisal. Following assessment appropriate therapies may include counselling, formal psychotherapy or behaviour modification techniques. As do other MDT members, psychologists will have a role in teaching patients and staff/informal carers and in research.

The physiotherapist

The physiotherapist like other therapists will offer traditional intervention when appropriate for conditions not linked with the patient's psychiatric state, as well as for those directly or indirectly attributable to the individual's mental health. In certain settings they may have a particularly valuable role in teaching relaxation techniques. They will have roles in teaching, advising and liaising with others – for example, on how to position or transport patients.

Other team members

Table 11.1 gives some idea of the possible range of disciplines involved with the MDT – and many more could probably be added to the list. It deliberately places the patient and informal carers at the head (although others are not intended to suggest any order of importance) as it is startling how often these most essential team members are relegated to the role of being passive recipients rather than active participants in the team decision-making process.

Many disciplines are important in particular cases but are not core members of the MDT in that they are not involved with all or most of the patients, such as dentists, chiropodists and opticians. Others are still fighting to be recognized as having a valuable contribution to make within the field of psychiatry, such as art, music or drama therapists. Even some mainstream professions are not always seen by colleagues as having a part to play – in some areas speech therapists would fall into this category.

Another group of staff that tend to have their value grossly under-estimated are the domestics and catering staff, despite being essential to hospital routine and also at times central in maintaining people in the community, under the titles of home helps and meals on wheels services. Volunteers are similarly undervalued, but are often necessary if individual patient programmes are to be followed through, and on a broader level voluntary bodies have played a massive role in developing services for mentally ill people on both local and national scales. Such groups include the National Schizophrenia Fellowship and MIND, for example.

The speech therapist

It would, of course, be unfair to exclude the speech therapist from this discussion of the MDT, although obviously their role is addressed throughout this volume. It is surprising that so few speech therapists do work in MDTs within psychiatry when other professions are so firmly established. Their role may cover traditional/conventional therapy, assessment of communication to assist in making diagnoses (this may include audiometric assessment if other resources are not available), teaching relating to general communication skills and needs, teaching and advising on individual cases, and research. Some general suggestions on the teaching role of the speech therapist are made in Gravell (1988).

SKILL MIX

The possibility of role conflict has been referred to elsewhere in this chapter and at other points in the volume. There has recently been much debate on the question of skill mix and the delineation of professional boundaries. Fussy *et al.* (1988) say 'we are all aware that we each secretly believe that our discipline has the most to offer. Therefore the members of MDTs may all be doing what they think is appropriate for the patient's needs, but it may not be coordinated in a common goal'. While it is debatable how far this can be taken – few speech therapists would argue they were more crucial to the patient than the nursing staff or the psychiatrist, for instance – there is an element of truth. Certainly attention needs to be given to the question of professional boundaries, but it seems logical to do this within a multidisciplinary forum – either in a particular team or through interdisciplinary discussion. A single profession cannot know where role blurring is creating problems for other disciplines, and often professionals are unaware of the specific skills of others and so have inappropriate expectations. It must be recognized ultimately that while each profession 'has its essential function' it has also 'its necessary overlap with others' (Younghusband Report, 1959). Some skills are and need to be shared – such as listening, group work and so on.

It is quite possible that role blurring can lead to great stress in individual team members and this will affect in turn patient care. Perhaps ultimately certain grey areas will only be possible to discuss and allocate in each MDT, taking into account not only professional skills but the skills, interests and experience of each member.

EVALUATING TEAM-WORK

Undoubtedly team-work is a buzz word in medical fields, and a great deal of lip service is paid to it, often without much practical evidence of a team existing in a particular area. One reason for this may well be that little attention has been paid to evaluating the MDT approach formally. Each profession should be assessed, according to Downham and Walker (1976), by their effectiveness 'according to the standard of their service when it reaches the patient'. This should also be applied to the MDT – after all, why invest time and energy in attended meetings, reporting and taking joint decisions if there is no ultimate benefit to the patient or the overall service?

Evaluating team-work is not, however, an easy task. It may be that evaluation is in relation to declared standards and whether or not these are achieved – which can be a rather circular approach if the team sets its own standards. Other measures may be indirect or subjective, such as whether members attend meetings regularly and feel positive about the MDT, can discuss failures openly and ask advice (and accept it!). More direct patient-oriented measures may be used, such as records/ monitoring, existence of high levels of therapeutic input and use of innovative approaches to treatment. Individual professional records may be valuable, for example indicating whether a patient improves more quickly or achieves a higher level if other members of the team are backing up that discipline's work. The MDT may be evaluated in relation to its effects on issues like staff recruitment and turnover, but a nominal team approach does not mean a staff group is in fact functioning as a team and this must be considered if turnover is high.

It is easy to rely on subjective opinions that a team works well, but some objective criteria are important not least in order to justify to administrators and professional hierarchies that working through an MDT can be an efficient and effective use of time.

REFERENCES

Davies, N. (1981) Social work, in *Handbook of Psychiatric Rehabilitation Practice* (eds J. K. Wing and B. Morris), Oxford University Press, Oxford, pp. 56–61.

Downham, D. J. and Walker, P. R. (1976) The role of the adminstrator, in *Comprehensive Psychiatric Care* (ed. A. A. Baker), Blackwell Scientific Pubications, London, pp. 141–64.

Drake, W. (1981) The community psychiatric nurse, in *Handbook of Psychiatric Rehabilitation Practice* (eds J. K. Wing and B. Morris), Oxford University Press, Oxford, pp. 37–8.

Finlay, L. (1988) *Occupational Therapy Practice in Psychiatry*, Croom Helm, London.

Fox, E. M. (1985) Community resources and the dementing patient. *Geriatric Medicine*, April,

Fussy, I., Cumberpath, J. and Grant, C. (1988) The application of a behavioural model in rehabilitation, in *The Rehabilitation of the Severely Brain Injured Adult*, (eds I. Fussy and G. Muir Giles), Croom Helm, London.

Gostin, L. (1983) *A Practical Guide to Mental Health Law*.

Gravell, R. E. (1988) *Communication Problems in Elderly People: Practical Approaches to Management*, Croom Helm, London.

Gray, A. (1982) The challenge of multidisciplinary work. *College of Speech Therapists Bulletin*, p. 358.

Hume, C. and Pullen, I. (1986) *Rehabilitiation in Psychiatry: An Introductory Handbook*, Churchill Livingstone, Edinburgh.

Mental Health Act (1983) HMSO, London.

O'Sullivan, D. (1988) *The Hallmark of a Team: Workshop*, APSA Conference, Swansea.

Pollock, L. (1986) The multidisciplinary team, in *Rehabilitation in Psychiatry:*

An Introductory Handbook, (eds C. Hume and I. Pullen), Churchill Livingstone, Edinburgh, pp. 126–48.

Ramsden, A. (1981) The role of the nurse in a hospital rehabilitation unit, in *Handbook of Psychiatric Rehabilitation Practice*, (eds J. K. Wing and B. Morris), Oxford University Press, Oxford, pp. 31–2.

Royal College of Nursing (1981) *Towards Standards: A Discussion Document*, RCN, London.

Shadden, B. B., Raiford, C. A. and Shadden, H. S. (1983) *Coping with Communication Disorders in Aging*, CC Publications, Tigard, Oregon.

Squires, A. and Wardle, P. (1988) To rehabilitate or not? in *Rehabilitation of the Older Patient*, (ed. A. Squires), Croom Helm, London.

Willson, M. (1981) Occupational therapy, in *Handbook of Psychiatric Rehabilitation Practice*, (eds J. K. Wing and B. Morris), Oxford University Press, Oxford, pp. 41–7.

Younghusband Report (1959) HMSO, London.

12

Conclusion: the state of the art

Jenny France and Rosemary Gravell

Communication is central to people's ability to take part in and enjoy a satisfactory life. The loss of or failure to develop the skills necessary to communicate effectively has enormous impact on individuals, their families, and indeed on a wider social scale. When this is due to a mental disorder people face very particular and distressing difficulties in the way others approach them and in the degree of support society is prepared to offer. Sadly the communicative needs of this population have been neglected in the past, partly because professionals have failed to appreciate these needs and partly because mentally disordered people have often been consigned on diagnosis to being 'no-hopers'. Recent years have bought many changes in general rehabilitation work and in particular in the way communication is at last being given the importance it merits in terms of assessment, diagnosis and management. At the forefront of this movement has been the speech therapist.

This volume has attempted to provide an overview of communication disorders in that proportion of the population who make use of psychiatric services, to offer suggestions and guidance in working with these groups and to stress throughout the centrality of the team approach. However, a book of this size cannot hope to do justice to a topic as far reaching as communication and mental disorder and does not pretend to be a comprehensive text – it offers an introduction and those interested in the field are advised to make use of the reference lists provided. Perhaps more importantly there is the need to talk to others in the field, learn from their experiences and one's own, and to evaluate both experiential and book-based learning with a critical eye.

It is worth drawing attention to a few areas outside this volume's scope which are of particular importance. Many of these stem from general social issues which have ramifications for all groups within society, not least the mentally disordered population. One such issue in the UK is the increase over recent years in the number and size of ethnic minority groups. There are obvious language barriers to consider, but more difficult to address in planning intervention are the more subtle cultural and racial differences that will exist – for example in non-verbal communication. There may also be differences in those who come forward for psychiatric help and in the presenting symptoms. The authors strongly suspect, for example, that there are large numbers of people from ethnic minorities who do not use the available resources within psychiatry.

Another issue is the rapid ageing of the population, which this volume has touched upon, but which in relation to mental health care needs more detailed attention than can be offered here. At the other end of the age scale psychiatric teams are becoming increasingly aware of what can be done during childhood and adolescence to support those diagnosed as suffering from mental illness or mental handicap, and to help them develop within their potential, rather than assuming their illness or handicap prevents any useful intervention.

There has been a great deal of stress over recent years on women in society and this is very much an area of concern in mental health. There are, as was seen in Chapter 1, more women than men affected by mental illness. This has important implications for a society in which it is still the woman who tends to bring up the children either within a family setting or as a single parent. Attention needs to be given to the question of how mental illness in the mother affects children and the family as a whole.

A topic that has been mentioned in several places in this book is that of resettlement of mentally disordered people from long-stay institutions to live in the community. This has meant that those who received rehabilitation input in hospitals, as a 'captive' audience, are moving into situations where, while the skills are needed more, the support offered is less. There are difficulties for health care workers of all professions in keeping tabs on this dissipating population, who often will not seek help by the very nature of their condition, as it limits their insight and motivation. All these issues are general concerns for the speech therapist and all the other professions and organizations working in the field or psychiatry.

Research has not been addressed in detail in this volume, although research findings have of course been used to support and explain points throughout. However, it is a next step from this general introduction to look at the research needs in the field. Research goes on into causes and cures for mental disorder, but in the lack of a definitive answer treatment must also go on, adapting to findings and utilizing innovative ideas as it grows and develops. Part of this process must be continuous evaluation of the methods of assessment and intervention currently used with different groups and subgroups of this population. This is true for all disciplines, but is crucial to speech therapists as relative new-comers to the field who need to prove themselves both to other professions and indeed within their own. It does not seem a helpful approach to withdraw from the field before there has been opportunity to evaluate properly whether one's role is worthwhile or, indeed, worthless. Nor does it seem sensible to dismiss *all* interventions that might be considered if one, two or more do not prove to be of value with a particular client group. All this does mean, and rightly so, is that there must be well-planned and carefully executed ongoing clinical research and that findings should be shared and publicized.

One aspect of evaluating the role of the speech therapist will involve looking at how best to deliver a service not just to hospital-based clients/patients, but also to those already in or soon to be moved to the community. Quality assurance should be high on the agenda of all health care workers and the state of play at present is that a great deal more education, preparation and discussion is needed to ensure the optimal use of professional time towards the optimal health – physical and mental – of the population.

Education is needed to teach all the professions about each others' roles and to address, within that brief, first the essentials. Too often esoteric pieces of research or small projects will be discussed and reported before there is a basic knowledge of the different disciplines' skills and abilities. There does seem to have been increasing acceptance of the speech therapist within psychiatric teams, although there will always be teams that exist only in name and recognize only the very traditional professions. Education is needed also within speech therapy to draw attention to this area of work and, within it, to highlight the aspects that are of particular relevance to the speech therapist as specialist – childhood and adolescence, hearing impairment, mental handicap and so on.

In conclusion it is fair to say that much more research and evaluation is needed in the field, opportunities often sadly limited by funding, but that this is an area which is developing rapidly. Creative and innovative methods of work can be the first to suffer in a highly budget-conscious environment, but they do not have to be. We believe that those already in the field are enthusiastic, motivated and determined to look objectively at interventions, such as those described throughout this volume, and to ensure that this population receives the best possible care. The challenge is to assess and then to meet the needs of those whose communication is impaired by mental disorder, to reject paths that prove inappropriate or ineffective, and to refine and develop a quality service. It is not an easy challenge to meet, but if it can be done the quality of life of many people will be immeasurably improved.

Index